Pathogenesis of Functional Bowel Disease

TOPICS IN GASTROENTEROLOGY

Series Editor: **Howard M. Spiro, M.D.**
Yale University School of Medicine

COLON
Structure and Function
Edited by Luis Bustos-Fernandez, M.D.

KEY FACTS IN GASTROENTEROLOGY
Jonathan Halevy, M.D.

MEDICAL ASPECTS OF DIETARY FIBER
Edited by Gene A. Spiller, Ph.D., and Ruth McPherson Kay, Ph.D.

MODERN CONCEPTS IN GASTROENTEROLOGY
Volume 1: Edited by Alan B. R. Thomson, M.D., Ph.D.,
L. R. DaCosta, M.D., and William C. Watson, M.D.
Volume 2: Edited by Eldon Shaffer, M.D.,
and Alan B. R. Thomson, M.D., Ph.D.

NUTRITION AND DIET THERAPY
IN GASTROINTESTINAL DISEASE
Martin H. Floch, M.S., M.D., F.A.C.P.

PANCREATITIS
Peter A. Banks, M.D.

PATHOGENESIS OF FUNCTIONAL BOWEL DISEASE
Edited by William J. Snape, Jr., M.D.

A Continuation Order Plan is available for this series. A continuation order will bring delivery of each new volume immediately upon publication. Volumes are billed only upon actual shipment. For further information please contact the publisher.

Pathogenesis of Functional Bowel Disease

Edited by
William J. Snape, Jr., M.D.

Director
Inflammatory Bowel Disease Center
Harbor–UCLA Medical Center
Torrance, California
and Professor of Medicine
University of California–Los Angeles
Los Angeles, California

Plenum Medical Book Company
New York and London

Library of Congress Cataloging in Publication Data

Pathogenesis of functional bowel disease / edited by William J. Snape, Jr.
    p.   cm. — (Topics in gastroenterology)
  Includes bibliographical references and index.
  ISBN-13: 978-1-4684-5696-7   e-ISBN-13: 978-1-4684-5694-3
  DOI: 10.1007/978-1-4684-5694-3

  1. Irritable colon — Pathogenesis. 2. Gastrointestinal system — Diseases — Pathogenesis. I. Snape, William J. II. Series.
  [DNLM: 1. Gastrointestinal Diseases — etiology. 2. Gastrointestinal Diseases —
physiopathology. 3. Gastrointestinal Motility. WI 100 P2945]
RC862.I77P37 1989
616.3′42071 — dc20
DNLM/DLC   89-16047
for Library of Congress   CIP

© 1989 Plenum Publishing Corporation
Softcover reprint of the hardcover 1st edition 1989

233 Spring Street, New York, N.Y. 10013

Plenum Medical Book Company is an imprint of Plenum Publishing Corporation

Contributors

Thomas P. Almy, Departments of Medicine and Community and Family Medicine, Dartmouth Medical School, Hanover, New Hampshire 03756

Haile T. Debas, Department of Surgery, University of California–San Francisco, San Francisco, California 94143

Wylie J. Dodds Department of Radiology, Medical College of Wisconsin, Milwaukee, Wisconsin 53226

Andre Dubois, Laboratory of Gastrointestinal and Liver Studies, Digestive Diseases Division, Department of Medicine, Uniformed Services University of the Health Sciences, Bethesda, Maryland 20814

Joseph E. Geenen, Department of Medicine, St. Luke's Hospital, Racine, Wisconsin 53403

Kenneth W. Heaton, University Department of Medicine, Bristol Royal Infirmary, Bristol BS2 8HW, England

Walter J. Hogan, Department of Medicine, Medical College of Wisconsin, Milwaukee, Wisconsin 53226

Paul E. Hyman, Division of Pediatric Gastroenterology, Harbor–UCLA Medical Center, Torrance, California 90502

John E. Kellow, Department of Medicine, Royal North Shore Hospital, St. Leonards, New South Wales 2065, Australia

M. A. K. Khalil, Digestive Diseases Research Group, Division of Gastroenterology, University of Ottawa, Ottawa Civic Hospital, Ottawa, Ontario K1Y 4E9, Canada

C. D. Lind, Department of Internal Medicine, Division of Gastroenterology, University of Virginia Medical Center, Charlottesville, Virginia 22908

R. W. McCallum, Department of Internal Medicine, Division of Gastroenterology, University of Virginia Medical Center, Charlottesville, Virginia 22908

Emeran A. Mayer, Division of Gastroenterology, Harbor–UCLA Medical Center, Torrance, California 90509

Sean J. Mulvihill, Department of Surgery, University of California–San Francisco, San Francisco, California 94143

Sidney F. Phillips, Gastroenterology Unit and Digestive Diseases Care Center, Mayo Clinic, Rochester, Minnesota 55905

Helen Raybould, Center for Ulcer Research and Education, Veterans Administration Medical Center, and Department of Medicine, University of California–Los Angeles, Los Angeles, California 90073

N. W. Read, Department of Human Gastrointestinal Physiology and Nutrition, Royal Hallamshire Hospital, Sheffield S10 2TN, England

James C. Reynolds, Department of Medicine and Physiology, Hospital of the University of Pennsylvania, Philadelphia, Pennsylvania 19104

Joel E. Richter, Section on Gastroenterology, Department of Medicine, The Bowman Gray School of Medicine, Wake Forest University, Winston-Salem, North Carolina 27103

William J. Snape, Jr., Inflammatory Bowel Disease Center, Harbor–UCLA Medical Center, Torrance, California 90502; and Department of Medicine, University of California–Los Angeles, Los Angeles, California 90073.

Wei Ming Sun, Department of Human Gastrointestinal Physiology and Nutrition, Royal Hallamshire Hospital, Sheffield S10 2TN, England

Yvette Taché, Center for Ulcer Research and Education, Veterans Administration Medical Center–West Los Angeles, and Department of Medicine and Brain Research Institute, University of California–Los Angeles, Los Angeles, California 90073

W. G. Thompson, Digestive Diseases Research Group, Division of Gastroenterology, University of Ottawa, Ottawa Civic Hospital, Ottawa, Ontario K1Y 4E9, Canada

William E. Whitehead, Division of Digestive Diseases, Francis Scott Key Medical Center, and Department of Medicine, The Johns Hopkins University School of Medicine, Baltimore, Maryland 21218

Foreword

In their second year in medical school, students begin to learn about the differences between "disease" and "illness." In their studies of pathology they learn to understand disease as pertubations of molecular biological events. And we clinicians can show disease to them by our scans, lay it out even on our genetic scrolls, and sometimes even point out the errant nucleotide.

Disease satisfies them and us; at Yale, lectures on the gastrointestinal tract run from achalasia to proctitis. There is, alas, little mention of functional bowel disease or of the irritable or spastic colon, for that is not easy to show on hard copy. Functional bowel disease represents "illness," the response of the person to distress, to food, to the environment, and to the existential problems of living.

In real life such matters are most important. Richard Cabot first found out at the Massachusetts General Hospital almost a century ago that 50% of the patients attending the outpatient clinic had "functional" complaints. The figure had grown to over 80% when the very same question was reexamined 60 years later.

Yet we rarely talk to students about irritable bowel because the intensive care units, which the hospitals have become, admit no one who is vertical; only the horizontal can get through the doors. But students do live in the real world, and some of them—more of them, now that they spend time in the outpatient areas—ask me about the "irritable bowel." I tell them what I have learned and try to emphasize that some physicians regard functional bowel disease as a specific neurobiological event, triggered by inherent but errant neural impulses, like epilepsy, whereas others—and I side with them—look on the irritable bowel as simply an illness, like blushing or weeping or some other autonomic response to daily life.

But now I can keep silent. I'll simply send the medical students to this fine compendium which you are about to read, for it tells almost everything there is to know not only about the irritable colon, but about the "irritable gut."

Dr. Snape and his colleagues have laid out a veritable feast for practitioners, academicians, medical students, and other physicians, who will find the information which follows of inestimable value. While I might not dignify "functional bowel disease" with the title of "disease," still I find all the arguments summarized in this book valid and I am happy indeed to include it in our series.

Howard M. Spiro, M.D.

New Haven, Connecticut

Preface

The functional bowel disorders encompass a large number of gastrointestinal symptoms that have no associated organic (anatomic) cause. These disorders are considered in this book as disturbances of visceral neural function and/or discoordination of smooth muscle contraction.

Functional bowel disease constitutes a major component of the office practice of general internists and gastroenterologists.[1,2] Both physicians and patients are frustrated by the vague symptoms of abdominal pain and altered bowel habits that comprise the functional bowel syndrome. Many physicians have difficulty establishing the diagnosis and initiating effective treatment. Patients often feel that their physicians do not understand their disease and consequently do not provide compassionate or effective care. These perceptions lead to a group of peripatetic patients who, dissatisfied with their medical care, move from doctor to doctor seeking relief.

Until recently, the understanding of the pathogenesis of functional conditions was imprecise due to the lack of specific techniques to measure gastrointestinal motor function. The development of new technologies to study neuromuscular control of the gastrointestinal tract has enabled clinical investigators to better understand disturbances in gastrointestinal motility. The enhanced ability to study motility has led to a resurgence of interest in patients who have the nonspecific symptoms of the functional bowel syndrome. The increase in clinical investigation of bowel function provided the data base for this book.

This book encapsulates the recent advances in functional disease of the gastrointestinal tract. Eating and stress have been implicated as causes of the functional complaints. Recent studies have demonstrated that the central nervous system and the humoral–enteric neuropeptides can interact to regulate gastrointestinal motility and transit. The first several chapters provide a background for understanding the interaction between the afferent signals, which enter the central nervous system carrying signals from the external and visceral environment, and the efferent signals, which regulate the intestinal tract via the enteric nervous system. Alterations in central nervous system modulation of the release of the circulating gastrointestinal peptides and peptide neurotransmitters from the enteric nervous system may disturb the integrative controls of the bowel and cause symptoms in patients with functional bowel disease.

The next several chapters examine the role of diet and use of pharmaceutical agents, accepted accoutrements of Western civilization, in causing symptoms of functional bowel disease. Dietary practices can produce or relieve symptoms of functional bowel disease.

Side effects from the appropriate and inappropriate use of pharmaceutical agents also may cause the symptoms of functional bowel disease.

The remaining chapters of the book discuss the symptom patterns that are associated with motility disturbances in different anatomic regions of the gastrointestinal tract. Earlier studies focused on the role of the colon in producing the symptoms of the irritable bowel syndrome.[3] Recent evidence shows that functional bowel disease affects the entire gastrointestinal tract, not just the colon. The widespread presence of pathophysiologic abnormalities throughout the gastrointestinal tract explains the differences in symptoms and responses to therapy that occur in patients with the irritable bowel syndrome.

It is only recently that changes in gastrointestinal motility have been linked to alterations in transit. Discussion of the link between transit and motility is interspersed in the book in order to clarify the etiology of the altered bowel habits of patients with functional bowel disease. Each author discusses treatment of the symptoms in the context of the pathophysiology that leads to the symptom.

The authors of this text provide the scientific data to construct the conceptual foundation upon which further knowledge can be added. A better understanding of the pathophysiology will provide the opportunity to create models that explain the cause of symptoms and stimulate the development of new therapy. Hopefully, these advances will allow greater success in the treatment of symptoms of the different types of functional bowel disease.

REFERENCES

1. Mendeloff A: Epidemiology of the irritable bowel syndrome. Pract Gastroenterol 3:12–25, 1979
2. Almy TP: Digestive disease as a natural problem II. A white paper by the American Gastroenterological Association. Gastroenterology 53:821–824, 1967
3. Bockus HL, Bank J, Wilkinson SA: Neurogenic mucous colitis. Am J Med Sci 176:813–829, 1928

Contents

Pathogenesis of Functional Bowel Disease

Historical Perspectives of Functional Bowel Disease

Thomas P. Almy

A 31-year-old white housewife complained of persistent diarrhea for 18 months. Her stools were semiliquid to mushy, and often contained visible mucus but never blood. They were passed from three to eight times daily, but never at night; and though often accompanied by great urgency, they were usually small.

Since the age of seven she had had irregular bowel movements, the stools being occasionally loose but usually in the form of small scybala. Lower abdominal griping pain often preceded the bowel movement, and was relieved by defecation. Frequent belching, postprandial fullness, and abdominal distention, as well as insomnia, frequent headaches, and premenstrual tension were acknowledged on direct questioning.

1. EVOLUTION OF CLINICAL CONCEPTS

From the early 19th century to the present, a history such as this has suggested to observant physicians an ill-defined class of persistent or recurrent, but nonlethal, gastrointestinal ailments now referred to as *functional disorders*. The syndromes described by Powell,[1] Clark,[2] and others in England were later reported in America by da Costa,[3] and by physicians caring for patients in health spas on the continent of Europe. In the early descriptions, attention focused on the passage of visible mucus in the stool (mucous disease of the colon[2]), particularly in the form of pseudomembranes or casts of the colonic lumen (membranous enteritis[3] or membranous colitis[4]). Yet the minute study of these membranes and of available tissue specimens yielded no understanding of the pathogenesis of these disorders. On the other hand, it soon became clear that they encompassed a much broader range of symptom patterns, referable to all levels of the gastrointestinal

Thomas P. Almy • Departments of Medicine and Community and Family Medicine, Dartmouth Medical School, Hanover, New Hampshire 03756.

tract, and associated with altered circulatory, respiratory, and genitourinary function as well as with emotional instability.

Over the years, neurosis in these patients has always been regarded by some physicians as in all probability a *consequence* of the long-standing distress occasioned by unremitting intestinal symptoms. Clinically detectable neurotic behavior, nevertheless, has been recognized so often, in well-studied cases, as *preceding* the onset of enteric symptoms that a majority have considered it a principal factor in etiology and pathogenesis.

The rubric of *functional disorders* has persisted as one of clinical convenience, signifying conditions recognizable only by symptom patterns corresponding to postulated disturbances of enteric physiology, but without *apparent* abnormalities of the structure, microbial environment, or biochemistry of the gut. As the concept is based in part on the exclusion of "organic" disease, the functional category has often been spurned as a "wastebasket diagnosis." Progress in understanding gastrointestinal disease and in the methods of laboratory diagnosis has led to the splitting off of several successive "functional" ailments that are now seen to have specific pathogenetic mechanisms, some of them treatable by simple and direct means. Thus, many cases of giardiasis, cholerogenous diarrhea, antral gastritis due to *Campylobacter pylori,* and intolerance of gluten, lactose, and other foods are no longer considered to have functional disorders, their underlying mechanisms having been specifically characterized.

In recent years, attention has returned to the positive characterization of at least one disorder, the irritable bowel syndrome (IBS), on the basis of typical symptoms.[5] Significant differences between groups of patients with IBS and those with "organic" conditions have been clearly shown, but the predictive value of the symptom complex is regarded by many as too low to justify an accurate clinical diagnosis, unless certain clinical features of organic conditions are shown to be absent.[6]

2. LIFE EVENTS, EMOTIONS, AND FUNCTIONAL DISORDERS

Over the last century and a half, clinical recognition of emotional lability in patients with functional disorders was paralleled by observations on bodily manifestations of emotion in humans and animals. Beaumont, in his studies of the exposed stomach of Alexis St. Martin, briefly noted that its mucosa became engorged at times of emotional arousal[7]; and many years later Pavlov showed conclusively that visceral function can be influenced by the complex integrative activity of the brain.[8] In the 1940s Wolf and Wolff,[9] Engel et al.,[10] and others, observing subjects with exposed gastric fistulas, demonstrated the sensitivity of the motility, secretion, and vascularity of the stomach to even minor life events when the latter were invested with emotional significance for the subject. The implications of these studies for the origins of dyspepsia in many patients were reinforced by subsequent demonstrations of the mechanisms of nausea[11] and of dysphagia[12] developing during emotional tension.

During the same period, several groups of investigators studied in greater depth the correlations between life situations, personality features, emotional conflicts, and colonic function, with particular reference to "mucous colitis." Bockus et al.[13] and Alvarez[14] described a range of psychoneurotic traits in patients with functional disorders. Alexander and other psychoanalysts found strong support, in selected cases, for a Freudian symbolic interpretation of the meaning of constipation and diarrhea.[15] In 1939 White et al.[16] published observations on 60 unselected patients with mucous colitis at a single clinic. In 53 of them, impressive temporal correlations were made between the onset and course of the illness and life events to which the patient was found to be psychologically vulnerable.

Meanwhile, the classic observations of Walter B. Cannon on the "emergency reaction" in terrified cats[17] had shown that the intestinal tract participates in the preparation of the animal for fight or flight. The cessation of rhythmic contractions of the opacified intestine, when in the darkened room the spread-eagled cat was confronted with a growling dog, coincided with other signs of defensive reaction, which included tachycardia, elevated arterial pressure, and erection of the hairs. (Cannon noted, interestingly, that "the tonic constrictions of the descending colon" were not inhibited during this reaction.) Thus, the notion that stressful life events, during which human beings might feel strong emotion, might temporarily alter the functions of the gut gained powerful support.

Conceived as part of the "emergency reaction," these phenomena were long thought to be due to the inhibitory action of adrenergic pathways in the autonomic nervous system, and to be evoked only under highly threatening circumstances. This belief has been reinforced by many subsequent clinical observations of human behavior under overwhelming stress, most recently in reports of the occurrence of IBS in acute form in patients with panic disorders, and the relief of both conditions by adequate dosage of psychoactive drugs.[18] But in the past 60 years, many human reactions failed to fit this model. White and Jones noted acute engorgement of the colonic mucosa (a "colonic blush") in a normal male subject who felt acute embarrassment when a female observer unexpectedly appeared[19]; and Friedman and Snape reported both blanching and hyperemia of children's colostomies following brief painful but noninjurious stimulation, or the expectation of repeated stimulation, of adjacent skin.[20] White and Jones were able to reproduce the proctoscopic features (spasm, mucosal engorgement, and hypersecretion of mucus) of patients with mucous colitis in human volunteers by topical or systemic administration of cholinergic agents.[19] When Cannon observed the engorgement and hypersecretion of the stomach that reflected periodic resentment in Tom, Wolf's fistulous subject, a consensus had developed that both sympathetic and parasympathetic pathways are involved, and that ordinary life events are significant, in the mechanism of functional disorders of the gut.

At that time the reports of clinicians, especially that of White et al.,[16] on large series of patients with functional disorders suggested that this mechanism is quite regularly involved in their causation. Observations of relevant physiologic changes linked to human emotion, nevertheless, had been made on relatively few persons, most of them either healthy or having other ailments. Almy, Kern, and their associates then undertook a lengthy series of experimental studies of the motility and vascularity of the sigmoid colon in healthy subjects and IBS patients. During sigmoidoscopic observation, seven normal volunteers who endured severe cold pain or self-inflicted compression of the head exhibited occlusive spasm and marked engorgement of the colon, together with facial pallor, sweating, sighing respirations, and elevated blood pressure. Five reported a brief but severe emotional conflict.[21] Other healthy persons responded similarly to interviews productive of manifest emotional tension.[22]

Similar "stress interviews" were conducted in IBS patients, focusing on life events emotionally disturbing to each, during continuous kymographic recording of motility in the lower sigmoid colon. Increased phasic contractions were noted during emotional arousal and "coping" behavior manifested by aggressive gestures and facial and verbal expressions of hostility and self-assertion.[23] On the other hand, whenever the patient indicated by speech, gestures, and other behavior feelings of guilt, depression, helplessness, and personal inadequacy, the phasic contractions were abruptly reduced or interrupted. All of the 11 instances of weeping observed during these studies coincided with this suspension of the usual phasic activity in the sigmoid. The hypermotile/coping pattern and the hypomotile/helpless pattern were of variable duration, and sometimes alternated in the same recording session.[24]

The gastrointestinal illness of one of the patients in this series was described at the beginning of this chapter. Her psychosocial history was obtained during the recording of her sigmoid motility. A portion of the tracing is shown in Fig. 1.

She was the second of five children of Roman Catholic parents. Her mother, prior to marriage a high school teacher, was strict but affectionate. Her father, a stockbroker's clerk, was emotionally labile and, when he drank to excess, abusive to his wife and children. Ten years before, having graduated from high school with honors, the patient left home, entered secretarial school, and afterwards was employed in a local bank in positions of increasing responsibility. She had few close friends and no serious suitors until she received the attentions of a junior executive 8 years older than herself. After long hesitation and much misgiving, but fearing the alternative would be spinsterhood, she accepted his proposal of marriage. The wedding was gay and somewhat bibulous, and on the wedding night she found her new husband, reeking of whisky, crude and insensitive. She recounted this discovery, to the implications of which she seemed so vulnerable, without tears but in a monotone expressive of helplessness and despair. During this time, wavelike contractions of the sigmoid were for the first time totally suppressed (see Fig. 1). When asked, at the conclusion of the interview, to date precisely the onset of her unremitting diarrhea, she replied that it had begun on her wedding night.

Clinical review of this entire series of IBS patients showed that "coping" behavior was described most often in patients whose usual complaint was constipation, whereas

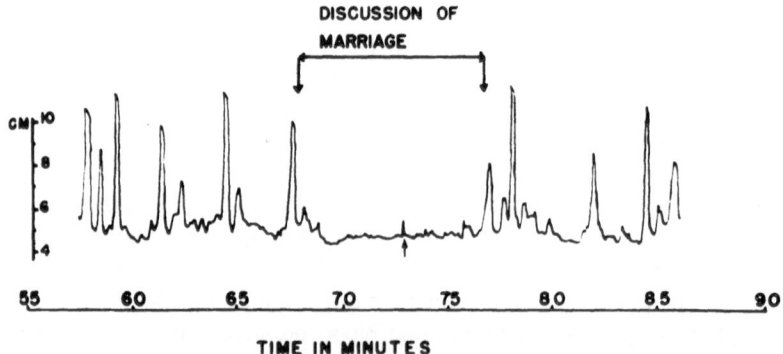

Figure 1. A portion of a continuous balloon kymograph recording from the sigmoid colon of the patient during an extended stress interview. At 73 min (short vertical arrow) the patient sobbed, "He drinks!"

"helpless" behavior was most often associated with painless diarrhea. In those whose emotional state and behavior varied between the two extremes, alternation of constipation and diarrhea was often impressive.[25] The consequences of these motor phenomena in the distal colon are revealed by their relationship to simultaneous motility in the more proximal colon—propulsion or retention of colonic contents will be determined, respectively, by aborad or orad *gradients* between proximal and distal segments. Thus, the activity of the (more often observed) distal sigmoid will appear to be the "paradoxical motility" described by Connell.[26] Others have regarded the sigmoid as a sphincteric zone.

Other investigators, most of them using more modern methods of recording motility, have confirmed the participation of the distal colon in the bodily reactions to stress. Grace et al. described several adult patients with exposed colostomies whose motility and vascularity underwent changes correlated with their ongoing emotional state.[27] Chaudhary and Truelove[28] and Wangel and Deller[29] observed striking changes in the intraluminal pressure in the distal colon in both healthy persons and IBS patients during stress interviews. The latter group also noted these phenomena in patients with a variety of other gastrointestinal diseases. In Chaudhary and Truelove's study, IBS patients showed increased sensitivity of the colon to stimulation by neostigmine[30]; and Kopel et al.[31] observed the same phenomenon in children with recurrent abdominal pain of presumed functional origin. Rubin et al. remarked, in children undergoing the cold pressor test, that those with abdominal pain showed slower-than-normal recovery of homeostatic pupillary reactivity following stress.[32] These findings together may indicate hyperactivity of the autonomic nervous system in patients with stress-related gastrointestinal disorders.

Whereas earlier workers in this field were principally concerned with the temporal correlation of emotions and enteric dysfunction, the attention of later investigators has been directed to the relationship of measurable personality traits to the spontaneous motility of the gut and its response to various stimuli. Whitehead et al.[33] compared normal subjects, predominantly constipated IBS patients, and IBS patients having diarrhea with respect to personality features and the motor responses of the rectum and anal sphincters to balloon distention of the rectosigmoid region. Both groups of IBS patients, as in other studies, had greater-than-usual degrees of anxiety, depression, and other traits. "Slow" contractions were more frequent in both groups of IBS patients than in normal persons, while only the greater frequency of "fast" contractions distinguished those with diarrhea from those with constipation.

Snape et al.[34] reported that the predominant frequency of myoelectrical rhythm at the rectosigmoid junction of IBS patients is 3 cycles/min (normal 6). Taylor et al.[35] confirmed this abnormality and found that it persists in the absence of symptoms and occurs equally in patients with constipation or diarrhea. In these studies the personality features of the patients were not defined. Latimer et al.,[36] confirming and extending these observations, found in "psychoneurotic controls" without a history of enteric symptoms, the same 3 cycles/min rhythm recorded in patients with IBS. They associated the myoelectrical phenomena not with the motility disorder, but with the underlying personality traits, of IBS patients. In their hands the colonic motility changes in the normal, IBS, and other psychoneurotic groups during "neutral" and "stressful" interviews were not significantly different despite great quantitative differences among individuals.

Welgan et al. recently recorded the intraluminal pressure and a basal electrical rhythm (BER) of the distal colon, in healthy subjects and in IBS patients under resting conditions and three kinds of experimental stress.[37] While motility was increased in both groups during stress, and their myoelectrical activity at rest did not differ, the proportion of 2–4 cycles/min activity increased during stress in IBS patients, but declined in the controls.

Kumar and Wingate, on the other hand, recorded the interdigestive myoelectrical activity of the upper small intestine in individuals exposed to standard, nonindividualized stressful stimuli. Abolition or irregularity of the migrating motor complexes was seen in 19 of 22 IBS patients but in only 1 of 10 healthy controls.[38] Their work confirms early indications that the small intestine participates in the pathophysiology of IBS. They suggested that its more regular motility patterns will allow easier identification of abnormalities than is possible in studies of colonic motility.

Recently, motility disturbances of the small intestine and the colon, analogous to those seen in normal human subjects and in IBS patients under stress, have been observed in a readily reproducible animal model. When Williams et al.[39] restricted with tape the movement of the upper body and forelimbs of laboratory rats, plasma levels of ACTH and of β-endorphin rose and the motility (transit) of the small intestine was inhibited while that of the colon was stimulated. The same changes in motility, together with retardation of gastric emptying, have been produced in dose-related fashion by systemic parenteral or intracerebroventricular administration of the neuropeptide corticotropin releasing factor (CRF) at levels characteristic of stress reactions.[40,41] CRF occurs both in the gut wall and in those areas of the brain affecting regulation of the autonomic nervous system; and the effects of stress on intestinal motility in the rat model of IBS are reported to be blocked by α-helical CRF, a competitive antagonist of the native hormone.[41] These findings may well lead to progressive clarification of the central control mechanisms involved in functional bowel disorders.

2.1. Critique

Of the studies recounted above, the earlier ones were seriously flawed as judged by modern standards of experimental design and instrumentation. Among other things, bias in the selection of subjects, the lack of appropriate controls, and the interpretation of physiological data by observers aware of the subjects' emotional reactions have served to limit confidence in their findings. The more recent reports involve much improved methodology, better controls, and more standardized stressful stimuli. At the same time, many will agree that stimuli become stressful, in all but extreme conditions, by virtue of the attitude and previous conditioning of the subject—factors that, together with the ongoing emotional state of the subject during the experiment, have been left out of account in most recent studies. In earlier reports, the most impressive physiological changes in the gut coincided very closely with externally visible manifestations of emotion, and often were just as fleeting.

2.2. Alternative Models of a Mind–Body Interaction

These varying approaches to the mechanisms of psychophysiological disorder can be represented by two disparate models.[42] In one, the "weeping" model, the physiological events underlying the symptoms of IBS and other functional disorders are, like blushing, weeping, and facial expressions, regarded as normal bodily manifestations of emotional tension. Those more familiar, easily visible signs of emotion often but not always coincide with the clinical symptoms of gut disorder. Within the limits of the experimental methods so far employed, the alterations in the gut during emotional arousal appear qualitatively similar in healthy persons and in IBS patients (though it should be noted that neither sigmoid hypomotility nor lacrimation has yet been described during experimental emotional conflict in normal subjects).

Meanwhile we have learned that about 30% of the healthy, uncomplaining population have clinically definable functional disorders, almost one-half of these having typical IBS.[43-45] These "nonpatients" with IBS outnumber by a factor of three or more those who have consulted a physician. In the "weeping" model, then, functional disorders are viewed as responses differing only in degree from the normal behavior of the gut during emotional conflict.

In both patients and healthy persons, the physiological changes induced by stressful stimuli in the laboratory were seldom accompanied by relevant symptoms. A mechanism of importance in producing constipation might have given rise to the symptom only if it persisted for much longer than the span of the experiment, and neither intestinal pain nor diarrhea has been noted during clearly visible alterations in motility. This suggests that many of the less severe or persistent episodes in patients with functional disorders go unrecognized by either patient or physician; and that the data on their clinical prevalence in the community, which have been cited above, as well as our clinical impressions of their persistence in individual patients, represent substantial underestimates.

The greater sensitivity, or perhaps only greater awareness, of the intestine during stress in patients with functional disorders is explained by some as the consequence of operant conditioning, or "visceral learning," dating from early youth. The childhood experience of receiving parental displays of affection after complaining of intestinal symptoms, it has been suggested, may lead later on to unconscious "selection" of abdominal distress as a means of evoking sympathy and comfort; or, in other words, to the ready adoption of the "sick role."[46] In recent studies, "patients" with IBS differed from "nonpatients" in that greater attention had been paid to these and other common symptoms in their youth, that they had more often been taken to the doctor for minor ailments, and that IBS had more often appeared in one or both parents.[47] As formal psychological assessments have so far revealed no major differences between "patients" and "nonreporters" of IBS,[48] the factor of health-seeking behavior may be of special importance in defining the borderline between health and illness.

For the clinician, the "weeping" model suggests that he or she explore the background of psychosocial vulnerability and illness behavior in the individual patient, and identifying the current life situations that precipitate or intensify distress, some of which may be correctable. Improved management in the future might involve the "unlearning" of uneconomical behavior patterns, as has been so far attempted by counseling or biofeedback. Alternatively, progress might come from growing knowledge of the complex neurotransmitter mechanisms activated during reactions to stress, as utilized in the current pharmacotherapy of panic disorders. By contrast, more minute study of the control mechanisms during rest, following meals, or administration of individual chemical agonists may prove less fruitful.

In the alternative concept of the functional disorders, the "epilepsy" model, its advocates view the patterns of psychophysiological phenomena as relatively fixed, and possibly inborn. The familial incidence of these disorders and their undoubted occurrence in early childhood may be attributable to nature more than nurture. They are often associated with well-defined categories of personality disorder—witness the high prevalence of depression, anxiety states, and somatization disorder in patients referred to digestive disease clinics with intractable IBS. In many patients, their individual symptom patterns are remarkably constant over long periods of time, and tend to recur in the same pattern after long symptom-free intervals. All of these facts together suggest that the underlying mechanisms are qualitative departures from the normal, analogous to the cerebral dysrhythmia of epilepsy, and that stress is significant only as a nonspecific trigger. To date, however, no clear-cut qualitative difference, or any unique quantitatively abnormal, physiological mechanism, has been demonstrated.

The experimental manipulation of psychophysiological events, and some of the more recent investigations of intestinal motility, give partial support to the "epilepsy" hypothesis. The motility changes induced by contrived stressors, in several widely separated laboratories focusing on different portions of the gut, were in no way specific to the stimulus employed, be it peripheral pain, hypoglycemia, mathematical calculations, video games, or stress interviews.[22,25,37,38] The higher prevalence of 2–4 cycles/min frequency of the BER in the distal colon in IBS has been found to be a relatively fixed characteristic of the patient, persisting through changes in symptom pattern and well into periods of clinical remission.[35] Latimer's finding of a similar spectrum of myoelectrical activity in psychoneurotic patients who have never complained of intestinal symptoms[36] can be interpreted as a physiological clue to innate susceptibility to IBS, not yet manifest clinically, analogous to the abnormal EEGs of many first-order relatives of epileptics. But against this hypothesis is the high overall prevalence of functional disorders, amounting to almost one-third of mankind in the Western world, as well as its highly variable course in most patients and the numerous examples of hectic variations in both symptom patterns and emotional states.

The Discovery of the "Little Brain." Recently, as the complexity of the neurohumoral control mechanisms in the gut has been revealed, the intramural ganglion networks have been recognized as a third component of the nervous system, the enteric nervous system (ENS) or the "little brain." Wood has compared the ENS, with its abundance of internal connections, to a well-programmed microcomputer,[49] capable of two-way communication with a mainframe (the "big brain") with which it is connected, or alternatively able to function without continuous mainframe control. This conception offers a theoretical basis for understanding the automaticity and intractibility of long-established functional disorders, in turn expressed by the "epilepsy" model. It invites pharmacologists to continue seeking to control the "little brain" by threshold-raising drugs analogous to anticonvulsants, but tailor-made for the ENS. To behavioral scientists it underscores the futility of simple counseling or insight-giving in persistent functional disorders, and suggests the greater promise of measures such as relaxation training and hypnosis.[50]

2.3. Widening Concepts of Mind–Body Interaction

For many decades, since Cannon's early studies with X-rays, those interested in the response of the intestine to stress have directed their attention chiefly to the motility of the gut. Such studies have helped in the understanding of several syndromes, but have shed little light on that of persistent, painless, voluminous, watery diarrhea. In recent years this problem has been addressed in terms of modern concepts of transport of water and electrolytes across the intestinal mucosa. In patients with IBS and diarrhea, Rask-Madsen and Bukhave[51] continuously perfused the jejunum and ileum with various concentrations of chenodeoxycholic acid, and found a net secretion into the lumen at concentrations that in normal subjects regularly allow net absorption, thus identifying the disorder as a secretory diarrhea. They found high concentrations of a prostaglandin (PGE_2) in the luminal fluid, a phenomenon also noted in some cases of diarrhea due to food intolerance. These findings have prompted the trial of indomethacin and other antiplatelet agents, which have been effective in controlling diarrhea in some patients. Though this mechanism might appear to lie outside the limits of psychophysiology, evidence that acetylcholine, serotonin, and other neurotransmitters in the ENS can stimulate the local release of prostaglandins suggests that this alteration in fluid transport may be yet another mechanism in the general adaptation to stress.

Furthermore, recent evidence that the lymphoid tissue of the intestinal wall is innervated by the "little brain," and that the lymphocytes and other immunocompetent cells have receptors for a variety of neurotransmitters, has further widened our concepts of the scope of neurohormonal influences on intestinal function[52]. For example, substance P is known to enhance proliferation of lymphocytes, stimulate synthesis of immunoglobulins, and cause release of histamine from the mast cells of the mucosa, with which substance P-containing nerve endings are in close apposition. While it remains to be demonstrated that these defense mechanisms of the host are also mobilized in humans under nonspecific stress, such a discovery will hardly surprise those clinically familiar with the psychophysiological aspects of illness.

3. CONCLUSION

More than a century of clinical and experimental study of common functional disorders of the gastrointestinal tract has yielded a train of evidence implicating psychophysiological mechanisms in their pathogenesis. Yet careful study of individual cases rarely reveals an instance in which such a mechanism is not intertwined with other influences on the gut by allergens, microorganisms, the products of fermentation of nutrients, environmental chemicals, and drugs that contribute to the manifestations of illness, and often interact with each other. For example, the response of the stomach to appetizing food, or even to atropine, may be modified by the emotional state of the subject.[53] In view of the nigh-universal capacity of the gut to react to stress, even the stress of disease of another cause, any gastrointestinal *illness* can be a combination of the effects of an "organic" with a "functional" disorder. Thus, a psychophysiological mechanism must be regarded as a common *factor* in the causation of illness, which is sometimes predominant but always worthy of attention.

REFERENCES

1. Powell R: On certain painful affections of the intestinal canal. Med Trans Coll Physicians 6:106–117, 1820
2. Clark A: Clinical illustrations of mucous disease of the colon from notes of various cases. Lancet 2:614–615, 1859

3. da Costa JM: Membranous enteritis. Am J Med Sci 62:321–338, 1871
4. White WH: A study of 60 cases of membranous colitis. Lancet 2:1229–1235, 1905
5. Manning AP, Thompson WG, Heaton KW, et al: Towards positive diagnosis of the irritable bowel. Br Med J 2:653–654, 1978
6. Kruis W, Thieme C, Weinzierl M, et al: A diagnostic score for the irritable bowel syndrome—its value in the exclusion of organic disease. Gastroenterology 87:1–7, 1984
7. Beaumont W: Experiments and Observations on the Gastric Juice, and the Physiology of Digestion. Plattsburg, FP Allen, 1833
8. Pavlov I: The Work of the Digestive Glands. English translation from the Russian by WH Thompson. London, C Griffin & Co, 1910
9. Wolf S, Wolff HG: Human Gastric Function. London, Oxford University Press, 1943
10. Engel G, Reichsman F, Segal HL: A study of an infant with gastric fistula. Psychosom Med 18:374–398, 1956
11. Abbot FK, Mack M, Wolf SG: The relation of sustained contraction of the duodenum to nausea and vomiting. Gastroenterology 20:238–248, 1952
12. Wolf S, Almy TP: Experimental observations on cardiospasm in man. Gastroenterology 13:401–421, 1949
13. Bockus HL, Bank J, Wilkinson SA: Neurogenic mucous colitis. Am J Med Sci 176:813–829, 1928
14. Alvarez WC: Nervous Indigestion. New York, Paul B Hoeber, 1930
15. Alexander F: Influence of psychologic factors upon gastrointestinal disturbances: Symposium, general principles, objectives, and preliminary results. Psychoanal Q 31:501–539, 1934
16. White BV, Cobb S, Jones CM: Mucous colitis. Psychosom Med Monogr #1, 1939
17. Cannon WB: The movements of the intestines studied by means of the roentgen rays. Am J Physiol 6:251–277, 1902
18. Lydiard RB, Laraia MT, Howell EF, et al: Can panic disorder present as irritable bowel syndrome? J Clin Psychiatry 47:470–473, 1986
19. White BV, Jones CM: The effect of irritants and drugs affecting the autonomic nervous system upon the mucosa of the normal rectum and rectosigmoid with special reference to "mucous colitis." N Engl J Med 218:791–797, 1938
20. Friedman MHF, Snape WJ: Color changes in the mucosa of the colon in children as affected by food and psychic stimuli, Fed Proc 5(pt II):30, 1946
21. Almy TP, Tulin M: Alterations in colonic function in man under stress: Experimental production of changes simulating the "irritable colon." Gastroenterology 8:616–626, 1947
22. Almy TP, Kern F, Tulin M: Alterations in colonic function in man under stress. II: Experimental production of sigmoid spasm in healthy persons. Gastroenterology 12:425–436, 1949
23. Almy TP, Hinkle LE, Berle B: Alterations in colonic function in man under stress. III: Experimental production of sigmoid spasm in patients with spastic constipation. Gastroenterology 12:437–449, 1949
24. Almy TP, Abbot FK, Hinkle LE: Alterations in colonic function in man under stress. IV: Hypomotility of the sigmoid colon and its relationship to the mechanism of functional diarrhea. Gastroenterology 15:95–105, 1950
25. Almy TP: Experimental studies on the "irritable colon." Am J Med 10:60–67, 1951
26. Connell AM: The motility of the pelvic colon. II: Paradoxical motility in diarrhea and constipation. Gut 3:342–348, 1962
27. Grace WJ, Wolf S, Wolff HG: The Human Colon. New York, Paul B. Hoeber, 1951
28. Chaudhary NA, Truelove SC: Human colonic motility: Comparative study of normal subjects, patients with ulcerative colitis, and patients with the irritable colon syndrome. III: Effects of emotions. Gastroenterology 40:27–36, 1962
29. Wangel AG, Deller DJ: Intestinal motility in man. III: Mechanisms of constipation and diarrhea with particular reference to the irritable bowel syndrome. Gastroenterology 48:69–84, 1965
30. Chaudhary NA, Truelove SC: Human colonic motility: Comparative study of normal subjects, patients with ulcerative colitis, and patients with the irritable colon syndrome. II: The effect of prostigmine. Gastroenterology 40:18–26, 1962
31. Kopel FB, Kim IC, Barbero GJ: Comparison of rectosigmoid motility in normal children, children with recurrent abdominal pain, and children with ulcerative colitis. Pediatrics 39:539–545, 1967
32. Rubin LS, Barbero GJ, Sibinga MS: Pupillary reactivity in children with acute abdominal pain. Psychosom Med 29:111–120, 1967

33. Whitehead WE, Engel BT, Schuster MM: Irritable bowel syndrome: Physiological and psychological differences between diarrhea-predominant and constipation-predominant patients. Dig Dis Sci 25:404–413, 1980

34. Snape WJ Jr, Carlson GM, Cohen S: Colonic myoelectric activity in the irritable bowel syndrome. Gastroenterology 70:326–330, 1976

35. Taylor I, Darby C, Hammond P: Comparison of rectosigmoid myoelectric activity in the irritable colon syndrome during relapses and remissions. Gut 19:923–929, 1978

36. Latimer P, Sarna S, Campbell D, et al: Colonic motor and myoelectrical activity: A comparative study of normal subjects, psychoneurotic patients and patients with irritable bowel syndrome. Gastroenterology 80:893–901, 1981

37. Welgan P, Meshkinpour H, Hoehler F: The effect of stress on colon motor and electrical activity in irritable bowel syndrome. Psychosom Med 47:139–149, 1985

38. Kumar D, Wingate DL: The irritable bowel syndrome: A paroxysmal motor disorder. Lancet 2:973–977, 1985

39. Williams CL, Villar RG, Peterson JM, et al: Stress-induced changes in intestinal transit in the rat: A model for irritable bowel syndrome. Gastroenterology 94:611–621, 1988

40. Lenz HJ, Burlage M, Raedler A, et al: Central nervous system effects of corticotropin-releasing factor on gastrointestinal transit in the rat. Gastroenterology 94:598–602, 1988

41. Williams CL, Peterson JM, Villar RG, et al: Corticotropin-releasing factor directly mediates colonic responses to stress. Am J Physiol 253:G582–586, 1987

42. Almy TP: The irritable bowel syndrome: Back to square one? (editorial) Dig Dis Sci 25:401–403, 1980

43. Thompson WG, Heaton KW: Functional bowel disorders in apparently healthy people. Gastroenterology 79:283–288, 1980

44. Drossman DA, Sandler RS, McKee DC, et al: Bowel patterns among subjects not seeking health care. Gastroenterology 83:529–534, 1982

45. Greenbaum DS, Abitz L, Van Egeren L, et al: Irritable bowel syndrome prevalence, rectosigmoid motility, and psychometrics in symptomatic patients not seeing physicians. Gastroenterology 84:1174, 1983 (abstr)

46. Whitehead WE, Winget C, Fedoravicius AS, et al: Learned illness behavior in patients with irritable bowel syndrome and peptic ulcer. Dig Dis Sci 27:202–208, 1982

47. Lowman BC, Drossman DA, Cramer EM, et al: Recollection of childhood events in adults with irritable bowel syndrome. J Clin Gastroenterol 9:324–330, 1987

48. Welch GW, Hillman LC, Pomare EW: Psychoneurotic symptomatology in the irritable bowel syndrome: A study of reporters and non-reporters. Br Med J 291:1382–1383, 1985

49. Wood JD: Enteric neurophysiology. Am J Physiol 247:G585–597, 1984

50. Whorwell PJ, Prior A, Colgan SM: Hypnotherapy in severe irritable bowel syndrome: Further experience. Gut 28:423–425, 1987

51. Rask-Madsen J, Bukhave K: The irritable bowel syndrome: The role of intestinal secretion, in Read NW (ed): Irritable Bowel Syndrome. New York, Grune & Stratton, 1985, pp 111–122

52. Bienenstock J, Perdue M, Stanisz A, et al: Neurohormonal regulation of gastrointestinal immunity. (editorial) Gastroenterology 93:1431–1434, 1987

53. Wolf S: The Stomach. London, Oxford University Press, 1965, pp 118–119

2

Role of Neural Control in Gastrointestinal Motility and Visceral Pain

Emeran A. Mayer and Helen Raybould

I. INTRODUCTION

Neural control mechanisms play a critical role in pain perception and modulation of gastrointestinal motility. However, little is known about the role of the nervous system in mediating symptoms in irritable bowel syndrome (IBS). Subsets of patients with the diagnosis of IBS have symptoms either of altered bowel habit (diarrhea and/or constipation) or of altered visceral sensation (pain, "gaseous distension"), or changes in bowel habits and visceral sensation can occur together. Current selection criteria (self-selection of health-seeking patient subset, diagnosis by exclusion, lack of distinct pathophysiological marker) result in a highly heterogeneous group of patients who share the following: (1) a high degree of psychoneuroticism; (2) symptoms are not local but affect the entire GI tract to various degrees; (3) GI symptoms are embedded in a matrix of symptoms of chronic pain and/or psychosocial distress.[1-3] Thus, careful questioning of IBS patients reveals pain in multiple sites, including headaches, back pain, muscle pain, and heartburn.[4-10] In addition, non-GI symptoms such as weakness, fatigue, palpitations, dizziness, perspiration, sweaty palms, brisk reflexes, dysuria, and dysmenorrhea are common in IBS.[1] Recent studies indicate that there is a disturbance in colonic electrolyte transport in certain patients with IBS. These common features suggest a more generalized systemic dysregulation that may be mediated in part by the autonomic nervous system.

In the following we discuss possible alterations in neural control mechanisms in IBS from three aspects. First, we summarize current knowledge about the role of neural control in visceral sensation, intestinal motility, and reflex pathways. Second, we present

Emeran A. Mayer • Division of Gastroenterology, Harbor–UCLA Medical Center, Torrance, California 90509.   *Helen Raybould* • Center for Ulcer Research and Education, Veterans Administration Medical Center, and Department of Medicine, University of California–Los Angeles, Los Angeles, California 90073.

current clinical evidence for altered pain perception in IBS. Third, using this background information, a model is proposed, which is consistent with reported abnormalities in visceral sensation and GI motility in IBS and which could explain symptoms of this syndrome.

This model proposes that the primary event in different forms of IBS is a centrally mediated downregulation of the threshold of afferent mechanisms within the gut. This results in inappropriate (pathological) pain and/or altered reflex mechanisms, involving motility. Even if the original central trigger does not persist, the network of peripheral and central motility reflexes operates on a newly established, inappropriate setpoint.

2. ROLE OF THE AUTONOMIC NERVOUS SYSTEM IN GI MOTILITY AND VISCERAL SENSATION

The GI tract has a dual extrinsic innervation through the parasympathetic and sympathetic nerves (Fig. 1). These autonomic nerve trunks contain efferent fibers that transmit information from the CNS to the viscera and afferent fibers that transmit information from the viscera to the CNS. Visceral afferents are one branch of the ubiquitous system of primary sensory afferents described for a variety of peripheral structures, such as skin, joints, and muscle. It has been suggested that the differences that exist in the afferent mechanisms of these different tissues can be explained solely by regional variations in structure of the tissue innervated, such as the smooth muscle type, collagen content, and compliance. Each sensory neuron has a single process arising from the cell body that divides into a peripherally and centrally directed fiber. The central terminals of vagal afferents terminate in the brain stem and the afferent fibers pass to the periphery in the vagus nerve. The central terminals of spinal afferents terminate in the dorsal horn of the spinal cord and the afferents pass to the periphery in the main sympathetic nerve trunks. However, pelvic afferents run to the periphery with the parasympathetic nerves innervating the pelvic viscera. The cell bodies of the vagal afferents lie in the nodose ganglion and the cell bodies of the spinal afferents lie in the dorsal root ganglia. Both sets of visceral afferents, those running with the parasympathetic and sympathetic nerves, participate in a number of reflexes and in visceral sensation.

Vagal preganglionic (efferent) neurons lie in the brain stem and synapse with neurons in the intrinsic plexuses; the postganglionic fibers then innervate the muscle, mucosa, or blood vessels. The preganglionic sympathetic fibers from the spinal cord synapse with the postganglionic fibers in the prevertebral (mesenteric) ganglia, which in turn synapse with the intrinsic plexuses. Thus, vagal and sympathetic inputs generally do not regulate effector function of muscle, mucosa, and blood vessels directly but modulate relatively autonomously functioning circuits within the intrinsic neural network, the enteric nervous system (ENS). In the following, we will describe the extrinsic sensory and motor innervation and the principal structure of the circuitry of the ENS. In particular, emphasis will be placed on the sensory innervation and its role in visceral sensation and reflex alterations in GI motility. The central regulation of autonomic function (central sympathetic and parasympathetic outflow) will be discussed in Chapter 4.

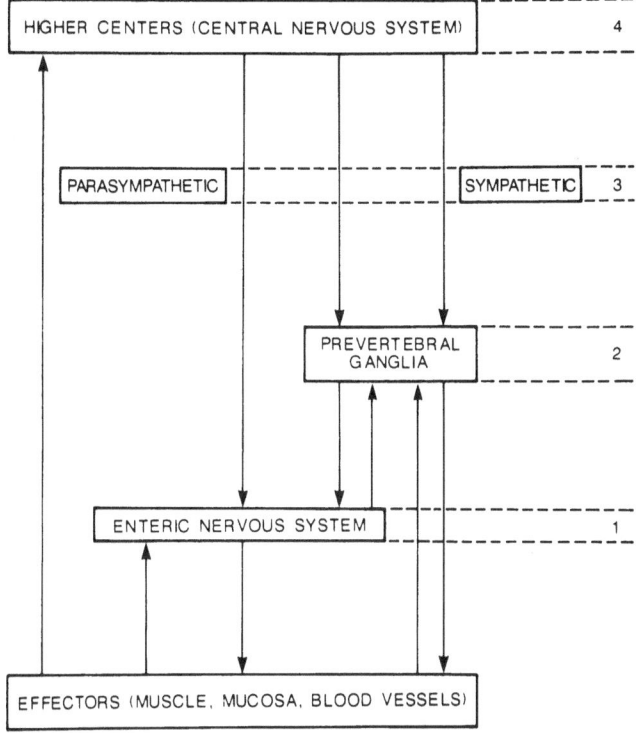

Figure 1. Schematic diagram showing control levels for neural regulation of GI effector function. The enteric nervous system integrates information from the periphery and the central nervous system and modulates effector function (1). In prevertebral ganglia (2), afferent inputs from the gut and descending inputs through the sympathetic branch of the autonomic nervous system are integrated into output which has primarily inhibitory effects on gut motility. Autonomic nuclei of sympathetic and parasympathetic nerves located in the brain stem (3) integrate inputs from the periphery and the cortex (4). Output reaches the gut via the parasympathetic and sympathetic nerves. Adapted from Davison.[5a]

2.1. Enteric Nervous System

A comprehensive discussion of this topic is beyond the scope of this chapter, and we will focus on aspects of the ENS relevant to afferent–efferent integration. Since the majority of structural and functional studies have been done in the small bowel, this information will be used as a model system for the entire GI tract.

Current concepts view the ENS not simply as a relay station for autonomic input to the GI tract but as an integrative system with structural and functional properties analogous to the CNS.[11,12] The circuitry of the ENS is able to generate stereotypic ("hardwired") patterns of electrical activity that regulate motility, secretion, blood flow, and other gut functions.[11–14] These intrinsic patterns are modulated by a variety of external inputs that reach the ENS either via extrinsic nerves or via hormones in the bloodstream.[15] Beside the autonomic input from the CNS, the ENS receives a multitude of inputs from sensory receptors within the gut wall. Visceral sensory input is processed in intrinsic networks within the ENS, prevertebral ganglia, spinal cord, and the CNS. External sensory input is processed within the CNS and integrated with visceral sensory input in the ENS (Fig. 2).

The principal architectural design of the ENS is a number of interconnected neuronal networks, or plexuses.[16,17] Two of these networks contain the majority of enteric ganglia, the myenteric plexus and submucous plexus. Even though the former is primarily concerned with regulation of intestinal motility, and the latter with mucosal function, there are a series of structural and functional connections between them. Among these connections are collaterals from spinal afferent terminals located in the mucosa which form connections with myenteric cholinergic motoneurons.[18,19] In addition, it has recently

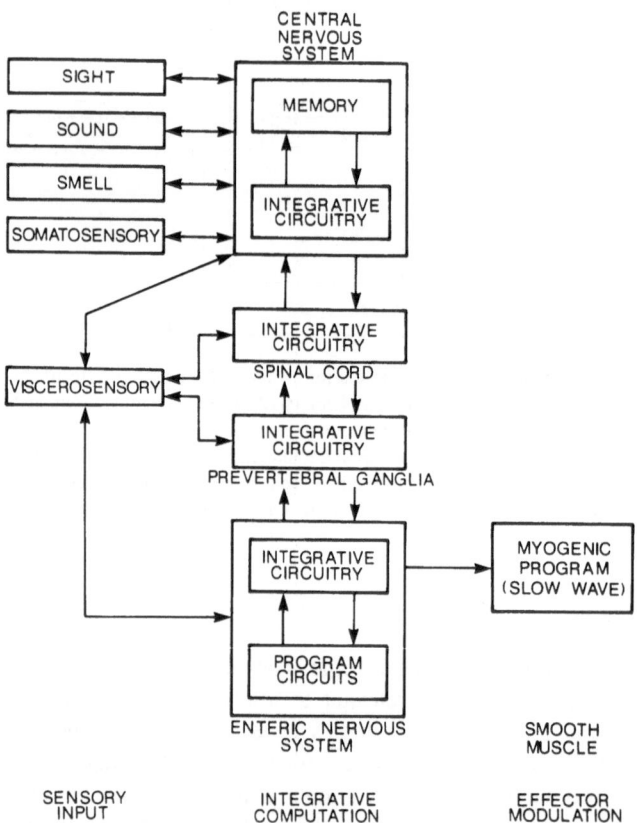

Figure 2. Schematic diagram illustrating the parallel processing of input from external sensory (sight, sound, smell, somatosensory) and from internal sensory (viscerosensory) sources, and from memory within separate integrative neural circuits of the central nervous system, the spinal cord, the prevertebral ganglia, and the enteric nervous system. Outputs from these different "channels" are integrated within the enteric nervous system. Enteric motoneurons are the final common pathway modulating intrinsic myogenic rhythmicity. Sensory input results both in conscious perception and in modulation of effector function via reflexes. Alterations in the threshold of afferent mechanisms may result in a resetting of connections within the entire computational network resulting both in inappropriate sensation (pain, satiety) and in dysmotility.

been shown that motor neurons located in the submucous plexus regulate electrical activity of the circular muscle of the canine colon.[20]

Neurons with nerve cell bodies located within the myenteric plexus show three basic types of projections: motoneurons which innervate the muscle layers, mechanosensitive neurons which synapse with postganglionic sympathetic neurons located in prevertebral ganglia, and interneurons which connect between myenteric neurons. In principle, longitudinal muscle throughout the GI tract is primarily under the control of cholinergic motoneurons. Regulation of longitudinal muscle contraction occurs via modulation of these cholinergic neurons. In contrast, circular muscle is also under significant control by noncholinergic, peptidergic nerves. In both instances, the basic functional unit for regulation of intestinal motility is a motoneuron with its cell body located in the myenteric plexus which innervates a group of muscle cells. Motoneurons which form the final common pathway for various inputs can be excitatory or inhibitory. Since enteric neurons innervate a multitude of smooth muscle cells through varicose processes given off along the course of an axon, and since smooth muscle cells are electrically coupled, 10 to 15 neurons can contribute to smooth muscle regulation recorded at a single point.[14] Analogous to the modulatory influence of extrinsic nerves on stereotypic patterns of electrical activity generated by the ENS, motoneurons modulate intrinsic rhythmic activity of smooth muscle cells. The type of modulation varies in different parts of the GI tract. In the stomach and colon, neuronal input can modulate both frequency of myogenic rhythm and amplitude of contractions,. In contrast, in the small intestine, the frequency of the myogenic rhythm is not under neural control.

Neurons in the ENS have been characterized by neurochemical and electrophysiological techniques.[11-13] Based on these studies, preliminary correlation between function and morphology has become possible. The traditional classification assumes cholinergic and noncholinergic excitatory motoneurons, and adrenergic and noncholinergic, nonadrenergic inhibitory motoneurons. However, similar to chemical coding of subpopulations of spinal afferents, enteric neurons show distinctive patterns of immunoreactivity for a variety of neuropeptides which are colocalized with classical neurotransmitters. Even though the functional importance of colocalization is poorly understood, immunohistochemical coding has allowed tracing of specific projections of enteric neurons.

It has been proposed that a "meshwork" of multipolar neurons with distribution around the entire gut circumference (basic peristaltic circuits) is modulated by inputs from monopolar excitatory and inhibitory neurons (Fig. 3). Even though the exact pattern of colocalized neuropeptides in this proposed model has not been determined, it appears that the predominant neuropeptides in the circumferential network, excitatory input neurons, and inhibitory input neurons are neurokinins, secrotonin, and opioids, respectively.[12]

Mechanosensitive elements which have their cell bodies within the ENS have been fairly well characterized. In contrast to functionally homogeneous peripheral terminals of spinal afferents, several functionally different mechanosensitive neurons, intrinsic to the ENS, have been described.[11] Slowly adapting mechanosensitive units respond to a transient distortion with a prolonged discharge, and frequency of stimulation is directly related to stimulus intensity. Fast-adapting mechanoreceptors give an intensity-dependent discharge at the onset of the stimulus which adapts rapidly to continued stimulation. A third type of unit discharges independent of the duration or intensity of stimulus and continues to discharge for many seconds after termination of the stimulus. These tonic-

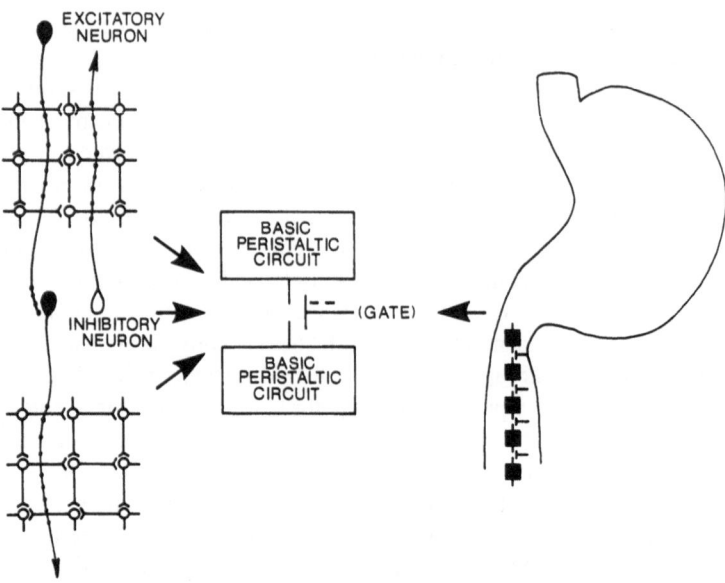

Figure 3. Schematic diagram illustrating the propagation of peristaltic activity via interconnected basic peristaltic circuits. The distance of propagation of electrical activity between networks of specified neurons is regulated by excitatory or inhibitory neurons, functioning as gates. Neurotransmitter candidates for neurons within basic peristaltic units are substance P, for excitatory neurons serotonin, and for inhibitory neurons galanin, purinergic substances, and opioids. Adapted from Wood.[12]

type units signal the occurrence of mechanical distortion with a stereotyped train of spikes. Experimental evidence suggests that these units are so-called AH/type 2 neurons previously identified in morphological studies. These multipolar neurons show a characteristic prolonged afterhyperpolarization; this property enables them to function as "gates" between inputs from their various processes. During hyperpolarization, the nerve cell body is "closed" for transmission of further input from its processes while integration of synaptic input at each process goes on. When the gate is open, integration of inputs from all processes occurs. It is conceivable, but not proven, that the response pattern of specific mechanosensitive neurons can be modulated by autonomic input.

Enteric inhibitory and excitatory motoneurons to intestinal muscle layers are activated via local reflex pathways, entirely contained within the wall of the intestine. Distension, by activating mechanosensitive afferent neurons, evokes polarized reflexes resulting in contraction on the orad and relaxation on the aborad side. This pattern of response constitutes the peristaltic reflex. Enteric excitatory reflexes can also be elicited by mechanical or chemical irritation of intestinal mucosa. It has been suggested that the distance over which the peristaltic reflex propagates along the intestine is determined by the state of the synaptic gates which connect basic peristaltic circuits.[12] Depending on the state of the synaptic gates, activation of mechanosensors would result in either a stationary, segmental contraction or a propagated contractile wave. It is unclear if these neurons receive direct input from extrinsic autonomic nerves. If they do, this would allow a significant regulatory input from the CNS on the propagation of intrinsic enteric reflexes (see below).

2.2. Visceral Afferent Mechanisms

Despite the results from experiments early in the century demonstrating the existence of visceral afferent pathways, the extent of the visceral sensory innervation was not appreciated until the work of light microscopists in the 1950s. This revealed that in the vagus, nonmyelinated afferent fibers were present in far greater numbers than efferent fibers. The vagal, splanchnic, and pelvic nerves have an afferent-to-efferent-fiber ratio of $9:1$, $3:1$, and $1:1$, respectively.[21] Both spinal and vagal visceral afferents subserve several functions: visceral sensation, modulation of efferent output by long (e.g., vag-ovagal) and short reflex loops (via the prevertebral ganglia or within the ENS), and local effector mechanisms at the peripheral terminal region. In contrast to vagal afferents, spinal afferents are also involved in the transmission of pain (Fig. 4).

Spinal and vagal afferents share the property of monitoring the mechanical state of the GI tract via mechanoreceptors. Subsets of vagal afferent fibers respond quite selectively to mechanical stimulation of the muscle and mucosa, or to chemicals in the lumen of the viscera.[21,22] In contrast, for the majority of spinal afferents innervating the GI tract it is not clear whether they respond specifically to a particular chemical or physical stimulus and whether this is linked to changes in function or sensation.[23-24] The response of hollow viscera to distension must be considered in relation to the pressure–volume curve, or "stiffness" of the respective part of the gut.[24] Most viscera are compliant within the physiological range of distension; further small increases in volume may result

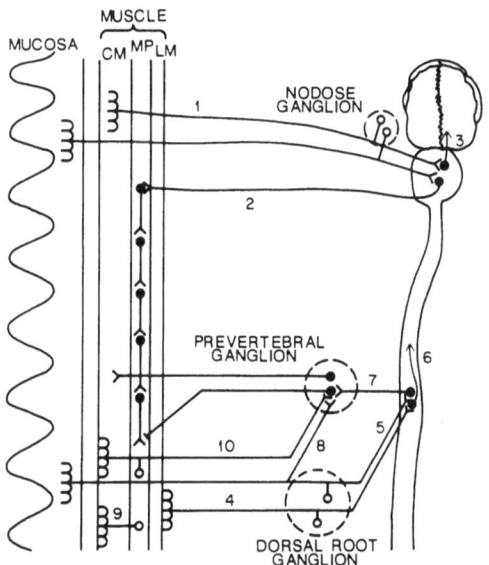

Figure 4. Schematic diagram illustrating major afferent pathways within the GI tract. *Vagal afferents* (1; upper half) have their nerve cell bodies in the nodose ganglion. Sensory structures are located within the mucosa and the muscle coat and record afferent signals via mechanoreceptors, chemoreceptors, osmoreceptors, and thermoreceptors. Ascending pathways to the central nervous system mediate conscious, nonpainful visceral sensation. Parasympathetic reflex loops are established via synaptic connections of vagal afferents with nerve cell bodies of vagal effector neurons (3) located in the brain stem. *Spinal afferents* (4; lower half) have their cell bodies in the dorsal root ganglion. Sensory structures are located in the mucosa, the muscle coat, and the mesentery and record afferent signals via non-specialized receptors sensitive to chemical and mechanical stimuli. The central terminals (5) synapse both with ascending pathways (6) mediating conscious visceral sensation (pain) and with preganglionic sympathetic neurons located within the spinal cord (7) mediating reflex regulation of motility. In addition, collaterals from spinal afferents (8) synapse with postganglionic sympathetic neurons located within the prevertebral ganglion to establish short sympathetic reflex loops. *Intrinsic mechanosensitive neurons* with their nerve cell bodies within the myenteric plexus have two projections (9, 10). They synapse either directly or via interneurons with enteric motoneurons (9) or with postganglionic neurons within the prevertebral ganglion (10). The three types of afferents mediate visceral sensation and establish reflex loops of varying length involving the central nervous system (1, 2), the spinal cord (3), the prevertebral ganglia (4–6), and the enteric nervous system (5). Adapted from Davison.[5a]

in sharp rises in pressure. Compliance, and hence the response of afferent endings, is dependent on smooth muscle tone and the degree of ongoing activity in efferent fibers. Insometric contractions will stimulate visceral mechanoreceptors even at low volumes. The rate of distension may also be an important determinant of the afferent response.

2.2.1. Vagal Afferent Innervation

The abdominal vagus innervates the esophagus, stomach, all parts of the small intestine, and the proximal two-thirds of the colon. Electrophysiological techniques have provided evidence for a variety of receptors including mechanoreceptors, chemoreceptors, thermoreceptors, and osmoreceptors in the GI tract.[21,22] Two types of mechanoreceptors have been located in the wall of the viscera: muscular and superficial. These receptors are stimulated by distension of the viscera or contraction of the smooth muscle in the receptive field and the response is very slowly adapting. It is generally assumed that the receptors lie ''in series'' with the smooth muscle fibers, although this has not been confirmed histologically. These receptors are ideally suited to provide information concerning events persisting for several hours, such as the volume and composition of GI contents. Superficial receptors are located in the mucosa or submucosa and are especially sensitive to stroking of the mucosa. Mechanoreceptors also respond to various chemicals, applied either to the lumen or in the blood, though it is unclear if this is secondary to reflex or local contractions of smooth muscle or to direct effects on the nerve endings.[25] There are also receptors resembling slowly adapting mechanoreceptors in the serosa and mesentery.

There are several types of chemoreceptors in the GI tract. Receptors such as glucoreceptors and acid receptors are specific for that particular stimulus, while others appear to act as nonspecific or polymodal receptors.[22] Vagal afferent fibers responding to acid, alkali, glucose, amino acids, and hypo- and hypertonic solutions have been described in several species. In addition, the intestine is innervated by thermal receptors, similar to cutaneous thermoreceptors.

2.2.2. Spinal Afferent Innervation

In contrast to vagal mechanoreceptors, mechanoreceptors in the spinal afferent pathway have their receptive fields in the mesentery or peritoneal ligament and/or the adjacent viscera.[23] They consist of several mechanoreceptive sites distributed along the course of the periarterial nerves innervating the viscera throughout the abdomen. These receptors give a slowly adapting discharge to probing (local pressure) of the receptive field and respond to distortion of the mesentery. Similar to their vagal counterparts, spinal mechanoreceptors also respond to visceral distension and contractions; the nature of the response to distension and in particular the threshold, varies between different parts of the GI tract. In general, spinal afferents respond to distension within physiological ranges.

Spinal mechanoreceptive units respond to injection of allogenic substances, such as bradykinin.[26,27] Bradykinin also stimulated discharge in mesenteric receptors, suggesting at least part of the response is a direct effect on nerve endings. However, muscular contraction probably contributes to the response in most situations. Mechanosensitive endings also respond to intraperitoneal or intraarterial KCl, HCl, hypertonic saline and to heating of the intestinal wall. Spinal afferents innervating the colon have been found to respond to distension, bradykinin, and ischemia, the latter potentiating the response of afferents to colonic distension.[27]

Nociceptive signals originating from the viscera are conveyed to the CNS by spinal afferent fibers. There has been some debate on the nature of the receptors mediating visceral pain and whether specific nociceptors exist within the intestine.[24,28] Although there is some evidence for specific nociceptors responding to supraphysiological pressures in the gallbladder[29] and for receptors sensitive only to ischemia in the heart,[30] in general the evidence from electrophysiological experiments as described above does not support the concept of a subset of receptors that respond only to supraphysiological levels of intraluminal pressure. For example, mechanoreceptors innervating the colon show a graded response to distension at physiological and supraphysiological levels.

It is evident from the discussion of the functional properties of vagal and spinal visceral afferents that they may subserve different functions. Both sets of visceral afferents may play a role in producing reflexes and sensations. The vagus nerve appears to contain fibers responsible for nonpainful sensations, and information important for digestive processes and maintenance of homeostasis. Spinal afferents, in addition to being involved in the generation of reflexes, play a crucial role in the mediation of visceral pain.

2.2.3. Neurochemistry of Visceral Afferents

Until recently, little was known of the transmitters that might be used by primary somatic and visceral afferent neurons. With the advent of radioimmunoassay and immunocytochemical methods and molecular biology, many biologically active peptides have been demonstrated in vagal and spinal visceral afferents. The evidence indicates that these peptides are synthesized within small-diameter afferent fibers, transported to their peripheral and central terminals and can be released at these sites.[31,32] Nerve cell bodies of the nodose ganglion have been stained in immunohistochemical studies with antibodies to substance P, cholecystokinin (CCK), vasoactive intestinal peptide (VIP), somatostatin, and calcitonin gene related peptide (CGRP). There is evidence for the transport of peptides within afferent fibers since immunoreactive material accumulates central to ligatures of nerve trunks. Immunoreactivities to CCK, substance P, VIP, bombesin/gastrin-releasing peptide, and CGRP have been demonstrated in dorsal root ganglia, though it is not clear if they are contained within visceral afferents. Immunohistochemical methods have shown that similar to the efferent nerves of the ENS, neuropeptides are localized in neurons with other neuropeptides and with classical transmitters, such as acetylcholine, noradrenaline, and serotonin. Recently it has been shown in guinea pig dorsal root ganglion that populations of neurons show defined patterns of colocalization of substance P, CGRP, CCK, and dynorphin.[33] Moreover, by examining coexistence of these peptides in peripheral fibers, each population of neurons had a distinctive pattern of termination, either to skin, blood vessels, viscera, or a combination of these sites. Combined release of coexisting peptides could result in complex effects at effector sites; little is known about the interactions between these peptides (Fig. 5).

The physiological significance of neuropeptides in peripheral and central terminals is not clearly defined. In central transmission of afferent information, neuropeptides may act as neurotransmitters within the spinal cord and brain stem.[32] Neuropeptides released from peripheral endings may function as neuromodulators (via autoreceptors on peripheral nerve endings) or as mediators of tissue responses (Fig. 5). Release of peptides from

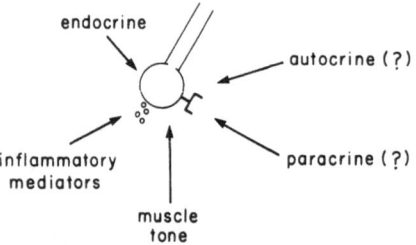

Figure 5. Modulation of peripheral terminals of spinal afferent nerves. Inflammatory mediators and muscle tone have been shown to increase the sensitivity to mechanical stimuli. Even though not proven, the presence of neuropeptide receptors on these terminals is consistent with the hypothesis that neuropeptides released from afferent terminals (autocrine) or associated nerve structures (paracrine) can modulate sensory function. Since opioids have been shown to modulate release of neuropeptides from peripheral terminals, circulating opioid peptides could also regulate sensory function by an endocrine mechanism.

peripheral afferent endings has been shown to contribute to local tissue reactions and to the modulation of postganglionic neurons in myenteric plexus and autonomic ganglia. The concept of afferent endings subserving efferent functions was first evaluated in skin.[34] In skin, electrical stimulation of the peripheral cut end of sensory fibers (antidromic nerve stimulation) results in vasodilatation and plasma extravasation. Substantial evidence supports the notion of the release of sensory neuropeptides (in this case, substance P) which results in vascular changes.[18] Spread of "flare" of the triple response of the skin is dependent on sensory innervation and has been explained by an axon-reflex arrangement.[24] However, neurophysiological evidence for the occurrence of these reflexes is scarce. Thus, afferent endings can subserve a sensory role and may also take part in control of local effector systems. In some regions of the GI tract, antidromic nerve stimulation results in plasma extravasation. In other regions, antidromic stimulation produces other types of responses, such as increased mucosal blood flow, mucosal bicarbonate secretion, local smooth muscle contraction, and activity of autonomic ganglia.[19] Since smooth muscle tone can influence the threshold for afferent function, modulations in the neuropeptide release from afferent nerve endings could allow changes in both motility and visceral sensation in a positive feedback mechanism.

2.2.4. Visceral Sensation

Visceral sensation can be subdivided into two functional categories: (1) nonpainful conscious sensation which provides the individual with vague, emotionally colored sensations about the state of the GI tract, such as fullness, hunger, satiety, or nausea, and (2) painful visceral sensation which informs the individual about potentially noxious events.

Stimuli that induce pain in the viscera are different from those that produce pain in somatic structures; abdominal viscera are ordinarily insensitive to stimuli that when applied to the skin evoke severe pain. Potentially painful stimuli to the viscera include irritation of the mucosa or serosa, gross distention of the viscus, torsion or traction on the mesentery, forceful contractions, particularly against immovable contents, anoxemia and necrosis and inflammation.[21–24]

It is generally (though by no means exclusively) believed that the skin, joints, muscle, and other somatic structures are innervated by a category of sensory receptors that respond specifically to intensities of stimulation within the noxious range. These are the somatic nociceptors whose adequate forms of stimulation are injury and potential damage.

Such a general category of nociceptors has not been identified in the viscera.[24,28] It is assumed that noxious and nonnoxious events are encoded by the intensity of discharge in the same population of primary afferent neurons. According to this intensity theory, discrimination between noxious and nonnoxious stimuli is achieved within the CNS.

There is a wealth of clinical and experimental evidence to suggest that visceral pain is mediated by afferents in sympathetic nerve trunks. Pseudoaffective responses to excessive distension of the gallbladder in experimental animals are only evoked if the splanchnic nerves are intact.[35] Clinical studies have shown that abdominal pain can be elicited by stimulation of sympathetic, but not parasympathetic nerves and is relieved only by section of sympathetic nerve trunks.[36]

Spinal afferents from intraabdominal viscera enter different segments of the spinal cord and though there is some degree of overlap, there is a rostrocaudal organization from different organs. Visceral afferents terminate in defined anatomical zones of the spinal cord dorsal horn, lamina I, V–VII, and X, a pattern of termination markedly different from somatic afferent neurons. It has been estimated that the number of visceral afferents terminating in the spinal cord at the level of the splanchnic nerves is small. This is surprising considering that noxious stimulation of the viscera produces not only pain but also many other more general symptoms such as increased sympathetic output and motor activity. The explanation lies in the convergence of visceral afferent input onto second-order neurons in the spinal cord that have a somatic input.[28,37] Electrophysiological recordings of neurons in the spinal cord have shown that there are two types: somatic neurons that receive an input solely from somatic structures and somatovisceral neurons that respond to somatic and visceral stimulation. Thus, visceral sensation can only be mediated via somatosensory pathways; there is no evidence for a pathway exclusively concerned with mediation of visceral sensation. It is interesting to note that the somatic input of these viscerosomatic neurons is mainly from nociceptive or multimodal cutaneous receptors and from subcutaneous structures, particularly muscle. These observations form the basis for explaining two well-known clinical observations: that visceral pain is poorly localized and diffuse and is frequently accompanied by autonomic and somatic reflexes. The referral of visceral pain to somatic areas is largely a consequence of activation of pathways normally involved in mediation of somatic nociceptive signals.[38]

Several teleological speculations can be made regarding the physiology of visceral sensation: first, the GI mucosa provides a huge interface with the environment, which is not only two orders of magnitude larger than the skin surface but also severalfold more permeable. Central conscious function would be overwhelmed if visceral sensation provided the same conscious discrimination of stimuli as the skin. Second, since injury and inflammation are relatively rare events within the GI tract, one could argue that a specialized set of afferent fibers for nociception is unlikely if adequate nociceptive information can be encoded by receptors that also signal physiological events.

2.3. Autonomic Efferent Innervation

2.3.1. Parasympathetic

In humans, the colon receives parasympathetic innervation via the vagus and pelvic nerves issuing from spinal roots S2 to S4 and connecting to the pelvic plexus.[39] The central regulation of the parasympathetic efferent output is discussed in Chapter 4 and will not be addressed here. In contrast to the cervical component which contains predominantly afferent fibers, the abdominal vagus contains more than 90% efferent fibers with their nerve cell bodies located in the medulla.[40] The pelvic plexus is a laminar plexus situated on either side of the rectum; from these ganglia originate nerve fibers which innervate the urogenital tract and the distal part of the colon and rectum.[40]

The parasympathetic innervation contains two distinct populations of preganglionic efferent axons, one connected with intramural cholinergic excitatory neurons, the other with intramural nonadrenergic, noncholinergic inhibitory neurons. The exact projection of parasympathetic fibers is only partly understood.[40] In addition to the fibers synapsing with intramural postganglionic neurons, branches of the upper and lower parasympathetic innervation run within the wall of the viscus (between the two muscle layers)[17] (Fig. 6). The physiological function of this circuitry is unknown.

2.3.2. Sympathetic

The sympathetic component of the ANS consists of neuronal pathways that emerge from the thoracic and lumbar parts of the spinal cord.[15,39] The preganglionic neurons are

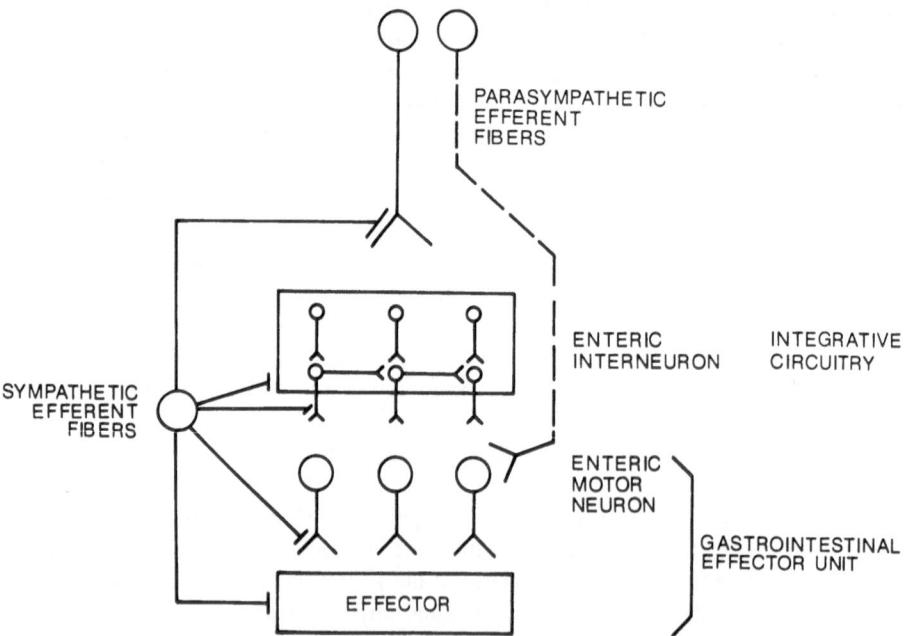

Figure 6. Schematic diagram illustrating the interface of sympathetic and parasympathetic branches of the autonomic nervous system with the gut. Autonomic nervous input does not regulate the effector (muscle) directly, but via modulation of the circuitry of the enteric nervous system. *Sympathetic* efferent fibers, mediating inhibitory effects on GI motility, modulate parasympathetic nerves, enteric interneurons, and motoneurons predominantly via presynaptic inhibition of neurotransmitter release. In sphincteric regions, sympathetic nerves also innervate the muscle directly. *Parasympathetic* efferent fibers interface with the circuitry of the enteric nervous system and possibly directly with motoneurons. Adapted from Wood.[12]

cholinergic and have their cell bodies in the intermedio-lateral columns of the spinal cord. Their processes run to the prevertebral ganglia within the spinal nerves. The fibers that run from these prevertebral ganglia to the gut form the mesenteric nerves and are non-radrenergic.[15,39] The celiac–superior mesenteric ganglia provide fibers to the stomach, small intestine, and proximal large intestine. The majority of the large intestine is innervated by fibers from the inferior mesenteric ganglia. The rectum receives fibers from the pelvic ganglia.

The majority of noradrenergic fibers interface with myenteric neurons (Fig. 6). Noradrenergic terminals ramify extensively among the ganglia of the myenteric plexus and also contribute to the internodal strands. Many of the varicose fibers run for long distances without branching. Dense pericellular rings of varicose noradrenergic axons are found around a small proportion of nerve cell bodies in the myenteric plexus.[41] These rings may represent a specialized input to some neurons, which perhaps differ in functional significance from the apparently more generalized input to the majority of myenteric neurons.[15,41] The major effect of noradrenergic nerves on the ENS is the inhibition of acetylcholine release from myenteric cholinergic neurons. This effect is mediated by α_2-receptors.[15,41]

In the human gut there is a sparse direct noradrenergic innervation of the muscle layers of the upper GI tract and a slightly denser innervation toward the distal large intestine.[41] In contrast, all sphincteric regions of the mammalian gut have a dense noradrenergic innervation. The origin of noradrenergic fibers supplying the sphincters seems to correspond with the sources of noradrenergic fibers to adjacent nonsphincteric muscle. Smooth muscle contains both α-excitatory and β-inhibitory receptors for catecholamines. With few exceptions, stimulation of the sympathetic nerve supply to sphincteric regions causes a constrictor effect mediated by α-receptor activation. Nonsphincteric muscle is inhibited when sympathetic nerves are stimulated in the presence of atropine in vitro.[15]

Subpopulations of noradrenergic neurons supply specific target tissues within the gut wall.[42,43] These subpopulations of neurons are characterized by specific patterns of colocalization of noradrenaline with various neuropeptides.[42,43] It is conceivable, but not proven, that differently coded noradrenergic neurons innervate myenteric neurons and sphincteric smooth muscle.

2.3.3. Intramural and Extramural Reflex Pathways

A principal concept in the regulation of GI function are neuronal reflex loops interconnecting sensory events (mechanical, chemical) with effector changes (contraction and relaxation of smooth muscle, secretion and absorption, blood flow). Besides the existence of classical synaptic connections between afferent and efferent neurons, two other mechanisms have been postulated[11,18,19]: (1) axon-reflex mechanism where stimulation of afferent nerve terminals results in antidromic excitation of collaterals (the subsequent release of neurotransmitters from the nerve terminals of the collaterals modulates muscle contraction either directly or via modulation of myenteric effector neurons) and (2) excitation of AH/type 2 neurons as discussed above.

In the following we discuss reflex mechanisms involving the efferent sympathetic and parasympathetic systems, and those involving collaterals of spinal afferents.

2.3.4. Parasympathetic Reflexes

These reflexes are mediated by vagal afferent fibers and the vagal motor nuclei within the brain stem and are discussed elsewhere. The predominant parasympathetic efferent output on GI motility is excitatory. Modulation of parasympathetic reflexes by spinal afferents has not been reported. One example of a parasympathetic reflex relevant to this discussion is the so-called gastrocolonic reflex.[44,45]

2.3.5. Sympathetic Reflexes

Postganglionic sympathetic neurons are the final common pathway integrating information coming from the periphery and the CNS. Most of the neurons located in the inferior mesenteric ganglion receive synaptic inputs from both peripheral and central origins[39]: from mechanoreceptors in the colon by axons running in the colonic nerves, and from preganglionic sympathetic neurons located in the spinal cord by axons running in the splanchnic nerves (Fig. 7).[39] There is little input from the inferior mesenteric ganglia to the gut via noradrenergic nerves in the resting individual. However, during afferent stimulation from within or from outside the GI tract the predominant effect of the noradrenergic input is inhibitory.

Complex reflex interactions are demonstrable between the gut and the prevertebral ganglia. Peripheral input consists of two types: (1) cholinergic neurons within the ENS which either are primary sensory neurons or receive synaptic input from mechanosensitive neurons (see above)[46,47]; and (2) collaterals from primary sensory nerves from the gut forming the substance P-immunoreactive intraganglionic networks.

A significant number of peripheral axons projecting to the interior mesenteric ganglion from the gut have their cell bodies within the gut wall.[15] It has been shown that these intestinofugal cholinergic neurons also contain several neuropeptides, including CCK, dynorphin, enkephalin, CGRP, and VIP.[43] Most of the preganglionic inputs to the inferior mesenteric ganglion are found to operate through the integration of subthreshold excitatory inputs to the postganglionic neurons.[47]

Collaterals from primary sensory nerves from the gut form the substance P-immu-

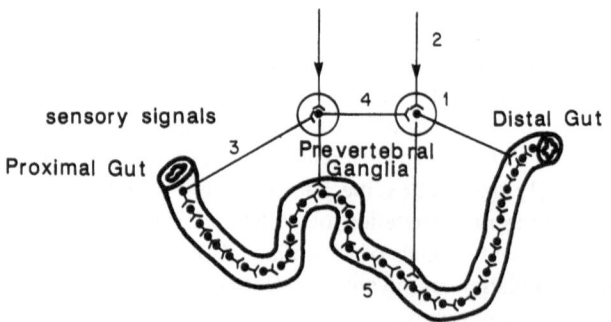

Figure 7. The role of prevertebral ganglia in short inhibitory reflex loops. In addition to input from preganglionic sympathetic nerves (2), nerve cell bodies of noradrenergic nerves (prevertebral ganglia; 1) receive input from mechanosensitive enteric neurons (3) and from neurons forming intermesenteric nerves (4). The processes of these noradrenergic nerves (5) interface with enteric circuits mediating inhibition of GI motility. Excitation of mechanosensitive neurons (proximal gut) result in aboral inhibition of motility (distal gut) via pathways 3–5. This circuitry enables bypass of the multisynaptic pathway of enteric neurons (5). Adapted from Kreulen and Szurszewski.[46]

noreactive intraganglionic networks. This network can modulate reflexes by raising the excitability of respective neurons. Experimental evidence exists for the possibility of such intraganglionic modulation operating like an axon reflex through a short loop system of collaterals from peripheral branches of primary sensory neurons with cell bodies in the dorsal root ganglia.

Several reflex loops involving postganglionic noradrenergic nerves have been characterized in the mammalian gut.[15] These inhibitory intestinointestinal reflexes are called peripheral or central depending on the involvement of synaptic connections with neurons located in the CNS or spinal cord. The afferent signal in these reflexes is distension (or mucosal irritation) of one part of the GI tract which leads to the inhibition of contractile propulsion in another. Reflexes involving noradrenergic excitation of sphincter regions can also be regarded as inhibitory since they oppose the normal movement of digestive fluids.[15] The intestinointestinal reflex has been shown to have a low-threshold component which involves a spinal pathway and a high-threshold component which runs through prevertebral ganglia.[15] Experimental evidence suggests that the spinal component of this reflex is under tonic restraint by descending central pathways.[15] The peripheral circuitry of the intestinointestinal reflex has been characterized in the guinea pig colon[46-48] (Fig. 7). In the inferior mesenteric ganglia of the guinea pig, processes of mechanosensitive cholinergic neurons located within the wall of the colon synapse with postganglionic noradrenergic neurons. Processes of the latter neurons have synapses with the same cholinergic neurons in the gut. Since the effect of noradrenergic input on cholinergic neurons is inhibitory, this circuitry provides a negative feedback loop for the regulation of peripheral synaptic input to neurons within the ganglia. This circuitry allows two types of regulation: (1) the mechanosensitivity of the afferent pathway is in part controlled by efferent noradrenergic neurons of the inferior mesenteric ganglion[48]; (2) a colo-colonic inhibitory reflex is established through which distension of one colonic segment leads to inhibition of another segment.[46]

Thus, in addition to intrinsic reflex pathways of the ENS, complex pathways involving prevertebral ganglia, the spinal cord, and the brain stem are involved in the regulation of intestinal motility. The complexity and interrelationship of various reflex pathways, including the intrinsic modulation of mechanoreceptor sensitivity, suggest that minor changes in specific afferent receptors would be reflected in generalized alterations in motility regulation.

2.4. Pain-Modulating Mechanisms

In addition to the modulatory influences of central mechanisms on visceral afferents involved in reflex pathways regulating motility, the CNS can also modulate afferent mechanisms involved in visceral pain perception. Humans have a series of pain-modulating mechanisms which allow the body to either increase or decrease the experience and reaction to pain.[49-53] Typical examples include the upregulation of nociception and local tissue reaction during inflammation,[49] and the downregulation of nociception during stressful situations.[52] Pain modulation is accomplished by central, spinal, and peripheral mechanisms.

Central mechanisms include modulation of pain perception and descending modulation of somatic and visceral sensory structures and pain transmission. Even though its precise role is incompletely understood, the cerebral cortex may participate not only in the discriminative aspects of pain perception (such as localization and estimation of stimulus strength) but also in the elaboration of the sensory experience of pain.[49] Descending pain-inhibiting systems which are activated by endorphins in the periaqueductal gray area of the CNS have been shown to play a crucial role in modulating pain perception during stress and central electrical stimulation.[52] A detailed discussion of this aspect is beyond the scope of this chapter and has been reviewed elsewhere.[49]

The modulation of peripheral sense organs by central mechanisms has been proposed since the early part of the century.[49] Well-documented examples outside of the GI tract include central modulation of the sensitivity of the muscle spindle, reflex activation of the middle ear muscles, and reflex changes in pupil size. Even though definitive experimental evidence for similar mechanisms is lacking for visceral sensors, such mechanisms have been suggested.[24] Since most visceral receptors are associated with GI muscle, contractions can modulate the excitability or may lead to excitation of visceral receptors, by changing visceral compliance or by altering the spatial arrangement of receptive structures and smooth muscle cells.[24] As discussed above, both tone and contractile activity of GI muscle are continuously modulated by neural influences from the ANS and ENS, which thereby are likely to modulate spinal afferents in analogy to the central modulation of muscle spindles. In addition, a role of inhibitory efferent supply to the viscera in inhibiting the urge to void or defecate has been suggested.[24] Voluntary or involuntary contractions may play a part in "recruiting" receptors to sense the degree of distension. This could be achieved by comparing afferent activity with the efferent command signal, in a manner similar to that proposed for proprioception.[24]

For somatosensory afferents several mechanisms have been suggested which lead to pathological pain perception. Even though not demonstrated experimentally, several of these mechanisms could also result in altered visceral sensation. These mechanisms include cross talk between high- and low-threshold afferent neurons and sensitization of afferent terminals. Such sensitization has been demonstrated after repeated stimulation or tissue damage.[49] In the skin antidromic stimulation of a nerve can sensitize afferent nerve endings in the nerve's peripheral distribution by an axon-reflex mechanism.[54] Other mechanisms of sensitization include chemical and thermal stimulation. For example, inflammatory mediators, potassium, bradykinin, and prostaglandin have all been shown to alter the sensitivity of afferent fibers.[49]

In somatosensory nociception it has been shown repeatedly that certain types of afferents can facilitate or inhibit pain-related mechanisms.[49] The convergence of various sensory inputs onto the same second-order neuron within the spinal cord plays a crucial etiologic role in this concept. Empirical evidence suggests that counterirritation of the skin, cutaneous electrical stimulation, and acupuncture can all inhibit the original pain experience stemming from injury or disease. Even though this concept had been suggested in form of the gate control theory by Melzack and Wall,[49,50,55] definitive experimental proof for the exact neural mechanism is currently lacking. However, the recent demonstration of an increased somatic pain threshold in IBS patients may be an example whereby increased visceral afferent input modulates transmission of somatic pain.[56]

Summary. The nervous regulation of intestinal motility is best described as a hard-wired circuitry of enteric neurons which are continuously modulated by parallel processed inputs from the intestinal lumen, the CNS, and from other somatic afferents (Fig. 2). Optimal regulation is achieved by integration of all sensory inputs and coregulation of a series of reflex loops of different length: from axon reflexes involving spinal afferent collaterals, and short intramural connections within the gut wall, over afferent–sympathetic reflex connections in prevertebral ganglia, to spinal and central reflexes. The recruitment of respective reflex loops depends partly on stimulus strength. These reflexes can have both stimulatory and inhibitory effects on GI motility. Considerable evidence suggests that the same afferent pathways are used for intestino-intestinal reflexes, and for conscious visceral painful and nonpainful sensations. There are several sites where modulating influences on both visceral sensation and reflexes can occur: at the mechanoreceptor or the intramural sensory neuron, at afferent–sympathetic synapses within prevertebral ganglia (inputs from both periphery and the CNS), in the spinal cord (descending inhibitory system, sensory inputs from the skin), and in the CNS (emotional and cognitive factors).

3. EVIDENCE FOR ALTERATION IN PAIN PERCEPTION (VISCERAL AND SOMATIC) AND COLONIC MOTILITY IN IBS

In the preceding section, evidence was provided to demonstrate that visceral afferent mechanisms play a crucial role in mediating both visceral sensation and reflex changes in GI motility. In the following section, current clinical and experimental evidence suggesting alterations in visceral afferent mechanisms resulting in pain and GI motility changes in patients with IBS is summarized.

3.1. Colonic Motility

Evidence has been provided to suggest that motility patterns in the entire GI tract, from the esophagus to the rectum, can be abnormal in IBS patients.[57] The majority of reported abnormalities have come from motility studies performed in the rectosigmoid area of different groups of IBS patients. These studies have not resulted in a consensus on alterations in colonic motility under basal conditions, during an emotive interview, following a meal, or in response to pharmacologic stimuli.[2] Differences of reported results may be secondary to differences in experimental protocols, or different subgroups of patients studied. However, despite these differences several investigators have reported independently decreased motor activity in diarrhea-predominant patients, increased motor activity in constipated patients, an increased contractile response to rectal distension in both groups of patients, an altered gastrocolonic reflex and an alteration in the predominant colonic slow-wave frequency.[2,58] In general, abnormal motility response to stimulants of colonic motility, such as neostigmine or CCK, has not been reported.[59]

Despite their inconsistencies, the reported abnormalities are consistent with alterations in reflex pathways modulating colonic motility. In contrast to traditional teachings, slow-wave frequency is also under neural control and reported alterations in the predominant frequency pattern could adequately be explained by alteration in neural control.

3.2. Visceral Sensation

Several symptoms suggest that alterations in visceral sensation are common among IBS patients. Typical symptoms are abdominal pain, a sensation of fullness or of gaseous distension, and a feeling of incomplete evacuation after defecation. As discussed above, these symptoms could result from a dysregulation of peripheral mechanisms of visceral sensation, from changes in descending modulating influences by the CNS, or by an alteration of the central pain experience. This dysregulation could result in changes in pain threshold and/or pain tolerance. In the following, we will discuss the available evidence for each of these possibilities.

Abdominal pain can be the only manifestation of IBS, or it can be associated with altered bowel habits.[60] Typically, abdominal pain is not a feature of patients who complain predominantly of diarrhea. The quality of pain is highly variable. It can be constant or intermittent, colicky, dull, sharp, and stabbing in nature. It may begin during or right after a meal, but more typically is most severe 1 to $1\frac{1}{2}$ hr postprandially. The location of the reported pain is classically distributed in the left iliac fossa or hypogastrium.[4] However, patients describe the pain as occurring at any site of the abdomen, even at extraabdominal sites such as the chest and back.[4-10]

Current evidence suggests that the stimulus for visceral pain in IBS patients is intestinal distension, even though compression of nonmuscular gut wall components has recently been suggested.[61,62] As discussed above, both distension and compression of the gut wall are appropriate stimuli for visceral mechanoreceptors. Considerable evidence suggests that the threshold for conscious perception of visceral sensation in the form of inappropriate visceral sensation or pain is altered in IBS.

The indirect evidence suggesting a causative role for intestinal distension in the pain of IBS may be summarized as follows: IBS patients frequently complain of gaseous distension and bloating with or without an objectively demonstrable increase in abdominal girth. These symptoms can be associated with pain. However, the quantity and quality of intestinal gas are the same as in normal subjects.[63,64] Inflation of air during sigmoidoscopy frequently reproduces the typical pain in IBS.[60] Two additional examples of chronic visceral pain in patients that are not considered to have IBS lend further support to the theory that visceral distension is a a major etiologic factor. A subgroup of patients formerly considered to have IBS was subsequently characterized as having lactase deficiency.[60] Pain in these patients is assumed to result from intraluminal fluid accumulation and colonic distension secondary to an increased osmotic load from unabsorbed lactose and its bacterial fatty acid metabolites. In patients with diffuse esophageal spasm, it has been demonstrated that pain episodes poorly correlate with episodes of spastic motility.[65-67] However, typical pain could be induced by balloon distension of the esophagus. The increased pain experience induced by balloon distension of a hollow viscus in IBS could result from several peripheral mechanisms. As discussed above, visceral mechanoreceptors are closely associated with GI muscle. If the normal interrelationship between gut wall tension and gut diameter in IBS is altered by a change in the muscular component, wall tension may be excessive at normal intraluminal volumes. Second, if compliance is normal, a lowered threshold for excitation of afferent terminals may explain distension-induced pain. Third, if both compliance and pain threshold are normal, intermittent episodes of functional luminal obstruction by muscular spasms could result in intermittent excessive increases in wall tension farther upstream, triggering pain. Alternatively, visceral pain in IBS may result from excitation of afferent nerve terminals located outside the muscle coat, such as the mesentery or the mucosa. To define the mechanism of pain and pain referral in patients with IBS, a series of studies was undertaken using balloon distension of the GI tract.[5,61,62]

Ritchie compared pain and gut wall tension in response to balloon distension in the sigmoid colon in 67 IBS patients and in control subjects.[61,62] Balloon inflation to different volumes was normally painless to a constant, maximum acceptable diameter: continued inflation eventually gave rise to pain without increasing diameter. Balloon inflation to 60 ml caused pain in 6% of controls and in 55% of IBS patients. Sigmoid diameter and estimated gut wall tension in the two groups were similar. The incidence of pain in relation to wall tension was increased nearly tenfold in the IBS group. In 6% of controls and in 50% of patients, pain occurred at balloon diameters that could still be increased by 10% or more with further inflation. These studies together with the above-cited clinical observations strongly suggest that certain patients with IBS have a lowered threshold for visceral pain perception which is independent of gut wall tension.

More recently, Ritchie concluded that pain in IBS is not due to gut wall tension but rather to mucosal or submucosal compression.[62] This conclusion was based on the finding that isometric contractions were usually associated with pain episodes. Earlier studies by Connell et al. and Holdstock et al. suggested also that abdominal pain episodes in patients with functional abdominal pain were associated with increased colonic or intestinal contractile activity. Harvey and Read reported that the typical postprandial pain pattern could be reproduced in 4 out of 20 patients with functional postprandial pain.[59] Similar to the situation in esophageal dysmotility patterns in the esophagus associated with pain, it is unclear if the observed contractile activity is a primary event or secondary to previous distension (see below). Since visceral mechanoreceptors can be stimulated by both types of stimuli, it is conceivable that the threshold to both distension and compression is altered or that there are subsets of patients with a specific alteration of one type of visceral sensation.

Several investigators have studied the correlation of site of the pain experience with intraluminal balloon distension. Balloon distension in the sigmoid colon resulted in pain that was felt in the hypogastrium in 40%, in one or both iliac fossae in 31%, in the rectum in 21%, and in extraabdominal sites in 8%.[61,62] Balloon distension at the splenic flexure reproduced the pain felt by the patients in the left upper quadrant of the abdomen, the precordium, and other areas, such as the left shoulder, neck, and arm.[6] Dawson compared the pain experience in response to balloon distension in various parts of the GI tract in 48 IBS patients and control subjects.[5] Control subjects reported pain in response to balloon distension of various parts of the colon primarily in the hypogastric and occasionally in the epigastric and periumbilical areas. In contrast, IBS patients felt pain in any segment of the abdomen. In a majority of patients distension-induced pain and spontaneous pain were similar. Control subjects did not experience pain at extracolonic sites, whereas in a large number of patients balloon distension in the colon reproduced spontaneous pain at many extracolonic sites such as shoulder, back, and thigh. Similar findings were obtained when balloon distension was employed in the esophagus and small bowel.

These findings suggest that the entire alimentary tract can potentially act as a trigger point for abdominal or referred pain in IBS patients and that more than one site may be implicated in an individual patient. In addition to the above-mentioned evidence for a lowered threshold for visceral pain perception in IBS patients, these findings are also consistent with an alteration in visceral pain discrimination and a facilitation of mechanisms resulting in referred pain. As discussed above, the two proposed mechanisms responsible for referred pain are the convergence of visceral and somatic afferents onto the same spinal second-order neuron, or the innervation of visceral and nonvisceral structures by processes of the same spinal afferent neuron. It has been proposed that excessive stimulation of spinal visceral afferents could result in retrograde excitation of the nonvisceral neuron resulting in referred pain.

3.3. General Pain Perception

Clinical evidence suggests that nonvisceral pain perception is altered in a significant number of IBS patients. When carefully questioned, patients complain of migraine headaches,[8] back pain, muscle pain, heartburn, and dyspareunia.[7,10] In seeming contrast to these clinical observations which are consistent with a generalized decreased pain threshold, Cook et al. recently reported that patients with chronic abdominal pain and predominant constipation of functional origin are less sensitive to low-intensity nonpainful stimuli and have a higher threshold for acute painful stimuli than normal subjects.[56] Pain tolerance and discrimination of skin stimuli in these patients were not significantly different from normal controls. This profile of nonvisceral pain sensation was similar to a group of Crohn's patients. No correlation between the responses to acute stimulation and the severity of spontaneous abdominal pain was found.

The available data do not allow a definitive conclusion about altered pain perception in IBS patients. However, they do suggest that in certain IBS patients a dissociation between visceral and nonvisceral pain perception may be present. Altered pain perception secondary to chronic pain or stress has been reported.[67-71] Several mechanisms, including increased endorphin release, have been suggested to explain this phenomenon.[49,52,71]

Summary. Substantial evidence indicates that IBS patients have abnormal visceral sensation and alterations in reflex mechanisms modulating GI motility. Abnormal visceral sensation can be associated with nonvisceral chronic pain syndromes, but is not part of a generalized increase in pain perception or decrease in pain tolerance. The inappropriate sensations of fullness, distension, and pain are likely secondary to excitation of spinal and vagal mechanoreceptors in the gut unrelated to persistent changes in gut wall compliance.

4. PROPOSED MODEL FOR ALTERATIONS IN VISCERAL SENSATION AND GI MOTILITY IN IBS

Based on the clinical and experimental evidence reviewed above, a model is proposed which could explain the changes in visceral sensation and dysregulation in intestinal motility seen in IBS patients. In addition, it would be consistent with the existence of subgroups of IBS and with the frequently observed extraintestinal manifestations.

This model assumes that a dysregulation in parasympathetic and/or spinal afferent mechanisms is the central element resulting (1) in inappropriate transmission of afferent signals to the CNS (fullness, pain) and (2) in increased input into various reflex loops modulating motility. In addition, the ubiquitous distribution of spinal afferent innervation within the body would add extravisceral pain syndromes to the model. Alternatively, the convergence of visceral and somatic afferents in the spinal cord could account for extravisceral manifestations. In the absence of known peripheral factors resulting in an upregulation of visceral afferents in IBS (such as inflammation), central modulating influences via the ANS on afferent mechanisms are likely to be the initiating event. Neuropeptide release and peptide receptors on free afferent nerve endings may play a role in mediating the upregulation.

The ANS interfaces at several different locations with the neuronal network composed of the ENS, the prevertebral ganglia, and the spinal cord. Even though not proven, substantial epidemiological and clinical evidence suggests stressfully perceived life situations and the individual emotional reactions as a ubiquitous finding among IBS patients. Even if this central stimulus does not persist, the rearrangement of setpoints for the various interconnected reflex pathways may result in persisting, self-sustained dysregulation of visceral sensation and motility.

REFERENCES

1. Weiner H: The functional bowel disorders. in Weiner H, Baum A (eds): Perspectives in Behavioral Medicine—Eating, Regulation and Dyscontrol. New Jersey, Lawrence Erlbaum, 1988, pp 137–161
2. Latimer P: Functional Gastrointestinal Disorders. Berlin, Springer, 1983
3. Barsky AJ: Investigating the psychological aspects of irritable bowel syndrome. (editorial) Gastroenterology 93:902–904, 1987
4. Swarbrick ET, Hegarty JE, Bat L, et al: Site of pain from the irritable bowel bowel. Lancet (ii) 443–446, 1980
5. Dawson AM: Origin of pain in the irritable bowel syndrome, in Read NW (ed): Irritable Bowel Syndrome. New York, Grune & Stratton, 1985, pp 155–162
5a. Davison JSD: Innervation of the gastrointestinal tract, in Christensen J, Wingate DL, Wright PSG (eds): A Guide to Gastrointestinal Motility. Bristol, Wright & Sons, 1983, pp 1–47
6. Dworken HJ, Biel FJ, Machella TE: Supradiaphragmatic reference of pain from the colon. Gastroenterology 22:222–229, 1952
7. Rubin L, Wald A, Shuster MM: Unrecognized common features of the irritable bowel syndrome. Gastroenterology 76:1230, 1979 (abstr)
8. Watson WC, Sullivan SN, Corke M, et al: Globus and headache: Common symptoms of the irritable bowel syndrome. Can Med Assoc J 118:387–388, 1978
9. Kirsner JB, Palmer WL: The irritable colon. Gastroenterology 34:491–501, 1958
10. Whorwell PJ, McCallum M, Creed FH, et al: Non-colonic features of irritable bowel syndrome. Gut 27:37–40, 1986
11. Wood JD: Physiology of the enteric nervous system, in Johnson LR (ed): Physiology of the Gastrointestinal Tract. New York, Raven Press, 1987, pp 67–110
12. Wood JD: Neurophysiological theory of intestinal motility. Jpn J Smooth Muscle Res 23:143–186, 1987
13. Furness JB, Costa M: Transmitter chemistry of enteric neurons, in Furness JB, Costa M (eds): The Enteric Nervous System. Edinburgh, Churchill Livingstone, 1987, pp 55–89
14. Furness JB, Costa M: Influence of the enteric nervous system on motility, in Furness JB, Costa M (eds): The Enteric Nervous System. Edinburgh, Churchill Livingstone, 1987, pp 137–189
15. Furness JB, Costa M: Sympathetic influences on gastrointestinal function, in Furness JB, Costa M (eds): The Enteric Nervous System. Edinburgh, Churchill Livingstone, 1987, pp 200–238
16. Furness JB, Costa M: Arrangements of the enteric plexus, in Furness JB, Costa M (eds): The Enteric Nervous System. Edinburgh, Churchill Livingstone, 1987, pp 6–25
17. Furness JB, Costa M: Studies of neuronal circuitry of the enteric nervous system, in Furness JB, Costa M (eds): The Enteric Nervous System. Edinburgh, Churchill Livingstone, 1987, pp 111–136
18. Lembeck F, Gamse R: Substance P in peripheral sensory processes, in Porter R, O'Connor M (eds): Substance P in the Nervous System. London, Pitman, pp 35–49
19. Mayer EA, Raybould H, Koelbel CB: Neuropeptides, inflammation, and motility. Dig Dis Sci 33:71S–77S, 1988
20. Sanders KM, Smith TK: Enteric neural regulation of slow waves in circular muscle of the canine proximal colon. J Physiol (London) 377:297–313, 1986

21. Leek BF: Abdominal and pelvic visceral receptors. Br Med Bull 33:163–168, 1977
22. Mei N: Recent studies on intestinal vagal afferent innervation. Functional implications, in Kral JG, Powley TL, Brooks CM (eds): Vagal Nerve Function: Behavioral and Methodological Consideration. Amsterdam, Elsevier, 1983, pp 199–206
23. Morrison JFB: Splanchnic slowly adapting mechanoreceptors with punctate receptive fields in the mesentery and gastrointestinal tract of the cat. J Physiol (London) 233:349–362, 1977
24. Jaenig W, Morrison JFB: Functional properties of spinal visceral afferents supplying abdominal and pelvic organs, with special emphasis on visceral nociception. Prog Brain Res 67:87–114, 1986
25. Iggo A: Afferent C-fibres and visceral sensation. Prog Brain Res 67:29–38, 1986
26. Floyd K, Hick VE, Koley J, et al: The effects of bradykinin on afferent units in intra-abdominal sympathetic nerve trunks. Q J Exp Physiol 69:19–25, 1977
27. Haupt P, Janig W, Kohler W: Response pattern of visceral afferent fibers, supplying the colon, upon chemical and mechanical stimuli. Pfluegers Arch 398:41–47, 1983
28. Cevero F: Visceral nociception: Peripheral and central aspects of visceral nociceptive systems. Philos Trans R Soc London Ser B 308:325–337, 1985
29. Cevero F: Afferent activity evoked by natural stimulation of the biliary system in the ferret. Pain 13:137–151, 1982
30. Baker DG, Coleridge HM, Coleridge JCG, et al: Search for a cardiac nociceptor: Stimulation by bradykinin of sympathetic afferent endings in the heart of the cat. J Physiol (London) 306:519–536, 1980
31. Dockray GJ, Sharkey KA: Neurochemistry of visceral afferent neurones. Prog Brain Res 67:133–148, 1986
32. Salt TE, Hill RG: Neurotransmitter candidates of somatosensory primary afferent fibers. Neuroscience 10:1083–1103, 1983
33. Gibbins IL, Furness JB, Costa, M: Pathway-specific patterns of co-existence of substance P, calcitonin gene-related peptide, cholecystokinin and dynorphin in neurons of the dorsal root ganglia of the guinea pig. Cell Tissue Res 248:417–437, 1987
34. Lewis T: The blood vessels of the human skin and their responses. London, Shaw & Sons, 1927
35. Schrager VL, Ivy AC: Symptoms produced by distension of the gallbladder and biliary ducts. Surg Gynecol Obstet 47:1–13, 1928
36. White JC: Sensory innervation of the viscera. Studies on visceral afferent neurons in man based on neurosurgical procedures for the relief of intractable pain. Res Publ Assoc Nerv Res Ment Dis 23:373, 1943
37. Cervero F, Tattersall JEH: Somatic and visceral sensory integration in the thoracic spinal cord. Prog Brain Res 67:189–205, 1986
38. Ruch TC: Visceral sensation and referred pain, in Fullerton JF (ed): Howell's Textbook of Physiology. Philadelphia, Saunders, 1947, pp 385–401
39. Roman C, Gonella J: Extrinsic control of digestive tract motility, in Johnson LR (ed): Physiology of the Gastrointestinal Tract. New York, Raven Press, 1987, pp 507–554
40. Gabella G; Structure of muscles and nerves in the gastrointestinal tract, in Johnson LR (ed): Physiology of the Gastrointestinal Tract. New York, Raven Press, 1987, pp 335–382
41. Llewellyn-Smith IJ, Furness JB, O'Brien PE, et al: Noradrenergic nerves in human small intestine. Distribution and ultrastructure. Gastroenterology 87:13–529, 1984
42. Costa M, Furness JB: Somatostatin is present in a subpopulation of noradrenergic nerve fibers supplying the intestine. Neuroscience 13:911–920, 1984
43. Costa M, Furness JB, Llewellyn-Smith IJ: Histochemistry of the enteric nervous system, in Johnson LR (ed): Physiology of the Gastrointestinal Tract. New York, Raven Press, 1987, pp 1–40
44. Snape MJ Jr, Wright SH, Battle WM, et al: The gastrocolonic response: Evidence for a neural mechanism. Gastroenterology 77:1235–1240, 1979
45. Wiley J, Tatum D, Keinath R, et al: Participation of gastric mechanoreceptors and intestinal chemoreceptors in the gastrocolonic response. Gastroenterology 94:1144–1149, 1988
46. Kreulen DL, Szurszewski JH: Reflex pathways in the abdominal prevertebral ganglia; Evidence for a colo-colonic inhibitory reflex. J Physiol (London) 295:21–32, 1979
47. Weems WA, Szurszewski JH: Modulation of colonic motility by peripheral neural inputs to neurons of the inferior mesenteric ganglion. Gastroenterology 73:273–278, 1977
48. Szurszewski JH, Weems WA: Control of gastrointestinal motility in prevertebral ganglia, in Bulbring E, Shuba MF (eds): Physiology of Smooth Muscle. New York, Raven Press, 1976, pp 313–319

49. Perl ER: Pain and nociception, in Kandel ER (vol ed): Handbook of Physiology, The Nervous System (3). Baltimore, Williams & Wilkins, 1977, pp 915–972
50. Kelly DD: Central representatives of pain and analgesia, in Kandel ER, Schwartz JH (eds): Principles of Neural Science, ed 4. Amsterdam, Elsevier, 1985, pp 331–343
51. Fields HL, Basbaum AI: Endogenous pain control mechanisms, in Wall PD, Melzack R (eds): Textbook of Pain. Edinburgh, Churchill, Livingstone, 1984, pp 142–152
52. Cannon JT, Liebeskind JC: Analgesic effects of electrical brain stimulation and stress. Pain Headache 9:283–294, 1987
53. Devor M: The pathophysiology and anatomy of damaged nerve, in Wall PD, Melzack R (eds): Textbook of Pain. Edinburgh, Churchill Livingstone, 1984, pp 49–64
54. Fitzgerald M: The course and termination of primary afferent fibres, in Wall PD, Melzack R (eds): Textbook of Pain. Edinburgh, Churchill Livingstone, 1984, pp 34–48
55. Melzack R, Wall PD: Pain mechanisms: A new theory. Science 150:971–979, 1965
56. Cook IJ, van Eeden A, Collins SM: Patients with irritable bowel syndrome have greater pain tolerance than normal subjects. Gastroenterology 93:727–733, 1987
57. Cohen S, Soloway RD (eds): Functional Disorders of the GI Tract. Edinburgh, Churchill Livingstone, 1987
58. Sullivan MA, Cohen S, Snape WJ: Colonic myoelectrical activity in irritable-bowel syndrome. N Engl J Med 298:878–883, 1978
59. Harvey RE, Read AE: Effect of cholecystokinin on colonic motility and symptoms in patients with the irritable-bowel syndrome. Lancet (i) 7793;:1–3, 1973
60. Snape WJ Jr: Irritable bowel syndrome, in Cohen S, Soloway RD (eds): Functional Disorders of the GI Tract. Edinburgh, Churchill Livingstone, 1987, pp 69–93
61. Ritchie J: Mechanisms of pain in the irritable bowel syndrome, in Read NW (ed): Irritable Bowel Syndrome. New York, Grune & Stratton, 1985, pp 163–172.
62. Ritchie J: Pain from distension of the pelvic colon by inflating a balloon in the irritable colon syndrome. Gut 14:125–132, 1973
63. Fielding JF: A year in out-patients with the irritable bowel syndrome. Ir J Med Sci 146:162–166, 1977
64. Lasser RB, Bond JH, Levitt MD: The role of intestinal gas in functional abdominal pain. N Engl J Med 293:524–526, 1975
65. Vantrappen G, Janssens J: What is irritable esophagus. Gastroenterology 94:1092–1094, 1988
66. Richter JKE, Barish CF, Dalton CF, et al: On the mechanism of esophageal chest pain: Evidence for abnormal sensory perception. Dig Dis Sci 30:790, 1985
67. Madden J, Akil H, Patrick RL, et al: Stress-induced parallel changes in central opioid levels and pain responsiveness in the rat. Nature 265:358–360, 1977
68. Peters L, Maas, Petty D, et al: Spontaneous noncardiac chest pain. Evaluation by 24-hour ambulatory esophageal motility and pH monitoring. Gastroenterology 94:878–886, 1988
69. Cohen MJ, Nabiloff BD, Schandler SL, et al: Signal detection and threshold measures to loud tones and radiant heat in chronic low back pain patients and cohort controls. Pain 16:245–252, 1983
70. Hazouri LA, Mueller AD: Pain threshold studies on paraplegic patients. Arch Neurol Psychiatry, 64:607–613, 1950
71. Davis GC, Buchsbaum MS, Naber D, et al: Altered pain perception and cerebrospinal endorphins in psychiatric illness. Ann NY Acad Sci 398:366–372, 1982.

3

Effects of Psychological Factors on Gastrointestinal Function

William E. Whitehead

1. INTRODUCTION

Symptoms of psychological distress are seen in the majority of patients with gastrointestinal disorders, especially patients with irritable bowel syndrom (IBS) and "functional" dyspepsia. In irritable bowel syndrome, for example, 70% or more of patients recruited through medical clinics are found to score outside the normal range on standardized psychometric tests,[1-11] and 72–100% are reported to have psychiatric disorders.[2,12,13] A high proportion of patients with nonulcer dyspepsia[14] and nonspecific esophageal motility disorders[15] also are found to have psychiatric disorders. Psychological symptoms and abnormal personality traits are found with greater than expected frequency in peptic ulcer disease,[16-18] chronic vomiting,[19,20] and inflammatory bowel disease,[3,21] although the association of psychological distress with these disorders is less consistent[22] than for IBS and nonulcer dyspepsia.

What is the meaning of this association? At present, these correlations are not interpretable because there is no consensus about the mechanisms that could mediate the effects of personality traits or psychological symptoms on physiological responses in the gastrointestinal tract. Four mechanisms that could account for this association are described below, and the remainder of the chapter describes the evidence supporting each.

1. Gastrointestinal motility and secretion could be *directly* influenced by autonomic nervous system arousal associated with psychological symptoms of anxiety and depression or with psychological stress.[23] Maladaptive personality traits could lead people to experience such autonomic arousal more frequently.

2. Psychological stress could *indirectly* affect gastrointestinal motility and secretion through the agency of other behaviors such as air swallowing, smoking, dietary indiscretion, or aspirin abuse.

William E. Whitehead • Division of Digestive Diseases, Francis Scott Key Medical Center, and Department of Medicine, The Johns Hopkins University School of Medicine, Baltimore, Maryland 21218.

3. Personality traits could influence the perception and reporting of gastrointestinal symptoms without objectively modifying physiological responses.[24,25]

4. Learning through modeling and social reinforcement for somatic complaints could influence physiological responses and/or symptom reporting.[26]

Before discussing specific mechanisms that may mediate the effects of psychological variables on gastrointestinal physiology, studies on the incidence of psychiatric disorders and abnormal psychometric test scores in gastrointestinal disorders will be reviewed.

1.1. Psychiatric Diagnoses

Table I summarizes studies in which psychiatric diagnosis by DSM III criteria have been used to investigate psychopathology in functional gastrointestinal disorders. The base rates of these psychiatric diagnoses as determined by a household survey of 3481 randomly selected individuals conducted by the National Institute of Mental Health[27] are given in the last column. These studies may be summarized as follows:

1. Major depression appears to be overrepresented across gastrointestinal diagnoses.
2. Somatization disorder or hypochondriasis (the tendency to complain of multiple symptoms) may also be excessive by comparison to the ECA prevalence data.[27] However, the incidence of this disorder is surprisingly low by comparison with the psychometric test data reviewed below. This suggests that the operational criteria used to make the diagnosis may be inappropriately restrictive, leading to an underestimation of the incidence of somatization disorder.
3. Anxiety disorders including phobias are common in patients with functional gastrointestinal disorders, but their incidence does not differ from that in the general population.
4. There is no specific psychiatric disorder that is uniquely associated with any gastrointestinal disorder. Up to 53% of patients with each gastrointestinal disorder listed in Table I have no psychiatric disorder, and if one recruits patients with psychiatric disorders from the psychiatric clinic instead of the medical clinic, most do not have diagnosable gastrointestinal disorders.

1.2. Psychometric Testing

Psychometric tests do not demonstrate any specific pattern of psychological symptoms that are unique to patients with functional gastrointestinal disorders. Patients with

Table I. Psychiatric Diagnoses in Gastrointestinal Motility Disorders

Diagnosis	IBS	Nonspecific esophageal	Community
Major depression	20%	52%	4%
General anxiety disorder	14	36	25
Phobia	0	38	23
Somatization	20	20	0

nonulcer dyspepsia,[14,16] nonspecific esophageal motility disorders,[15] peptic ulcer disease,[16-18,28,29] inflammatory bowel disease,[3,21] and IBS[1-11] share features of elevated scores on depression, somatization, and anxiety subscales whether they are tested with the Minnesota Multiphasic Personality Inventory (MMPI), the Hopkins Symptom Checklist (SCL-90R), or other psychometric instruments. These psychological symptoms also do not distinguish patients with functional gastrointestinal disorders from patients with chronic pain[9] and other chronic illnesses believed to have a functional component.

Patients with different functional gastrointestinal disorders differ from each other primarily along the related personality dimensions of hostility and dependency. Clinic patients with IBS[1,4,11,30] and nonulcer dyspepsia[31] show elevated scores on hostility and do not describe themselves as dependent on others. In contrast, clinic patients with peptic ulcer disease are as a group shy, dependent on others, and lacking in self-confidence; they do not exhibit more hostility than controls.[18,29,32] Psychogenic vomiters are similarly found to be shy individuals who avoid confrontation.[19,20] Patients with inflammatory bowel disease are frequently described by their clinicians as dependent and unassertive,[33,34] although objective testing has not confirmed this.[6,35] These personality differences between patients with different functional gastrointestinal disorders are not found with enough consistency to serve as diagnostic markers, and their role if any in the development of functional gastrointestinal disorders is unknown. For a fuller discussion of psychometric studies of patients with functional gastrointestinal disorders, the reader is referred to Ref. 22.

1.3. Self-Selection Hypothesis

Recent studies suggest that the association between psychopathology and functional bowel disorders may be, in large part, an artifact of the tendency for more anxious and depressed people to visit a physician while well-adjusted people with the same bowel symptoms either treat themselves or ignore the symptoms. We[11] identified groups of women with IBS or lactose malabsorption by contacting the heads of church women's societies and charities and offering to pay the treasury of the organization for each woman participating. All the 149 women who volunteered were given a bowel symptom questionnaire, a breath hydrogen test for lactose intolerance, and a battery of psychometric tests that included the Hopkins Symptom Checklist, the MMPI, the Cornell Medical Index, and the Neuroticism–Extroversion–Openness Inventory. Those women in the community sample who had bowel symptoms but had not consulted a physician were compared to IBS patients and lactose malabsorbers seen in the medical clinic. Medical clinic patients had completed the same bowel symptom questionnaire and the Hopkins Symptom Checklist.

In this study women were classified as IBS only if they met restrictive diagnostic criteria intended to identify people with pain of colonic origin.[11] These criteria were negative physical examination and abdominal pain that is relieved by a bowel movement, plus at least two of the following: looser stools with the onset of pain, more frequent stools with the onset of pain, abdominal distension, mucus by rectum, and a feeling of incomplete evacuation. Women who satisfied conventional clinical criteria for IBS–abdominal pain plus constipation or diarrhea without evidence of another disease—but did not meet the restrictive diagnostic criteria for IBS given above were designated functional bowel disorder (FBD).

Women diagnosed as IBS were compared to women diagnosed as FBD in both the community and clinic samples in order to determine whether the more restrictive criteria identify a different group of patients than the vaguer conventional criteria.

The results are summarized in Fig. 1. The dependent measure is the global symptom index of the Hopkins Symptom Checklist; it represents the average severity of all psychological symptoms checked by the subject. It can be seen that IBS patients who had not consulted a physician were indistinguishable psychologically from women without bowel symptoms. However, women with IBS, FBD, and lactose malabsorption who had come to the medical clinic had significantly more psychological symptoms than women with the same diagnoses who had not consulted a physician. These findings, when taken together, suggest that psychological symptoms are unrelated to the development of the bowel symptoms that define IBS, but do contribute to the decision to see a physician. Similar results were obtained by Drossman et al.[36] when they compared IBS patients who had not consulted a physician and those who had.

Women diagnosed FBD in our study were found to have significantly more psychological symptoms than women who satisfied restrictive diagnostic criteria for IBS even among subjects who had not consulted a physician (Fig. 1). This occurred because a vague complaint of abdominal pain was related to psychometric measures of neuroticism. However, when subjects reported that their pain was relieved by defecation, the correlation with neuroticism disappeared. Thus, the use of more restrictive diagnostic criteria does identify a psychologically distinct group of subjects.

We[31] have also compared psychological symptoms in medical clinic patients with upper gastrointestinal symptoms to women in the community who had the same symptoms but did not consult a physician. Here the comparison was hampered by the absence of any generally accepted definition for nonulcer dyspepsia. We had included nine upper gastrointestinal symptoms in the bowel symptom questionnaire used in our IBS study de-

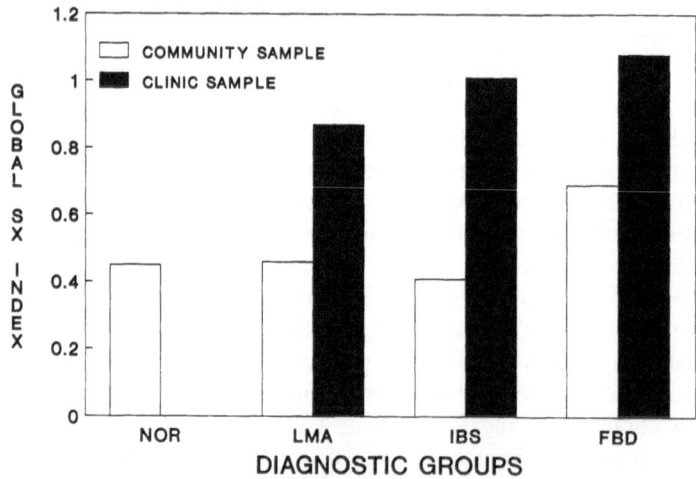

Figure 1. Comparison of women with gastrointestinal symptoms for which they have not consulted a physician (community sample) to medical clinic patients with the same symptoms. NOR, normal controls; LMA, lactose malabsorbers; IBS, irritable bowel syndrome defined by restrictive diagnostic criteria (see text); FBD, functional bowel disorder defined by abdominal pain plus altered bowel habit but not meeting restrictive diagnostic criteria for IBS.

scribed above. These were nausea, vomiting, indigestion, belching acid into the mouth, excessive belching of gas, visible distension of abdomen, excessive stomach rumbling, loss of appetite, and gastrointestinal reactions to foods. After eliminating all women in the community sample who had consulted a physician for any gastrointestinal symptom and all women who had less than two upper gastrointestinal symptoms, we used a covariance analysis to compare the two samples with respect to scores on the Hopkins Symptom Checklist. The use of total number of upper gastrointestinal symptoms as a covariate satistically equated the two groups for number of upper gastrointestinal symptoms. Lactose malabsorbers were also excluded.

The results of this analysis showed that the clinic sample had significantly higher scores on every subscale of the Hopkins Symptom Checklist except obsessive compulsive trait and interpersonal sensitivity. This greater level of psychological distress in clinic patients as compared to physician nonconsulters with the same number of upper gastrointestinal symptoms suggests that most of the reported association between nonulcer dyspepsia and psychopathology is an artifact of self-selection for treatment by more neurotic individuals. Talley et al.[37] have reported similar results in their comparison of clinic attenders and nonattenders with upper gastrointestinal symptoms, and a study[38] of peptic ulcer patients who were selected by random sampling rather than through medical clinic attendance failed to find the usual association between psychological abnormalities and peptic ulcer disease. Thus, self-selection for treatment by more psychologically distressed individuals may account for the previously published correlations between psychopathology and several gastrointestinal disorders.

2. DIRECT EFFECTS OF PSYCHOLOGICAL STRESS ON GASTROINTESTINAL PHYSIOLOGY

2.1. Esophageal Motility

The symptoms of diffuse esophageal spasm are reported to be more frequent when the patient is tired or anxious,[39,40] and the early literature on this disorder includes several well-documented demonstrations that stressful interviews intended to make the patient anxious can precipitate esophageal motor abnormalities.[41-43] Faulkner[44] published a particularly dramatic case example in which he repeatedly provoked and inhibited esophageal spasm in an impoverished patient by alternating discussion of his financial hardships with images of financial security. During discussions of financial hardship, the esophageal spasm was so great that it became impossible to withdraw the instrument (a rigid tube). More recently, investigators[45] have reported that loud noises elicit tertiary contractions in normal subjects. Richter's group[46] was unable to demonstrate tertiary contractions in response to loud noises or other stressors, but they did observe increased amplitude of swallow-elicited contractions during experimental stress.

2.2. Gastric Motility

Epidemiological evidence suggests that psychological stress contributes to the development of duodenal ulcers, and possibly also to gastric ulcers. Peptic ulcer disease is more common during wars than in peacetime and more common in urban than in rural areas.[47]

Peptic ulcers are also more common in stressful occupations such as policeman,[48] truck driver, and air traffic controller.[49] A greater number of stressful life events are reported by duodenal ulcer patients,[50,51] especially during the 6 months preceding onset of their ulcer symptoms or diagnosis.[18] In contrast to duodenal ulcer, some evidence suggests that psychological stress has a weaker effect[52] or no effect[53,54] on the development of gastric ulcers.

Psychological stress has repeatedly been shown to produce gastric ulceration in animals.[55–57] However, these experiments appear to be irrelevant to peptic ulcer disease in humans because 75% of peptic ulcers in humans occur in the duodenum and are associated with excess gastric acid secretion, whereas all the ulcers produced by experimental stressors in rats are gastric lesions, and they are associated with decreased acid secretion.[22]

In contrast to epidemiological studies, which generally support the hypothesis that psychological stress contributes to the development of peptic ulcer disease, experimental stress studies in humans have been unconvincing. The author has obtained statistically significant increases and decreases in gastric acid secretion in different groups of normal subjects, and studies of subjects with gastric fistulas have shown that emotional arousal produces changes in acid secretion that are consistent within subjects but vary widely between subjects.[22]

Gastric emptying is delayed following the stress of holding a hand in ice water.[58] Such stressors have been reported to be associated with both inhibition of antral motility[59] and increased amplitude of antral motility.[60]

2.3. Small Intestine

The experimental stress of a dichotic listening task, which involves paying attention to a different auditory message in each ear, is reported to reduce mouth-to-cecum transit time.[61] Other psychological stressors are reported to disrupt the rhythm of the migrating motor complex and to increase the frequency of abnormally propagated waves.[62] These stress-related effects on small intestinal motility may be relevant to IBS, which is frequently associated with upper gastrointestinal symptoms,[30] but they do not appear to aid our understanding of Crohn's disease.

2.4. Colon

From 50 to 85% of patients with IBS report that unusual psychological stress was associated with the onset or with exacerbations of symptoms of IBS.[6,63,64] However, psychological stress also affects people without chronic bowel symptoms; Drossman et al.[65] found that 47% of normal subjects reported that psychological stress caused increased abdominal pain and 68% reported that stress was associated with a change in bowel pattern. Comparable figures for IBS patients in their study were 69% who reported a stress-related exacerbation of pain and 85% who reported a change in bowel habits with stress.

Early laboratory studies by Almy and Tulin[66] demonstrated that colon motility and mucosal blood flow increased in response to fear arousal and experimentally induced pain. Their observation of stress-related increases in colon motility has been replicated by most other investigators[10,67,68] but not by Sarna.[69] In most of these investigations, normal control subjects also showed increases in colon motility in response to stress, although their responses were typically smaller than those seen in IBS patients.

The laboratory experiments reviewed above demonstrate that psychological stress and emotional arousal are associated with changes in the motility of the esophagus, small intestine, and colon, and probably also with changes in the motility of the stomach. Thus, psychological stress can have a direct effect on gastrointestinal physiology and thereby on the symptoms of functional gastrointestinal disorders.

It is paradoxical that all the physiological effects on the gastrointestinal tract that are attributed to stress are mediated by the parasympathetic nervous system (vagus or pudendal nerves), yet for both cardiovascular and electrodermal activity, stress responses are typically mediated by sympathetic nervous system arousal.

3. INDIRECT EFFECTS OF PSYCHOLOGICAL STRESS ON GASTROINTESTINAL PHYSIOLOGY

Peptic ulcer disease occurs more frequently in smokers than in nonsmokers[28,70,71] and smoking is associated with a reduced rate of healing and an increased frequency of recurrence of ulcers.[72] Alcohol ingestion stimulates gastric acid secretion, which is associated with the development of peptic ulcer disease.[28,73,74] Likewise, aspirin may cause erosions of the mucosa, and excess aspirin use is associated with the development of peptic ulcer disease.[75] The use of tobacco, alcohol, and analgesics may be correlated with the presence of anxiety or other psychological traits and may increase during periods of psychological stress. This has led to speculation that the correlation between stress and peptic ulcer disease may be mediated by the excessive use of these substances.

Walker et al.[28] reported the most comprehensive attempt to test this hypothesis. They first showed that patients with peptic ulcer smoked more cigarettes and consumed more alcohol and aspirins than nonulcer controls. However, when these behavioral variables were entered into a stepwise discriminant analysis along with 12 other variables reflecting psychological symptoms, family history of ulcer, and serum pepsinogen levels, the substance abuse variables did not emerge as independent predictor variables. This could have occurred because these variables were correlated with other variables that were stronger predictors of peptic ulcer disease than substance abuse. The intercorrelations between the substance abuse variables and other psychological variables were not reported but were described as not statistically significant at $p < 0.005$. The authors concluded that smoking, alcohol use, and aspirin use play relatively minor roles compared to the other variables they examined, and that these substance abuse variables did not mediate the effects of stress on peptic ulceration. A final decision on whether substance abuse makes an independent contribution to the development of peptic ulcer or mediates the effects of psychological stress will await replication of these results.

It has also been suggested that stress-mediated changes in air swallowing could contribute to the development of IBS.[76] It is known that anxiety is associated with an increased frequency of swallowing,[77] and that each swallow brings 2–3 ml of air into the stomach.[78] Some of this gas is carried into the small intestine and is swept down to the colon where it may produce symptoms of abdominal pain and bloating. The plausibility of this untested hypothesis is made greater by the fact that symptoms of belching and bloating are more common in IBS patients than in normal controls.[30,79]

Other life-style variables such as exercise and diet could mediate the effects of psychological traits on gastrointestinal physiology. Laxative abuse is recognized clinically as a cause of chronic constipation[80] and some have argued that food intolerance is a frequent cause of symptoms mimicking IBS.[81] Sedentary habits and a diet low in fiber are believed to contribute to constipation, although the evidence for fiber is not yet compelling since fiber supplementation has a variable effect on the symptoms of IBS.[82] The association of psychological traits with laxative use, diet, and exercise has not been investigated. However, many psychotropic drugs are anticholinergic and cause constipation as a side effect. Thus, psychotropic drug use represents a well-documented mechanism whereby psychopathology may indirectly influence gastrointestinal physiology.

4. EFFECTS OF PSYCHOLOGICAL TRAITS ON THE PERCEPTION AND REPORTING OF BOWEL SYMPTOMS

Ritchie[83] was the first to report that patients with IBS as compared to normal controls report pain at a lower threshold when the colon is distended with a balloon. This has become one of the most reliable observations made about IBS. It has been replicated by several other investigators,[1,84,85] although not by everyone.[2] Barish et al.[86] have extended these observations by showing that patients with nonspecific esophageal motility disorders also have a lower threshold for pain caused by distension of a balloon in the esophagus. Distention of a balloon in the gastrointestinal tract does not necessarily give rise to pain at the site of stimulation, however; Dawson and colleagues[87,88] have shown that visceral pain is poorly localized and that the clinical pain of IBS patients (typically lower abdominal pain) may be reproduced by stimulation at distant sites including the esophagus and small intestine.

Several hypotheses have been proposed to account for the lower pain threshold in IBS patients. Ritchie[89] himself proposed that the pain is produced by a bowel contraction that is elicited by balloon distension, while Kullmann and Fielding,[84] on the basis of physical examination findings of a tender colon on palpation, favor a change in receptor sensitivity as the explanation.

In contrast to these peripheral, physiological explanations for pain reports, Latimer[24] proposed that IBS patients may misperceive or mislabel as painful sensations that are within the normal range of intensity. He suggested that such misattributions were due to the personality trait of neuroticism.

Latimer's hypothesis grew out of a broader literature on psychosomatic disorders in which it has been noted that people are more likely to report somatic complaints and also more likely to consult a physician about somatic complaints when they are anxious or depressed.[24,90,91] Acute psychological stress has also been found to increase the frequency of somatic complaints, medical clinic visits, and disability days. Mechanic, the best-known spokesman for this type of research, hypothesized that anxiety, whether it be characterological or reactive to a specific situation, causes people to pay more attention to somatic sensations and suggests that this may give rise to the misattribution of illness to oneself.[92] His hypothesis is consistent with that of Latimer,[24] but goes beyond the balloon distension question to suggest a possible explanation for the tendency of IBS patients to make multiple psychosomatic complaints, to report that they have more other disorders, and to believe that their colds are more serious than those of other people.[93]

Cook et al.[8] tested the Latimer hypothesis by comparing IBS patients to normal controls and to patients with ulcerative colitis with respect to the threshold for pain due to electrical stimulation of the skin. Latimer's hypothesis would lead to the prediction that IBS patients would have lower pain thresholds for all types of aversive stimuli, and their pain threshold should be inversely correlated with psychometric measures of neuroticism. Neither prediction was supported. IBS patients had higher pain thresholds for electrical shock to the skin than did normals. Moreover, pain thresholds were unrelated to measures of neuroticism.

We have also tested the Latimer hypothesis and have come to similar conclusions. We compared tolerance for balloon distension of the colon to tolerance for holding a hand in ice water and to psychometric test data. As predicted, IBS patients had significantly lower thresholds than normals to report pain due to distension of the colon, but tolerance for holding a hand in ice water was not different from normal. Tolerance for balloon distension did not correlate with tolerance for ice water or with any of several psychometric measures. Thus, the Latimer hypothesis[24] appears to be disconfirmed. However, the more general hypothesis proposed by Mechanic,[25,92] which is not specific to balloon distension of the colon, has not been disproved.

The data comparing clinic attenders with IBS to clinic nonattenders, which were reviewed earlier, are relevant to the Mechanic hypothesis: These studies[11,36] showed that anxiety and depression contribute to the decision to consult a physician, perhaps because people become more aware of gastrointestinal symptoms when they are psychologically distressed. However, these studies also demonstrate that the Mechanic hypothesis cannot account for all the bowel symptoms of IBS because clinic nonattenders reported bowel symptoms suggestive of IBS although they were not psychologically distressed as judged by multiple psychometric inventories. Thus, IBS appears to exist as a motility disorder independent of psychological traits.

5. SOCIAL LEARNING INFLUENCES ON GASTROINTESTINAL SYMPTOMS AND PHYSIOLOGY

Through biofeedback training, many gastrointestinal physiological responses can be brought under voluntary control. These include both secretory[94,95] and motor responses.[96,97]

Neal Miller[98] first proposed that social reinforcement in the form of increased attention for somatic complaints or avoidance of aversive work or social situations might substitute for electronic information feedback in biofeedback training and might lead to learned modifications in physiological responses. Such learning could be unintentional and could occur outside of awareness. We[99] amended this hypothesis slightly to suggest that physiological responses could be learned in this way only if the subject (or the people reinforcing the subject) was able to discriminate small changes in the physiological process; otherwise the subject would not be able to reliably associate the reinforcer to the physiological response. He might, however, learn to complain more frequently of somatic symptoms in a manner that produced reinforcement. Encouragement of the sick role during childhood and modeling of illness behavior could therefore contribute to the development of bowel symptoms at two levels: through learned alterations in physiological processes or through learned changes in the overt behaviors of reporting symptoms, consulting doctors, and so forth.

In our first attempt to test the social learning hypothesis, we[26] used a telephone survey to compare subjects with FBD to subjects who had been told by a physician or nurse that they had a peptic ulcer. These two disorders were selected for comparison because the underlying physiological responses that are the presumed basis for symptoms differ in their discriminability. Contractions of the distal colon, which may be the basis for abdominal pain in IBS, are easily perceived[1] whereas the changes in acid secretion or mucus, which are presumed to contribute to the development of peptic ulcers, are difficult or impossible to discriminate.[100] We predicted that colonic contractions would be more likely to come under the control of social reinforcers and therefore that IBS would be associated with a pattern of inappropriate illness behavior to a greater extent than would peptic ulcer disease.

We interviewed 832 people and identified 67 with symptoms suggestive of FBD and 84 with peptic ulcer disease either currently or in the past. These groups were compared to each other and to subjects with neither disorder.

The questions used to define abnormal illness behavior are indicated on the abscissa in Fig. 2. These questions dealt mainly with the subject's response to having a cold because this is a common illness experience that has symptoms that are similar in objective severity for most people. Thus, differences between individuals as to how they coped with colds might reflect differences in illness behavior.

As shown in Fig. 2, subjects with FBD were significantly more likely than controls to report that they had more colds, they felt that their colds were more serious than those of other people, and they were more likely to consult a physician rather than to treat

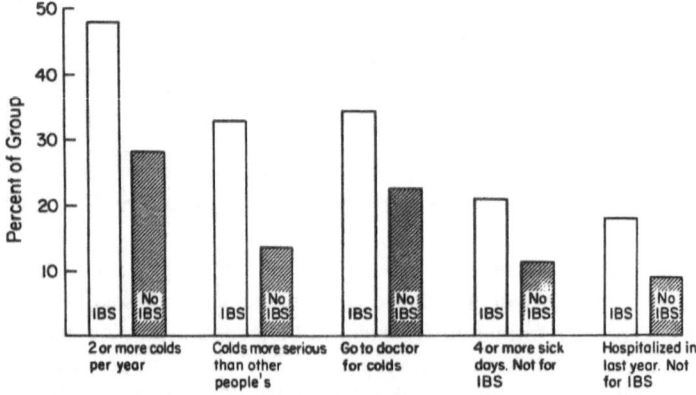

Figure 2. Comparison of 67 patients with FBD (labeled IBS here) to 765 subjects not meeting criteria for FBD. All subjects were interviewed by telephone. Questions that defined illness behavior are given on the abscissa. Ordinate is the proportion of each group responding affirmatively.

themselves. Subjects with FBD were also more likely to miss work due to illness, to make multiple visits to a physician's office, and to have been hospitalized for a nongastrointestinal disorder. Subjects with a history of peptic ulcer disease did not differ from asymptomatic controls in this regard.

These differences in reported illness behaviors associated with FBD were not attributable to anxiety and depression. Self-reported anxiety and depression were significantly more common in both FBD subjects and subjects with peptic ulcer disease and did not differentiate between them.

Illness behavior appeared to be due primarily to a childhood history of reinforcement for somatic complaints: Women with FBD were significantly more likely than controls or people with peptic ulcer to report that when they had a cold as a child their parents gave them toys, gifts, or treat foods such as ice cream. These data suggest that a history of childhood reinforcement for somatic complaints contributes to the development of FBD but not to peptic ulcer. By implication, these data also suggest that changes in gastrointestinal physiology and not just changes in symptom reporting were learned since one would otherwise expect the subjects with peptic ulcer disease to exhibit as much illness behavior and as much of a history for social reinforcement for somatic complaints as we found in subjects with FBD.

These results on childhood social learning have now been replicated by two other research groups. Lowman et al.,[101] in interviews conducted with IBS patients and healthy controls, found that more of the IBS patient group had been exposed during childhood to adult models with chronic bowel symptoms and had been encouraged to adopt the sick role when bowel symptoms occurred. Talley et al.[37] used a questionnaire to compare patients with FBD to healthy controls. The questionnaire included the question, "When you had a cold as a child, did your parents give you toys, gifts, or treat foods such as ice cream?" In agreement with our earlier findings, patients with FBD were significantly more likely to endorse this item.

The findings from these retrospective studies suggest that childhood social learning does play a significant role in the development of FBD and probably also IBS. However, it has not yet been established whether this learning occurs at the physiological level (altered colonic motility) or only at the behavioral level. Possible biases associated with retrospective reporting are also a concern. Answers to these questions await a prospective study.

6. CONCLUSIONS AND IMPLICATIONS FOR TREATMENT

The most important advance of the last decade that has been made in our understanding of the psychophysiology of functional gastrointestinal disorders is the recognition that medical clinic patients are not representative of all individuals with similar gastrointestinal symptoms. Clinic attenders consistently have more psychological symptoms than nonattenders. Moreover, people who satisfy restrictive diagnostic criteria for IBS but have not consulted a physician have no more psychological symptoms than individuals without bowel symptoms. This suggests that there is no inherent relationship between IBS and psychological traits and that the impression that there is such a relationship is an artifact—

people with bowel symptoms who are also neurotic are more likely to consult a physician than are people with the same bowel symptoms who are psychologically well adjusted.

The implication of these findings for the treatment of IBS is that those patients who consult a physician about IBS symptoms are very likely to have two disorders: a motility disorder and an independent psychiatric disorder, which in approximately half of the cases is severe enough to warrant referral to a psychiatrist or psychologist. This implies that gastroenterologists should routinely administer psychometric tests such as the Hopkins Symptom Checklist[102] to identify patients who may require referral.

6.1. Stress

Laboratory experiments and epidemiological studies demonstrate that psychological stressors can directly affect gastrointestinal motility and contribute thereby to exacerbations of bowel symptoms. This appears to be a biological property of the bowel rather than a psychological trait since psychological stress is only one of several stimuli to which IBS patients show a greater motility reaction than normal controls. These stimuli include balloon distension of the rectum,[1] food stimulation,[103] injections of cholecystokinin,[104] and circulating reproductive hormones or prostaglandins associated with menstruation.[105]

Because psychological stress can cause exacerbations of bowel symptoms in IBS patients even if they are psychologically healthy,[65] stress-management training can be helpful to most of them. Stress-management training is a relatively simple psychological treatment whose goals are to identify the situations to which the individual reacts and to teach him or her ways of coping with these situations that reduce the intensity of the reaction. Many different techniques are used to teach coping, ranging from biofeedback training to teaching relaxation of the muscles of the forehead and warming the hands, to cognitive changes in the attitude toward or the appraisal of the stressful situation.[106,107] Controlled studies have shown these techniques to be effective for the management of bowel symptoms in IBS as outlined below.

Svedlund et al.[108] compared a form of brief psychotherapy (average of 7.4 contact hours) to an attention-placebo treatment in 101 patients with FBD. Their treatment was described as teaching more effective ways of coping with stressful situations associated with exacerbations of bowel symptoms. The active treatment was associated with significantly greater improvements in abdominal pain and stool frequency at follow-up visits 6 and 12 months after treatment.

Whorwell et al.[109] compared treatment with hypnotic suggestions to relax and to reduce colonic motility, to an attention placebo. Hypnotherapy was associated with greater improvement in bowel symptoms and feelings of well-being during treatment, but follow-up was not reported.

Behavioral treatments that combined forehead EMG and skin temperature biofeedback training with cognitive restructuring have also been compared to no-treatment groups or periods without treatment in the same subjects.[106,107] These studies likewise support the efficacy of a stress-management treatment.

Most gastroenterologists will not find it to be cost-effective to provide stress-management training themselves. A more practical approach is to establish a gastrointestinal pain clinic with the help of a psychologist consultant or to refer these patients to a psychologist. Nurses can provide stress-management training if appropriately trained and supervised by a psychologist.

Earlier in this chapter, I reviewed evidence that anxiety or psychological stress may exert indirect effects on gastrointestinal symptoms via changes in other behaviors such as air swallowing in IBS, or ingestion of aspirin, tobacco, and alcohol. The data are inconclusive. If it is proved that they play a role in functional gastrointestinal disorders, then treatments directed at decreasing these behaviors would be rational.

6.2. Effects of Psychological Traits on Perception and Reporting of Gastrointestinal Symptoms

The available evidence suggests that the lower pain threshold seen in patients with IBS is not due to a neurotic tendency to mislabel normal sensations from the bowel as painful. However, the more general hypothesis proposed by Mechanic,[25,92] that psychological stress causes people to attend to and report more bodily sensations, was supported: Both we[11] and Drossman's group[36] found that medical clinic attenders were more psychologically distressed than clinic non-attenders with the same bowel symptoms, and we inferred that this occurs because psychological traits such as anxiety and depression influence the decision to seek medical care for symptoms that others ignore or treat themselves. The implications of this self-selection hypothesis have been dealt with previously; it was suggested that all patients with symptoms of IBS be tested for psychological dysfunction and referred for treatment when appropriate.

6.3. Learned Illness Behavior

The available evidence, all of which is based on retrospective reports about childhood experiences, suggests that encouragement of the sick role for gastrointestinal complaints and possibly also modeling of illness behavior by parents, predispose people to notice and to report more gastrointestinal symptoms, to take more disability days for these symptoms, and to consult physicians more often. It is likely that this predisposition interacts with other variables such as anxiety or social skills deficits in such a way that the predisposed individual is more likely to engage in illness behavior during periods when he or she is anxious, when his or her social or occupational skills are inadequate for the situation, or when the situation is conducive (e.g., during military service). These interactions have not been studied. Additional research is needed to confirm the social learning hypothesis prospectively and to investigate interactions with other psychosocial variables.

In another context,[22] we have discussed methods of identifying patients whose symptoms appear to have been learned and maintained by social reinforcement. The treatment of these patients is difficult, in part because it is very threatening to them to be confronted with the role of social reinforcement in their illness. Treatment must usually involve seeing the patient's family along with him or her and is best done by a psychologist or psychiatrist.

One can be more optimistic about prevention than about treatment. Most parents are eager to be better parents, and in fact the reinforcement of somatic complaints in children is usually perceived by the parent as kindness and nurturance. It seems likely that public education efforts that point out to young parents possible adverse health outcomes associated with encouraging the sick role would change the behavior of enough people to have an impact on the incidence of FBD.

REFERENCES

 1. Whitehead WE, Engel BT, Schuster MM: Irritable bowel syndrome: Physiological and psychological differences between diarrhea-predominant and constipation-predominant patients. Dig Dis Sci 25:404–413, 1980
 2. Latimer P, Sarna S, Campbell D, et al: Colonic motor and myoelectric activity: A comparative study of normal subjects, psychoneurotic patients, and patients with irritable bowel syndrome. Gastroenterology 80:893–901, 1981
 3. West KL: MMPI correlates of ulcerative colitis. J Clin Psychol 26:214–229, 1970
 4. Wise TM, Cooper JN, Ahmed S: The efficacy of group therapy for patients with irritable bowel syndrome. Psychosomatics 23:465–469, 1982
 5. Hill OW, Blendis L: Physical and psychological evaluation of "non-organic" abdominal pain. Gut 8:221–229, 1967
 6. Esler MD, Goulston KJ: Levels of anxiety in colonic disorders. N Engl J Med 288:16–20, 1973
 7. Palmer RL, Stonehill E, Crisp AH, et al: Psychological characteristics of patients with the irritable bowel syndrome. Postgrad Med J 50:416–419, 1974
 8. Cook IJ, Van Eeden A, Collins SM: Patients with irritable bowel syndrome have greater pain tolerance than normal subjects. Gastroenterology 93:727–733, 1987
 9. Blanchard EB, Radnitz CL, Evans ED, et al: Psychological comparisons of irritable bowel syndrome to chronic tension and migraine headache and non-patient controls. Biofeedback Self-Regul 11:221–254, 1986
10. Welgan P, Meshkinpour H, Beeler M: The effect of anger on colon motor and myoelectric activity in irritable bowel syndrome. Gastroenterology 94:1150–1156, 1988
11. Whitehead WE, Bosmajian L, Zonderman AB, et al: Symptoms of psychologic distress associated with irritable bowel syndrome: Comparison of community and medical clinic samples. Gastroenterology 95:209–714, 1988
12. Liss JL, Alpers D, Woodruff RA Jr: The irritable colon syndrome and psychiatric illness. Dis Nerv Syst 34:151–157, 1973
13. Young SJ, Alpers DH, Norland CC, et al: Psychiatric illness and the irritable bowel syndrome: Practical implications for the primary physician. Gastroenterology 70:162–166, 1976
14. Magni G, diMario F, Bernasconi G, et al: DSM-III diagnoses associated with dyspepsia of unknown cause. Am J Psychiatry 144:1222–1223, 1987
15. Clouse RE, Lustman PJ: Psychiatric illness and contraction abnormalities of the esophagus. N Engl J Med 309:1337–1342, 1983
16. Sjordin I, Svedlund J, Dotevall G, et al: Symptom profiles in chronic peptic ulcer disease. A detailed study of abdominal and mental symptoms. Scand J Gastroenterol 20:419–427, 1985
17. Feldman M, Walker P, Green JL, et al: Life events, stress, and psychosocial factors in men with peptic ulcer disease. A multidimensional case-controlled study. Gastroenterology 91:1370–1379, 1986
18. Magni G, Salmi A, Paterlini A, et al: Psychological distress in duodenal ulcer and acute gastroduodenitis. A controlled study. Dig Dis Sci 27:1081–1084, 1982
19. Hill OW: Psychogenic vomiting. Gut 9:348–352, 1968
20. Rosenthal RH, Webb WL, Wruble LD: Diagnosis and management of persistent psychogenic vomiting. Psychosomatics 21:722–730, 1980
21. McMahon AW, Schmitt PT, Patterson JF, et al: Personality differences between inflammatory bowel disease patients and their healthy siblings. Psychosom Med 35:91–103, 1973
22. Whitehead WE, Schuster MM: Gastrointestinal Disorders: Behavioral and Physiological Basis for Treatment. New York, Academic Press, 1985
23. Almy TP, Rothstein RI: Irritable bowel syndrome: Classification and pathogenesis. Annu Rev Med 38:257–265, 1987
24. Latimer PR: Irritable bowel syndrome: A behavioral model. Behav Res Ther 19:475–483, 1981
25. Mechanic D: Social psychologic factors affecting the presentation of bodily complaints. N Engl J Med 286:1132–1139, 1972
26. Whitehead WE, Winget C, Fedoravicius AS, et al: Learned illness behavior in patients with irritable bowel syndrome and peptic ulcer. Dig Dis Sci 27:202–208, 1982

27. Robins LN, Helzer JE, Weissman MM, et al: Lifetime prevalence of specific psychiatric disorders in three sites. Arch Gen Psychiatry 41:949–958, 1984
28. Walker P, Luther J, Samloff IM, et al: Life events stress and psychosocial factors in men with peptic ulcer disease: II. Relationships with serum pepsinogen concentrations and behavioral risk factors. Gastroenterology 94:323–330, 1988
29. Lyketsos G, Arapakis G, Psaras M, et al: Psychological characteristics of hypertensive and ulcer patients. J Psychosom Res 26:255–262, 1982
30. Dotevall G, Svedlund J, Sjodin I: Symptoms in irritable bowel syndrome. Scand J Gastroenterol 79(suppl): 16–19, 1982
31. Whitehead WE, Bosmajian L, Costa P, et al: Relationship of upper gastrointestinal symptoms to psychological distress. Gastroenterology 94:A494, 1988
32. Christodoulou GN, Gargoulas A, Papaloukas A, et al: Primary peptic ulcer in childhood. Acta Psychiatr Scand 56:215–222, 1977
33. Ecklenberger D, Overbeck G, Biebl W: Subgroups of peptic ulcer patients. Psychosom Res 20:490–499, 1976
34. Engel GL: Studies of ulcerative colitis. III. The nature of the psychologic processes. Am J Med 17:231–256, 1955
35. Helzer JE, Stillings WA, Chammas S, et al: A controlled study of the association between ulcerative colitis and psychiatric diagnoses. Dig Dis Sci 27:513–518, 1982
36. Drossman DA, McKee DC, Sandler RS, et al: Psychosocial factors in irritable bowel syndrome: A multivariate study. Gastroenterology 92:1374, 1987
37. Talley NJ, Phillips SF, Melton LJ, et al: A controlled study of psychosocial factors in presenters and nonpresenters with functional bowel disease (FBD). Gastroenterology 94:A454, 1988
38. Pfeiffer CJ, Fodor J, Geizerova H: An epidemiologic study of the relationships of peptic ulcer disease in 50 to 54 year old urban males with physical, health, and smoking factors. J Chronic Dis 26:291–302, 1973
39. Henderson RD: Motor Disorders of the Esophagus, 2. Baltimore, Williams & Wilkins, 1980
40. Earlam R: Clinical Tests of Oesophageal Function. New York, Grune & Stratton, 1975
41. Jacobson E: Spastic esophagus and mucous colitis: Etiology and treatment by progressive relaxation. Arch Intern Med 39:433–445, 1927
42. Rubin J, Nagler R, Spiro HM, et al: Measuring the effect of emotions on esophageal motility. Psychosom Med 24:170–176, 1962
43. Wolf S, Almy TP: Experimental observations on cardiospasm in man. Gastroenterology 13:401–421, 1949
44. Faulkner WB Jr: Severe esophageal spasm: An evaluation of suggestion-therapy as determined by means of the esophagoscope. Psychosom Med 2:139–140, 1940
45. Stacher G, Steinringer H, Blau A, et al: Acoustically evoked esophageal contractions and defense reaction. Psychophysiology 16:234–241, 1979
46. Young LD, Richter JE, Anderson KO, et al: The effects of psychological and environmental stressors on peristaltic esophageal contractions in healthy volunteers. Psychophysiology 24:132–141, 1987
47. Pflanz M: Epidemiological and sociocultural factors in the etiology of duodenal ulcer. Adv Psychosom Med 6:121–151, 1971
48. Richard WC, Fell RD: Health factors in police job stress, in Kroes WH, Hurrell JJ (eds): Job Stress and the Police Officer: Identifying Stress Reduction Techniques. HEW Publ NIOSH 76-187. Washington, DC, US Government Printing Office, 1975, pp 73–84
49. Grayson RR: Air controllers syndrome: Peptic ulcer in air traffic controllers. Ill Med J 142:111–115, 1972
50. Cobb S, Rose RM: Hypertension, peptic ulcer, and diabetes in air traffic controllers. J Am Med Assoc 224:489–492, 1973
51. Davies ET, Wilson AT: Observations on the life-history of chronic peptic ulcer. Lancet 2:1353–1360, 1937
52. Sapira JD, Cross MR: Pre-hospitalization life change in gastric ulcer (GU) vs duodenal ulcer (DU). Psychosom Med 44:121, 1982
53. Piper DW, Greig M, Shinners J, et al: Chronic gastric ulcer and stress. Digestion 18:303–309, 1978
54. Thomas J, Greig M, Piper DW: Chronic gastric ulcer and life events. Gastroenterology 78:905–911, 1980
55. Weiss JM: Somatic effects of predictable and unpredictable shock. Psychosom Med 32:397–408, 1970

56. Weiss JM: Effects of coping behavior in different warning signal conditions on stress pathology in rats. J Comp Physiol Psychol 77:1–13, 1971
57. Weiss JM: Effects of coping behavior with and without a feedback signal on stress pathology in rats. J 0Comp Physiol Psychol 77:22–30, 1971
58. Thompson EG, Richelson E, Malagelada JR: Perturbation of upper gastrointestinal function by cold stress. Gut 24:277–283, 1983
59. Stanghellini V, Malagelada JR, Zinsmeister AR, et al: Stress-induced gastroduodenal motor disturbances in humans: Possible humoral mechanisms. Gastroenterology 85:83–91, 1983
60. Hoelzl R, Schroeder G, Keifer H: Indirect gastrointestinal motility measurement for use in experimental psychosomatics: A new method on some data. Behav Anal Modif 3:77–97, 1979
61. Cann PA, Read NW, Brown C, et al: Irritable bowel syndrome: Relationship of disorders in the transit of a single meal to symptom patterns. Gut 24:405–411, 1983
62. Kumar D, Wingate DL: The irritable bowel syndrome: A paroxysmal motor disorder. Lancet 2:973–977, 1985
63. Chaudhary NA, Truelove SC: The irritable colon syndrome: A study of the clinical features, predisposing causes, and prognosis in 130 cases. Q J Med 31:307–323, 1962
64. Hislop IG: Psychological significance of the irritable colon syndrome. Gut 12:452–457, 1971
65. Drossman DA, Sandler RS, McKee DC, et al: Bowel patterns among subjects not seeking health care. Gastroenterology 83:529–534, 1982
66. Almy TP, Tulin NM: Alterations in colonic function in man under stress. I. Experimental production of changes simulating the "irritable colon". Gastroenterology 8:616–626, 1947
67. Welgan P, Meshkinpour H, Hoehler F: The effect of stress on colon motor and electrical activity in irritable bowel syndrome. Psychosom Med 47:139–149, 1985
68. Narducci F, Snape WJ Jr, Battle WM, et al: Increased colonic motility during exposure to a stressful situation. Dig Dis Sci 30:40–44, 1985
69. Sarna S, Latimer P, Campbell D, et al: Effect of stress, meal and neostigmine on rectosigmoid electrical control activity (ECA) in normals and in irritable bowel syndrome patients. Dig Dis Sci 27:582–591, 1982
70. Wormsley KG: Smoking and duodenal ulcer. Gastroenterology 75:139–152, 1978
71. Fielding JE: Smoking: Health effects and control. N Engl J Med 313:491–498, 1985
72. Korman MG, Hansky J, Eaves ER, et al: Influence of cigarette smoking on healing and relapse in duodenal ulcer disease. Gastroenterology 85:871–874, 1983
73. Piper DW, Nasiry R, McIntosh J, et al: Smoking, alcohol, analgesics, and chronic duodenal ulcer. A controlled study of habits before first symptoms and before diagnosis. Scand J Gastroenterol 19:1015–1021, 1984
74. Paffenbarger RS, Wing AL, Hyde RT: Chronic disease in former college students. XIII. Early precursors of peptic ulcer. Am J Epidemiol 100:307–315, 1974
75. Piper DW, McIntosh JH, Ariotti EE, et al: Analgesic ingestion and chronic peptic ulcer. Gastroenterology 80:427–432, 1981
76. Calloway SP, Fonagy P, Pounder RF: Frequency of swallowing in duodenal ulceration and hiatus hernia. Br Med J 285:23–24, 1982
77. Fonagy P, Calloway SP: The effects of emotional arousal on spontaneous swallowing rates. J Psychosom Res 30:183–188, 1986
78. Calloway DH: Gas in the alimentary canal, in Code CF (ed): Handbook of Physiology: Section 6. Alimentary Canal: Volume 4. Motility. Washington, DC, American Physiological Society, 1969, pp 2839–2859
79. Manning AP, Thompson WG, Heaton KW, et al: Towards positive diagnosis of the irritable bowel. Br Med J 2:653–654, 1978
80. Thayer WR Jr, Denucci T: Cathartic colon, in Kirsner JB, Shorter RG (eds): Diseases of the Colon, Rectum, and Anal Canal. Baltimore, Williams & Wilkins, 1988, pp 578–579
81. Hunter JO, Jones VA: Studies of the pathogenesis of irritable bowel syndrome produced by food intolerance, in Read NW (ed): Irritable Bowel Syndrome. New York, Grune & Stratton, 1985, pp 185–190
82. Heaton KW: Role of dietary fiber in irritable bowel syndrome, in Read NW (ed): Irritable Bowel Syndrome. New York, Grune & Stratton, 1985, pp 203–222
83. Ritchie J: Pain from distension of the pelvic colon by inflating a balloon in the irritable colon syndrome. Gut 14:125–132, 1973

84. Kullmann G, Fielding JF: Rectal distensibility in the irritable bowel syndrome. Ir Med J 74:140–142, 1981
85. Sun WM, Read NW: Anorectal manometry and rectal sensation in patients with the irritable bowel syndrome. Gastroenterology 94:A450, 1988
86. Barish CF, Castell DO, Richter JE: Graded esophageal balloon distension: A new provocative test for non-cardiac chest pain. Dig Dis Sci 31:1292–1298, 1986
87. Swarbrick ET, Hagerty JE, Bat L, et al: Site of pain from the irritable bowel. Lancet 2:443–446, 1980
88. Moriarity KJ, Dawson AM: Functional abdominal pain: Further evidence that the whole gut is effected. Br Med J 284:1670–1672, 1982
89. Ritchie J: Mechanisms of pain in the irritable bowel syndrome, in Read NW (ed): Irritable Bowel Syndrome. New York, Grune & Stratton, 1985, pp 163–172
90. Tessler R, Mechanic D: Psychological distress and perceived health status. J Health Soc Behav 19:254–262, 1978
91. Wooley SC, Blackwell B, Winget C: The learning theory model of chronic illness behavior: Theory, treatment, and research. Psychosom Med 40:379–401, 1978
92. Mechanic D: Adolescent health and illness behavior; Review of the literature and a new hypothesis for the study of stress. J Hum Stress 9:4–13, 1983
93. Whitehead WE, Winget C, Fedoravicius AS, et al: Learned illness behavior in patients with irritable bowel syndrome and peptic ulcer. Dig Dis Sci 27:202–208, 1982
94. Welgan PR: Learned control of gastric acid secretions in peptic ulcer patients. Psychosom Med 36:411–419, 1974
95. Whitehead WE, Renault PF, Goldiamond I: Modification of human gastric acid secretion with operant-conditioning procedures. J Appl Behav Anal 8:147–156, 1975
96. Whitehead WE, Drescher VM: Perception of gastric contractions and self-control of gastric motility. Psychophysiology 17:552–558, 1980
97. Bueno-Miranda F, Cerulli M, Schuster MM: Operant conditioning of colonic motility in irritable bowel syndrome (IBS). Gastroenterology 70:867, 1976
98. Miller NE: Learning of visceral and glandular responses. Science 163:434–435, 1969
99. Whitehead WE, Fedoravicius AF, Blackwell B, et al: Psychosomatic symptoms as learned responses, in McNamara JR (ed): Behavioral Approaches in Medicine: Application and Analysis. New York, Plenum Medical, 1979, pp 65–99
100. Enck P, Whitehead WE: Gastrointestinal disorders, in Blechman EA, Brownell KD (eds): Handbook of Behavioral Medicine for Women. New York, Pergamon Press, 1988, pp 178–194
101. Lowman BC, Drossman DA, Cramer EM, et al: Recollection of childhood events in adults with irritable bowel syndrome. J Clin Gastroenterol 9:324–330, 1987
102. Derogatis LR: SCL-90-R: Administration, scoring, and procedures manual—II. Towson, Md, Clinical Psychometric Research, 1983
103. Sullivan MA, Cohen S, Snape WJ Jr: Colonic myoelectrical activity in irritable-bowel syndrome: Effective eating and anticholinergics. N Engl J Med 298:878–883, 1978
104. Harvey RF, Read AE: Effect of cholecystokinin on colonic motility and symptoms in patients with the irritable bowel syndrome. Gut 13:837–838, 1972
105. Whitehead WE, Schuster MM, Cheskin LJ, et al: Exacerbations of irritable bowel syndrome during menses. Gastroenterology 94:A495, 1988
106. Neff DF, Blanchard EB: A multi-component treatment for irritable bowel syndrome. Behav Ther 18:72–83, 1987
107. Blanchard EB, Schwarz SP: Adaptation of a multi-component treatment program for irritable bowel syndrome to a small group format. Biofeedback Self-Regul 12:63–69, 1987
108. Svedlund A, Sjodin I, Ottosson J-O, et al: Controlled study of psychotherapy in irritable bowel syndrome. Lancet 2:589–592, 1983
109. Whorwell PJ, Prior A, Faragher EB: Controlled trial of hypnotherapy in the treatment of severe refractory irritable-bowel syndrome. Lancet 2:1232–1234, 1984

4

Central Control of Gastrointestinal Transit and Motility by Brain–Gut Peptides

Yvette Taché

1. INTRODUCTION

In 1820, the French physiologist Jean Georges Cabanis reported the influence of the brain over gastrointestinal function as follows: "A vigorous and healthy man has just eaten a good meal; in the midst of this feeling of well-being the foods that are at the moment carried to the various parts of the organism are energetically digested, and the digestive juices dissolve them easily and quickly. Should this man receive a bad news, or should sad and baneful passions suddenly arise in his soul, his stomach and intestines will immediately cease to act on the foods contained in them. The very juice in which the foods are already almost entirely dissolved will remain as though struck by a moral stupor and . . . digestion will cease entirely . . ."[1]

This early prescientific recognition of emotionally related disturbances of gastrointestinal function was substantiated 30 years later by William Beaumont's observations made on his fistulous patient, Alexis St. Martin,[2] and in 1906 by Cannon's experimental report that cats exposed to a barking dog have diminished gastric motor activity.[3] Other experimental studies published during the first half of this century established specific brain structures influencing gastrointestinal motor function based on alteration of motility following electrical stimulation or lesions of various brain areas.[4]

More recently, the availability of electrophysiological and sensitive neuroanatomic tracing techniques and the characterization of a large number of peptides in brain structures identified to influence gastrointestinal motility have given new input to investigate the neuroanatomical pathways and brain chemical messengers involved in the central nervous system (CNS) regulation of gastrointestinal motor function.

Yvette Taché • Center for Ulcer Research and Education, Veterans Administration Medical Center–West Los Angeles, and Department of Medicine and Brain Research Institute, University of California–Los Angeles, Los Angeles, California 90073.

This chapter will briefly review the neuroanatomical basis for brain regulation of gastrointestinal motor function and summarize the state of knowledge on the CNS action of peptides to alter gastrointestinal transit and motility and their possible role in stress-induced alteration of gut motor function.

2. CENTRAL NERVOUS STRUCTURES INFLUENCING GASTROINTESTINAL MOTILITY

Experiments using electrical or chemical stimulation or electrical lesioning of specific brain structures along with retrograde tracing techniques have brought important information on nuclei influencing gastric and small intestinal motility and afferent, efferent gastrointestinal projections.[4] There is relatively limited information about brain structures influencing colonic motility outside of the reports of Rostad in the cat[5] and as to whether the same brain sites influencing gut motility are also involved in modulating gastric emptying, intestinal and colonic transit.

Brain areas that are most commonly found to influence gastrointestinal motility are the nucleus tractus solitarius, dorsal motor nucleus of the vagus, nucleus ambiguus, hypothalamus, periaqueductal gray, and cerebral cortex.[4] Differences have been reported in the nature of the gut response following electrical stimulation of these brain nuclei. The disparity of the results may be related to differences in species, stimulation parameters, lesion size, animal preparation including anesthesia, or motility recording techniques, or a combination of these factors. The more recent use of chemical stimulation of these nuclei via injection of endogenous ligands or their agonists or antagonists, when available, has provided more specific information about the neurochemical substrate that may be involved in the central regulation of gut motor function.

2.1. Hypothalamus

2.1.1. Lateral Hypothalamus

Earlier reports consistently established that electrical stimulation of the lateral hypothalamus elicited an increase in gastric motility in the cat,[6] rat,[7] and rabbit[8] that is abolished by vagotomy and atropine. A recent study in anesthetized cats further demonstrated that electrical stimulation of the lateral hypothalamus produced a marked stimulus-bound increase in the amplitude of antral contractions assessed by miniature force transducers. The motor response to stimulation of the lateral hypothalamus was vagally and cholinergically mediated and purely motor since there was no change in gastric acid secretion.[9] Electrical stimulation of the lateral hypothalamus associated with flight or fear behavioral changes produces a vagal and cholinergic dependent increase in intestinal and colonic motility in the cat.[6] By contrast, electrical stimulation of the ventral part of the lateral hypothalamus in the medial forebrain bundle, which elicits a defense reaction in cats, is associated with the inhibition of gastric, small intestinal, and colonic motility.[6]

Chemical stimulation of the perifornical and medial forebrain bundle of the lateral hypothalamus by microinjection of the benzamide drugs increased gastric emptying in the guinea pig.[10] Other sites in the vicinity of the active sites were ineffective.[10] Microinjection of thyrotropin-releasing hormone (TRH) into the lateral hypothalamus also stimulated intestinal transit in the rat.[11]

2.1.2. Ventromedial Hypothalamus

Electrical stimulation of the ventromedial hypothalamus has been reported to predominantly cause inhibition of gastric motility in rats and rabbits,[7,8] and to increase colonic motility in the cat.[5] Chemical stimulation of the ventromedial hypothalamus by baclofen ($GABA_B$ agonist) resulted in a stimulation of gastric motility characterized by an increase in tone and long-lasting elevated amplitude of rhythmic contractions.[12] The gastric contractile response to ventromedial injection of baclofen is site specific and mediated by vagal cholinergic efferent fibers.[12] The receptor through which baclofen is acting is unclear since both muscimol ($GABA_A$ agonist) and GABA were ineffective when tested under the same conditions.[12]

Destruction of the ventromedial hypothalamus in rats caused a syndrome characterized by increasing obesity usually associated with hyperphagia which has been related to acceleration of daytime gastric emptying occurring after the lesions.[13]

2.1.3. Paraventricular Nucleus

Electrical stimulation of the medial parvicellular portion of the paraventricular nucleus of the hypothalamus increases the amplitude of gastric contractions in rats. The stimulatory effect is no longer observed following vagotomy.[14]

2.2. Medulla Oblongata

2.2.1. Dorsal Motor Nucleus of the Vagus

Gillis's studies in the cat have demonstrated that neurons in the dorsal motor nucleus that project to the stomach are located at the rostral portion of the nucleus.[15,16] Moreover, electrical stimulation of these neurons elicited a pronounced and selective stimulation of antral and pyloric contractions which is mediated by ipsilateral vagal fibers.[15-17] Chemical stimulation of the dorsal motor nucleus of the vagus using L-glutamic acid or the tripeptide TRH led to stimulation of gastric motility in cats and rats[14,18-20] whereas microinjection of oxytocin inhibited gastric contractility in rats.[14]

2.2.2. Nucleus Ambiguus

Electrical stimulation of the nucleus ambiguus increases contractility in the body, corpus, pylorus, and proximal duodenum in cats, an effect that is abolished by vagotomy.[21] Left-sided stimulation elicited greater duodenal but not gastric contractile response as compared with the right side.[21] Chemical stimulation of the nucleus ambiguus by microinjection of bicuculline ($GABA_A$ antagonist) markedly increased antral and pyloric contractions which were abolished by microinjection of muscimol ($GABA_A$ agonist) into the same site in cats.[22] The stimulatory effect is vagally mediated.[22] Bicuculline microinjected into the dorsal motor nucleus of the vagus was ineffective.[22] These results suggest that in cats, $GABA_A$ receptors in the nucleus ambiguus exert an inhibitory tone on the parasympathetic outflow regulating gastric motility. Microinjection of TRH into the nucleus ambiguus was recently reported to increase gastric contractions in rats.[23]

3. CNS ACTION OF PEPTIDES TO INFLUENCE GASTROINTESTINAL MOTILITY AND TRANSIT

Since 1970 when the first peptide was characterized in the brain, over 60 biologically active peptides have been detected in the CNS using immunohistochemical, chemical, and more recently recombinant DNA technology.[24] A number of these peptides and their receptors are densely localized in hypothalamic and medullary nuclei found to influence gastrointestinal motility.[25-27] Moreover, during the last decade, neuropharmacological studies initiated by Smith et al.,[28] Burks,[29] and Bueno and Ferre[30] have revealed that specific peptides injected in picomolar amount into the cerebrospinal fluid induced marked and prolonged stimulation or inhibition of gastrointestinal transit and alteration of gut motility in various animal species. Since peptides delivered into the CSF could rapidly diffuse into the peripheral blood,[31-33] CNS sites of action were further established for these peptides by the facts that similar responses (1) were not mimicked by the peripheral route of administration, (2) are reproduced by microinjection into the brain parenchyma, and/or (3) are maintained following peripheral injection of peptide antibody that will neutralize any active material leaking through the arachnoid villi into the blood. Further studies have established neurohumoral pathways involved in peptide action and in some cases brain sites mediating their effect. An important piece of missing information for most of these centrally active peptides is, however, the demonstration of their physiological relevance. The lack of specific peptide antagonists and the difficulty of assessing their possible brain release in relation to physiological neural stimuli eliciting alteration of gut motor function have impeded the generation of such knowledge.

3.1. CNS Action of TRH to Stimulate Gastrointestinal Motor Function

TRH is a triamino-acid hypothalamic releasing peptide first established to play a physiological role in the pituitary secretion of TSH. However, it became evident that TRH was localized in extrahypothalamic brain structures and exerted CNS actions unrelated to its endocrine effects.[34] Horita et al.[28] were the first to demonstrate that TRH acts in the brain to stimulate colonic motility. Since then, several groups of investigators have established that TRH is a potent centrally acting stimulant of gastrointestinal motor function.[35]

3.1.1. Gastrointestinal Transit

3.1.1a. Gastric Emptying. Intracisternal injection of TRH or the stable TRH analogue RX 77368 induces a dose-related and rapid onset stimulation of gastric emptying of a nonnutritive, methylcellulose solution in conscious rats (Fig. 1). The mechanism of action is CNS and vagally mediated, expressed through peripheral cholinergic receptors and not related to the stimulation of the pituitary–thyroid axis.[36]

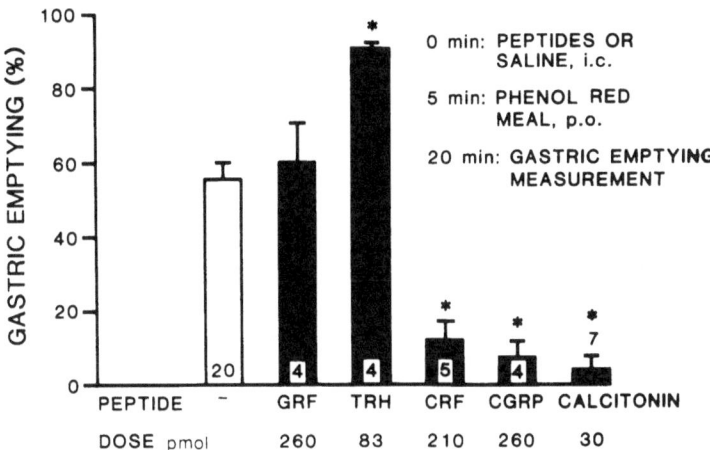

Figure 1. Effects of intracisternal injection of peptides on gastric emptying of a liquid noncaloric phenol red solution in conscious, 24-hr-fasted rats. Each column represents mean ± S.E. of the number of rats indicated at the base of the column. *$p < 0.05$ as compared to control group. GRF, growth hormone-releasing factor; TRH, thyrotropin-releasing factor; CRF, corticotropin-releasing factor; CGRP, calcitonin gene-related peptide.

3.1.1b. Intestinal Transit. Intestinal transit, measured by the distance of a charcoal marker injected into the lumen distal to the gastroduodenal junction, is enhanced in rats by microinjection of TRH into the medial septum, medial hypothalamus, and lateral hypothalamus.[11] Other hypothalamic or extrahypothalamic sites were inactive.[11] Intracerebroventricular injection of TRH inhibited neurotensin-induced delay in intestinal transit in the rat.[37] By contrast in mice, intracerebroventricular injection of large doses of TRH decreased gastrointestinal transit of a charcoal meal administered perorally.[38] It is not known whether the inhibitory effect observed in mice is related to species difference or experimental conditions, in particular the large dose of peptide used (Table I).

3.1.1c. Colonic Transit. TRH injected into the lateral ventricle of rabbits causes a marked increase in colonic transit, colonic fluid content, and subsequent diarrhea production.[39,40] The effect of TRH on colonic transit was not reversed by adrenergic blockade or by atropine at a dose that completely suppressed associated changes in colonic contractility.[39] Antiserotonin compounds such as cyproheptadine, cinanserin, and xylamidin, opiate antagonist, and vagotomy combined with sacral cord transection completely reversed the increase in colonic transit, fluid accumulation, and diarrhea production elicited by central administration of TRH.[39,40] These data indicate that diarrhea produced by central injection of TRH results not from the increase in colonic motility but rather from fluid accumulation in the colon following serotonin release. Similarly in conscious cats, intracerebroventricular injection of TRH induced defecation with an average latency of 30–90 sec.[41]

3.1.2. Gastrointestinal Motility

3.1.2a. Gastric Motility. In conscious or urethane-anesthetized rats implanted with extraluminal force transducers in the gastric corpus, injection of TRH or RX 77368 into

Table I. CNS Action of Peptides to Influence Gastrointestinal Transit in Experimental Animals[a]

Peptides	Gastric emptying	Intestinal transit	Colonic transit	Gastrointestinal transit
TRH	↑ rat (0.028–0.28)[36]	↑ rat (0.28–28)[11]	↑ rabbit (28)[70] ↑ cat (280)[41]	↓ mice (8.2–28)[38]
Bombesin	↓ rat (0.06–0.6)[126] ↓ dog (12)[71]	↓ rat (0.06–0.6)[126]	↑ rat (0.6)[126] ↓ mice (0.006–0.6)[131]	↓ rat (0.06–2)[129]
Calcitonin	↓ rat (0.003–0.03)[138]	↓ rat (0.1–1)[139]	0 rat (0.1–1)[139]	
CGRP	↓ rat (0.002–0.2)[148]	↓ rat (0.1–1)[139]	0 rat (0.1–1)[139]	
CRF	↓ rat (0.06–1)[67,68,70] ↓ dog (12)[71]	↓ rat (1–2)[68,70]	↑ rat (0.1–2)[68,70]	
Neurotensin	↓ dog (12)[71]	↓ rat (0.5–1)[111]		
Opiate agonists				
μ	↓ rat (0.01–0.12)[109]	↓ rat (0.06–0.6)[113]	↓ rat [108]	↓ mice (0.07–0.7)[106,107]
δ		0 rat (17)[113]		
κ		0 rat (5)[113]		0 mice (5–50)[107]

[a] ↑, increase; ↓, decrease; 0, no effect; numbers in parentheses are doses in nmoles per animal injected into the CSF or specific brain nuclei, followed by reference numbers.

CSF at the level of the cisterna magna elicited a rapid-onset, long-acting increase in the amplitude and, to a lesser extent, frequency of gastric phasic contractions.[42] In the rabbit and sheep, intracerebroventricular injection of TRH also produced marked stimulation of the amplitude of antral contractions.[43,44] Intravenous injection of the peptide was ineffective.[42,43] Further studies aiming at identifying brain sites of action of TRH were performed in rats using microinjection of TRH or RX 77368 (0.5–100 pmol) into selective medullary nuclei. Responsive sites eliciting increase in gastric contractility have been localized in the dorsal motor nucleus of the vagus, nucleus tractus solitarius, and nucleus ambiguus whereas the hypoglossal nucleus and area postrema were inactive.[14,19,23] Recent studies in the cat have confirmed that TRH microinjected into the dorsal motor nucleus of the vagus increases antral and pyloric motility and gastric intraluminal pressure.[18,20] Microinjection into the nucleus tractus solitarius, hypoglossal nucleus, and area postrema had no effect.[18]

The stimulation of gastric motility elicited by CSF or dorsal vagal complex injection of TRH or RX 77368 was abolished by vagotomy or atropine in rats and cats.[14,18,19,23,42] These data added to electrophysiological evidence that CSF injection of TRH stimulates cervical or gastric vagal efferent discharges[45,46] indicate that TRH acts by activating excitatory vagal pathways composed of preganglionic cholinergic fibers synapsing with myenteric neurons that excite gastric smooth muscle.[35]

3.1.2b. Intestinal Motility. Electromyographic activity of the duodenum was also found to be stimulated by intracerebroventricular injection of TRH in rats. The response appears rapid in onset and confined to the proximal duodenum, whereas midjejunum and midileum contractility was not altered.[47] The stimulatory effect is abolished by vagotomy or atropine treatment and not modified by hypophysectomy, cervical cord transection, or 6-hydroxydopamine treatment.[47] Intracerebroventricular injection of TRH facilitated the occurrence of prolonged phases of duodenal activity in sheep[43] and stimulated motor activity of the small intestine in rabbits.[44] By contrast in cats, preliminary evidence indicates that dorsal motor nucleus injection of TRH did not alter duodenal motility.[18]

3.1.2c. Colonic Motility. TRH injected into the CSF at the level of either the lateral ventricle, third ventricle, or cisterna magna produced within 2 min a long-lasting contractile response of both longitudinal and circular muscle of the proximal colon and cecum as measured by manometry or strain gauges sutured to the colon in conscious or anesthetized rabbits.[28,44] No effect was obtained when the peptide was administered intravenously at doses up to 100-fold higher than those for the CNS.[28,44] The role of the parasympathetic nervous system in mediating the activation of large intestine motility was substantiated by the inhibition of colonic response to TRH following vagotomy, atropine, or ganglionic blockade by tetraethylammonium, hexamethonium, or chlorisondamine.[28,44] By contrast, blockade of opioid receptors by naloxone or suppression of the sympathetic nervous system activity produced by cervical cord transection or guanethidine did not alter TRH response on the large intestine.[40,44]

3.1.3. Physiological Role of Brain TRH in the Regulation of Gut Motor Function

Growing anatomical and neuropharmacological evidence supports a possible physiological role of TRH present in the brain medulla in the vagal stimulation of gastrointestinal motor function. TRH-immunoreactivity is localized in brain stem nuclei that are involved in the regulation of autonomic function. In particular, 65% of total medullary TRH is concentrated in the dorsal motor nucleus of the vagus, nucleus tractus solitarius, and nucleus ambiguus.[48,49] TRH receptors are abundantly distributed in the dorsal vagal complex.[50,51] Such distribution of the peptide and its receptors is well correlated with site of origin of vagal preganglionic neurons to the stomach localized in the dorsal motor nucleus and nucleus ambiguus and site of termination of vagal afferent pathways in the nucleus tractus solitarius.[52-54] In addition, neuropharmacological studies clearly demonstrate that TRH injected into the CSF acts in the brain to stimulate gastric, intestinal, and colonic motor activity and transit through vagal-dependent pathways in several experimental animals including rabbits, rats, cats, and sheep (Fig. 2). TRH sites of action localized in the dorsal motor nucleus of the vagus in rats and cats are well correlated with peptide distribution and anatomical projections to the gastrointestinal tract. Moreover, cold exposure associated with the release of brain TRH in the rat[55,56] mimics the effects of central injection of TRH as shown by the increase in gastric contractility[57-60] and emptying[61,62] and marked watery fecal excretion.[63,64] The development of specific TRH antagonists will be very useful to further establish the physiological role of medullary TRH in relation to vagal excitatory outflow to the gut. TRH or the stable TRH analogue, RX 77368, represents the only peptide acting centrally to induce a vagally mediated

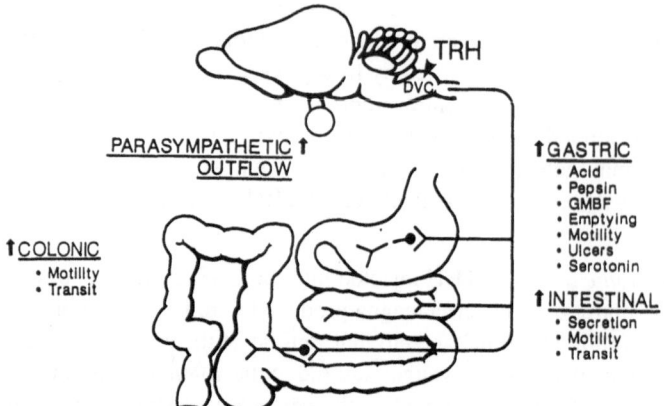

Figure 2. Summary of CNS-mediated stimulatory actions of TRH on gastrointestinal function in experimental animals. DVC, dorsal vagal complex; GMBF, gastric mucosal blood flow. For references, see review by Taché et al.[35]

stimulation of gastrointestinal motility and transit and appears as a useful chemical tool to elucidate central vagal excitatory pathways regulating gut motor function.

3.2. CNS Action of Corticotropin-Releasing Factor (CRF) to Alter Gastrointestinal Motor Function

CRF is a 41-amino-acid peptide characterized in 1981 and established to play a physiological role in the regulation of pituitary ACTH secretion.[65] The implications of central CRF in mediating some of the stress response have triggered interest in the CNS action of the peptide to influence gastrointestinal function.[66]

3.2.1. Gastrointestinal Transit

3.2.1a. Gastric and Intestinal Transit. Several groups of investigators have recently reported marked alterations of gastrointestinal transit elicited by central injection of CRF in rats, mice, and dogs. In rats, intracisternal or intracerebroventricular injection of CRF or related amphibian peptide (e.g., sauvagine) induced a long-lasting, dose-related, and potent inhibition of gastric emptying of a nonnutrient liquid meal[67-70] (Fig. 1) and a modest decrease in small bowel transit.[68,70] Tested under the same conditions, the other releasing factor, growth hormone-releasing factor (GRF), was inactive (Fig. 1). Peptide action is CNS mediated through brain sites yet to be localized.[67] CRF induced inhibition of gastric emptying and intestinal transit was not altered by hypophysectomy or adrenalectomy indicating that the alterations of gastrointestinal transit are not secondary to systemic endocrine effects associated with peptide administration.[67,68] Mediation through the autonomic nervous system was demonstrated by the reversal of CRF effects on gastric emptying and intestinal transit by pretreatment with the ganglionic blocker chlorisondamine, vagotomy, or noradrenergic blockade.[67,68] In dogs, CRF injected into the third ventricle delayed gastric emptying of a liquid protein meal[71] and did not modify gastric emptying of a saline solution when injected into the lateral ventricle.[72] In mice, intracerebroventricular injection of CRF increased gastric emptying of a milk meal.[73,74] To what extent the opposite effects of central CRF on gastric emptying in mice versus rats and dogs are related to species differences or the nature of the meal (caloric versus noncaloric) remains to be established.

3.2.1b. Colonic Transit. Intracerebroventricular injection of CRF in rats stimulates colonic transit and fecal pellet output.[68,70] The mechanisms through which central CRF stimulates colonic motility are unrelated to activation of the pituitary–adrenal axis inas much as hypophysectomy or adrenalectomy did not alter CRF action. CRF effect was abolished by ganglionic blockade and vagotomy but not by noradrenergic or opioid antagonists, suggesting that CRF stimulates large bowel transit by stimulating sacral parasympathetic outflow.[68]

3.2.2. Gastrointestinal Motility

3.2.2a. Gastric Motility. Intracisternal injection of TRH or 2-deoxyglucose-induced stimulation of gastric motility was dose dependently inhibited by injection of CRF into the cisterna magna of urethane-anesthetized rats acutely implanted with strain gauges.[75] The inhibitory effect of centrally injected CRF is centrally mediated and selective toward central vagal stimulation of gastric motility since intracisternal CRF did not alter intravenous carbachol-stimulated gastric motility.[75] In fasted dogs, antral mechanical activity is characterized by an "activity front" (gastric MMC) that lasted 20 min and occurred at 85- to 107-min intervals.[76] An immediate suppression of the cyclic activity fronts of the antrum occurred following intracerebroventricular injection of CRF. The activity fronts were replaced for several hours by irregular contractions of small amplitude.[76] By contrast, gastric motility elicited by intravenous injection of motilin was not altered.[77] In fed sheep, intracerebroventricular injection of CRF elicited complete suppression of antral motor activity for a duration that is dose related (1–2 hr).[43] No significant change in gastrointestinal motility was observed when the peptide was given intravenously in doses efficient given centrally in rats, dogs, or sheep.[43,75,76] These results show that CRF acts centrally on brain sites that remain to be localized to inhibit gastric motility in various animal species. The mechanism through which central CRF conveys alteration of motility has been related to the abolition of cyclic variations of plasma motilin in fasted dogs whereas plasma variations of somatostatin were not altered.[77]

3.2.2b. Intestinal Motility. Intracerebroventricular injection of CRF in fasted dogs at low doses that abolished the antral cyclic activity front did not alter the pattern of MMC in the proximal jejunum.[76,77] Higher doses of CRF delayed the occurrence of MMC in the proximal duodenum for 4–5 hr.[76] In sheep, central injection of CRF inhibited the duodenal motor activity observed after feeding.[43]

3.2.3. Role of Central CRF in Mediating Alterations of Gastrointestinal Transit Elicited by Stress

CRF is well established to mediate part of the endocrine, behavioral, and cardiovascular responses to stress.[65,78–80] Convergent information suggests that central CRF may also be involved in triggering gastrointestinal dysfunction elicited by stress exposure in experimental animals. First, CRF-immunoreactivity and receptors have been localized in hypothalamic and medullary nuclei regulating visceral function.[81-83] Second, although stimulus-specific gastrointestinal patterns occurred in response to exposure to different stressors, such as cold exposure which elicits an increase in gastric motility in rats and mice[57-60] and emptying,[61,74] most stress models including, panic, noise, wrap restraint, ether exposure, or water swim associated with the release of CRF[64] inhibit gastrointestinal motility[84-88] and transit of a nonnutrient liquid meal[64,70,87,89,90] in rats and dogs. In humans, painful stimuli applied to one hand, labyrinthine stimulation, or mental stress also inhibited the incidence of fasting migrating motor complex and postprandial gastrointestinal motility pattern[91-94] and gastric emptying.[94-96] Stress reportedly increases colonic motility, mouth-to-cecum transit time, and fecal output in experimental animals[63,64,70,90] and in humans particularly in patients with irritable bowel syndrome[97-99] except in one study.[100] Similar alterations of gastrointestinal transit (inhibition of gastrointestinal motility and emptying and stimulation of colonic transit) are reproduced by intracerebroventricular injection of CRF in the rat and dog.[67,68,70,75-77,88] Moreover, both stress- and central CRF-induced alterations of gastrointestinal and colonic transit occur independently from activation of the pituitary–adrenal axis.[64,67,68] Lastly, the CRF antagonist α-helical CRF9–41, injected intracerebroventricularly at a dose that effectively antagonized the effects of exogenous CRF on gastrointestinal transit, completely prevented restraint-[70,101] or abdominal surgery (Fig. 3)-induced inhibition of gastric emptying and restraint-induced increase in large intestinal transit.[70,101] The stimulation of fecal pellet output was significantly diminished by central injection of the CRF antagonist.[70,101]

Taken together, this neuroanatomical and neuropharmacological evidence supports a role of endogenous brain CRF in triggering the inhibition of gastric emptying and stimulation of large intestinal transit elicited by restraint. Further studies assessing whether the CRF antagonist reversed gastrointestinal motor alterations elicited by different stressors are required to provide more conclusive information on the relevance of endogenous CRF in various models of stress.

3.3. CNS Action of Opioid Peptides to Inhibit Gastrointestinal Motor Function

Optiates were among the first drugs established to have a CNS site of action to alter gastrointestinal motility.[29] They have long been known for their potent effects on gut motility and used since antiquity as a treatment of diarrhea. The relative importance of the central, spinal, and peripheral components as well as subtypes of opioid receptors involved has been extensively evaluated by Burks et al.[29,102] and other investigators[103] using the neuropharmacological approach of injecting prototype receptor agonists or endogenous peptides directly into the CNS. Electrophysiological studies provided further evidence of central opioid modulation of gastric function by demonstrating that single-unit neurons in the dorsal motor nucleus of the vagus responding to gastric distension can be modulated by iontophoretic application of an opioid agonist and antagonist.[104]

3.3.1. Gastrointestinal Transit

Intracerebroventricular injection of the μ receptor agonists morphine, dermorphin, phenazocine, or DAGO (D-Ala^2,N-methyl-Phe^4,Gly^4-ol-enkephalin) consistently delayed

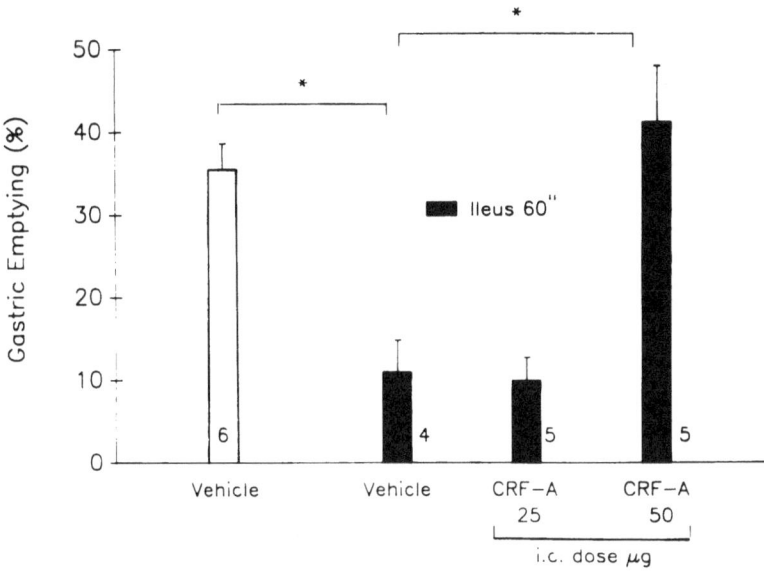

Figure 3. Reversal of postoperative gastric ileus by intracisternal injection of CRF antagonist [CRF-A; α-helical CRF(9–41] in 24-hr-fasted rats. Rats under ether anesthesia were injected intracisternally with vehicle or CRF antagonist (25 or 50 μg/rat) and subjected to sham operation (open bar) or ileus (laparotomy followed by 60-sec handling of the cecum and closing the incision), then methylcellulose solution was given by gavage and gastric emptying measured 20 min. Each column represents mean ± S.E. of the number of rats indicated at the base of the column.

gastric emptying, intestinal and gastrointestinal transit in mice[105–108] and rats.[105,109–112] The antipropulsive effect of μ agonists was reversed by naloxone and vagotomy.[108] By contrast, the κ agonists ketacyclazocine, ethylketacyclazocine, nalorphine, or U-50,488H (*trans*-3,4-dichloro-*N*-methyl-*N*-[2-(1-pyrolidinyl)-cyclohexyl]-benzeneacetamide methanesulfonate) or the highly selective cyclic enkephalin analogues DPLPE (D-Pen^2,L-Pen^5-enkephalin) and DPDPE (D-Pen^2, D-Pen^5-enkephalin) were inctive.[105–107] Further studies have established that the periaqueductal gray matter is a site of action of the antitransit effect of opiates. The μ receptor agonist FK 33824 [D-Ala^2,*N*-Me-Phe^4,Met(O)^5-ol-enkephalin] and β-endorphin strongly inhibited intestinal propulsion when microinjected into the periaqueductal gray matter whereas the selective δ receptor agonist DALA (D-Ala^2,*N*-Met^5-enkephalinamide) and the κ ligand dynorphin were inactive.[113] Taken together, these results suggest that the centrally mediated inhibitory action of opiates on gastrointestinal transit involve primarily μ but not δ or κ receptor populations.[107,113] Whether β-endorphin is acting on μ or ε receptors needs to be clarified.

Porreca et al.[114] reported the first experimental evidence that the spinal cord is a separate independent site of action for opiates to influence gastrointestinal transit. Intrathecal injection of morphine inhibits gastrointestinal transit in mice even following spinal cord transection.[114] These results were extended to rats,[115] although another report did not confirm the antitransit effect of intrathecal morphine in rats.[116] Using selective opioid receptor agonists injected intrathecally in mice, the μ agonists DAGO and morphine were found to be more potent than the δ agonists DPLPE and DPDPE; the κ agonist U-50,488H was less potent.[107] These results suggest that the antitransit effect of opiates at the spinal levels may be conveyed by activation of both δ and μ receptors.[102,107]

Morphine injected into CSF in rats, mice, or guinea pigs reduced fecal output and completely antagonized castor oil-induced diarrhea in rats.[108] The antidiarrheal effect of morphine was abolished by vagotomy.[108]

3.3.2. Gastrointestinal Motility

A less clear picture can be drawn concerning the effects of central injection of opiates on gastrointestinal motility. Alteration of motility pattern in response to opiates appears to vary according to the nutritional state of the animal (fasted or fed), part of the gut (stomach, intestine, or colon), subtypes of receptors stimulated (μ, δ, or κ), site of drug delivery (brain or spinal cord), and species studied.

3.3.2a. Gastric and Intestinal Motility. Intracerebroventricular injection of the μ agonists morphine, fentanyl, or dermorphin and the δ agonist DADLE restored the fasted pattern "MMC" in the duodenum 40 min after injection in fed rats[117,118] and inhibited reticular contractions and stimulated duodenal motility in fed sheep.[119] Similarly, in fed dogs, intracerebroventricular injection of DALAMIDE (D-Ala,Met^5-enkephalinamide), a mixed μ/δ receptor agonist, immediately restored the intestinal fasted pattern. In contrast, DADLE did not influence gastrointestinal motility.[120] The intracerebroventricular/intravenous potency ratio suggests a central site of action.[120]

In fasted state, intracerebroventricular injection of morphine decreased the frequency of contractions in the small intestine 30 min after drug injection in rats.[112] The jejunum appears to be more sensitive to the inhibitory effect of morphine.[112] A decrease in the motility index is also induced in fasted dogs following intracerebroventricular injection of DALAMIDE, but the effect is observed mostly in the stomach and not in the jejunum.[120] By contrast, the κ agonist ethylketazocine injected intracerebroventricularly enhanced the amplitude of contractions in the reticulum and duodenum in sheep.[119]

Intrathecal injection of fentanyl or DADLE did not affect the fed pattern of the small bowel in rats.[117] Dermorphin induced a fasting pattern in the duodenum.[118]

3.3.2b. Colonic Motiity. Intracerebroventricular injection of DADLE or fentanyl did not alter colonic motility in the rat,[117,121] whereas in fasted or fed dogs DADLE, but not DALAMIDE, produced a short and immediate period of contractile activity.[120]

Intrathecal injection of dermorphin or fentanyl inhibited contractile activity of both the proximal and distal colon at a dose ineffective intravenously in dogs and rats.[117,118,121] In contrast, intrathecal injection of DADLE produced an immediate increase in colonic motility in the rat at a dose inactive given subcutaneously.[117,121]

3.3.3. Physiological Role of Brain Opioid Peptides in the Regulation of Gastrointestinal Motor Function

The anatomical distribution of endogenous opioid peptides and their specific receptors in the brain,[122] added to neuropharmacological studies establishing a centrally mediated effect of μ opioid receptors on gastrointestinal transit and motility, substantiate a possible influence of brain opioid pathways on gut function. Blockade of opiate receptors by peripheral injection of naloxone accelerates colonic transit in humans, suggesting a tonic inhibitory role of opioids in the regulation of colonic transit.[123] Although naloxone is known to cross the blood–brain barrier and block central opioid receptors, no clear conclusions can be drawn regarding a central opioid involvement since alterations of motility may also result from an action of naloxone on peripheral opioid receptors in the gut. Preliminary evidence indicates that intracerebroventricular injection of naloxone did not alter the gastrointestinal and colonic myoelectrical profile in fasted rats, suggesting that central opioid peptides do not exert an inhibitory tone.[124] Further studies are required to evaluate the influence of specific opiate antagonists delivered into the CSF or specific brain nuclei on physiopathological stimuli associated with alterations of gastrointestinal transit.

3.4. CNS Action of Bombesin to Inhibit Gastrointestinal Motor Function

Bombesin is a 14-amino-acid peptide originally characterized from frog skin and later characterized in mammalian gut as a 27-amino-acid named gastrin-releasing peptide (GRP). GRP shares full homology with the C-terminal biologically active fragment of bombesin. Central action of bombesin to influence gut function was first established by the report of its potent inhibitory effect on gastric acid secretion in the rat.[125] Bombesin was subsequently demonstrated to alter gastrointestinal transit.[126] Bombesin-like peptides and specific receptors have been localized in the brain area related to regulation of visceral function.[127,128]

3.4.1. Gastrointestinal Transit

Bombesin injected intracerebroventricularly delays gastric emptying of a noncaloric solution, small intestinal transit, and stimulates large intestinal transit and fecal excretion in rats.[126] Bombesin-induced delay in gastric emptying was vagally mediated.[126] Bombesin injected into the third ventricle delays gastric emptying of a peptone meal in dogs.[71] Intracerebroventricular or intrathecal bombesin-induced inhibition of gastrointestinal transit in mice and rats was reversed by hypophysectomy and adrenalectomy but not by opiate blockade.[129–131] The inhibition of gastrointestinal transit by bombesin given intracerebroventricularly in mice was more potent as compared to bombesin given intrathecally or opiates given intracerebroventricularly.[131] After spinal cord transection, the inhibitory effect of intracerebroventricular injection of bombesin persisted whereas that of intrathecal injection disappeared. Thus, it is likely that intrathecal bombesin does not act directly through spinal outflow but is activating a supraspinal center to influence gastrointestinal transit.[131]

3.4.2. Gastrointestinal Motility

Central injection of bombesin stimulates gastrointestinal motility. Microinjection of bombesin into the tractus solitarius of fasted rats increases within 1–2 min postinjection both tonic and phasic gastric intraluminal pressure without concomitant change in arterial pressure. The gastric response to centrally injected bombesin was reversed by vagotomy combined with spinal cord transection.[132]

The frequency of duodenal activity was also increased by intracerebroventricular injection of bombesin into fasted rats. The motility pattern was characterized by the production of rapid and small-amplitude contractions. In the jejunum the nature of the motor response is related to the dose of peptide.[133,134] An inhibitory effect was elicited by small doses and a stimulatory effect by higher doses.[134] Although the stimulation of gastrointestinal motility contrasts with the inhibitory effect on transit in response to central injection of bombesin, it has been suggested that such a pattern of motility may be nonpropulsive.

3.5. CNS Action of Calcitonin to Inhibit Gastrointestinal Motor Function

Growing evidence indicates that calcitonin, a 32-amino-acid peptide hormone involved in the regulation of calcium, may also act as a neurotransmitter in the brain. Specific receptors for calcitonin have been characterized and localized in high concentrations in the hypothalamus.[135] Recent molecular biological studies do not support the generation of calcitonin from the calcitonin gene present in neural tissue.[136] Although calcitonin exerts potent centrally mediated actions on gastrointestinal function,[137] the presence of an endogenous ligand for calcitonin receptors in the brain is still to be elucidated.

3.5.1. Gastrointestinal Transit

Intracerebroventricular or intracisternal injection of salmon calcitonin dose dependently delayed gastric emptying of a noncaloric liquid solution and delayed small intestinal transit whereas the large bowel transit was not modified.[138,139] A dose as low as 30 pmole inhibited gastric emptying by 92% (Fig. 1). The inhibitory effect on gastric and small intestinal transit is mediated by the autonomic nervous system through a mechanism that remains to be established since neither adrenalectomy, hypophysectomy, vagotomy, nor the noradrenergic blocking agent bretylium altered peptide action.[139]

3.5.2. Gastrointestinal Motility

Bueno et al.[140] reported that intracerebroventricular injection of calcitonin 5 min before feeding reduced the frequency of reticular (forestomach) contractions observed during feeding in sheep. In fed dogs, they described a shortening of the postprandial disruption of the MMC pattern limited to the small intestine.[141] In the rat, they found that salmon calcitonin injected into the lateral ventricle or intrathecally disrupted the fed pattern elicited by a meal or pentagastrin infusion and restored within 5 min the MMC "fasted" motility pattern in the small intestine.[142–146] Peptide action was long-acting, observed at a dose as low as 83 fmole, and centrally mediated.[142,143] Calcitonin effects may involve changes in central calcium fluxes and vagal pathways since calcitonin-induced alterations of gastrointestinal motility were no longer observed after central injection of calcium gluconate,[142] the intracellular calcium antagonist TMB-8,[144] and vagotomy.[143] The fact that intracerebroventricular indomethacin, an inhibitor of cyclooxygenase with calcium antagonist properties, but not piroxicam, a selective inhibitor of cyclooxygenase, reversed the calcitonin effect on motility further substantiated that calcitonin action results from an effect on intracerebral calcium fluxes.[144,146]

3.6. CNS Action of Calcitonin Gene-Related Peptide (CGRP) on Gastrointestinal Motor Function

CGRP is a 37-residue peptide that was first identified by prediction of the tissue-specific RNA processing of the calcitonin gene in neural tissue.[136] CGRP-immunoreactivity and precursors as well as specific receptors have been localized in discrete populations of neurons in the hypothalamus and brainstem nuclei including the nucleus ambiguus.[135,147]

3.6.1. Gastrointestinal Transit

CGRP is a potent centrally acting inhibitor of gastric emptying of a liquid meal in the rat (Fig. 1).[139,148] Intracerebroventricular CGRP also decreased small intestinal transit but did not alter large intestinal transit.[139] CGRP action is mediated through the autonomic nervous system including the vagus and the adrenals.[139,148]

3.6.2. Gastrointestinal Motility

In sheep, intracerebroventricular injection of CGRP before feeding reduced the frequency of reticular contractions.[140] In fasted rats, intracisternal injection of CGRP resulted in rapid inhibition of phasic contractions of the antrum and corpus.[148] In fed rats, intracerebroventricular or intrathecal injection of CGRP changed the pattern of intestinal motility from fed to fasted MMC pattern within 5–10 min following intracerebroventricular injection and within 17–39 min following intrathecal injection.[145] The existence of a spinal site of action for CGRP was demonstrated by the persistence of CGRP action after intrathecal injection in spinal cord-transected rats.[145]

3.7. CNS Action of Neurotensin to Influence Gastrointestinal Motor Function

3.7.1. Gastrointestinal Transit

Cerebroventricular injection of neurotensin inhibited gastric emptying of a peptone meal in the dog[71] and intestinal propulsion in the rat.[111] In the rat, there is no tolerance to repeated central injection and no alteration of neurotensin's antipropulsive effect by naloxone.[111] A site of action for neurotensin-induced inhibition of intestinal propulsion has been localized in the dorsal portion of the periaqueductal gray matter.[111] Vagotomy blocked the intestinal action of neurotensin microinjected into the periaqueductal gray.[111]

3.7.2. Gastrointestinal Motility

Intracerebroventricular injection of neurotensin elicited a vagally mediated decrease in the gastric motility index in both fed and fasted dogs[149] and induced a vagally dependent decrease in the duration of the postprandial pattern of motility in the dog jejunum. In the fasted state, the peptide replaces the intestinal MMC pattern by phases of regular contractions.[149] Colonic motility was not altered under the same conditions. In the rat, neurotensin (12 pmol) injected into the lateral ventricle 1 hr after feeding restored the fasted pattern of motility in the duodenum–jejunum through vagally dependent pathways.[143] This effect is not reproduced by intravenous injection of 100-fold higher doses of the peptide.[143]

3.8. CNS Action of Other Peptides to Influence Gastrointestinal Motility

3.8.1. Cholecystokinin (CCK)–Gastrin

Microinjection of CCK or pentagastrin into the nucleus tractus solitarius elicited a prolonged decrease in the tonic gastric pressure without altering colonic pressure, heart rate, or arterial pressure in anesthetized rats.[150,151] The gastric response was abolished by vagotomy or ganglionic blockade.[151] In fasted or fed sheep, intracerebroventricular injection of CCK also resulted in a decreased amplitude[152] and frequency[153] of contractions of the rumen. CCK-induced hypomotility in the reticulorumen was blocked by central injection of naloxone.[153]

By contrast, the effects of intracerebroventricular injection of CCK on intestinal motility are stimulatory and the pattern of motor activity is characterized by a decrease in the frequency of MMC cycles in the small intestine and an increase in the intensity of spikes of duodenal contractions.[30]

3.8.2. Neuropeptide Y (NPY)

In fasted dogs, intracerebroventricular infusion of NPY elicited the abolition of phase III activity and phase II occurred throughout the stomach and small intestine.[154] This change in pattern of gastrointestinal motility was observed up to 5 hr following stopping the central infusion of NPY. In fed dogs, by contrast, intracerebroventricular infusion of NPY caused within 3–22 min the appearance of phase III-like activity in the stomach which propagated to the small intestine.[154] The effect of NPY in both fed and fasted dogs was CNS mediated, not altered by vagotomy,[154] and specific since motilin injected intrathecally or intracerebroventricularly did not alter the interdigestive MMC activity of the stomach and small intestine in conscious fasted dogs.[155]

3.8.3. Oxytocin

Rogers and Hermann[14] reported preliminary evidence that oxytocin microinjected into the dorsal motor nucleus of the vagus reduced whereas that of an oxytocin antagonist stimulated gastric contractions in fasted rats. The inhibitory effect of oxytocin was reversed by vagotomy and partly by atropine. These data suggest that oxytocinergic neurons may exert a tonic inhibitory effect on gastric motility through activation of the inhibitory vagal pathways.

3.8.4. Somatostatin

Somatostatin infusion into the lateral ventricle increased the frequency of MMC in the small intestine of fasted rats.[30]

3.8.5. Substance P

Substance P microinjected into the dorsomedial nucleus tractus solitarius elicited a dose-related decrease in tonic gastric pressure and inhibited phasic contractions.[156] When injected into CSF, substance P did not alter the fed pattern of intestinal activity but shortened the duration of the intestinal postprandial pattern in the rat.[143]

4. SUMMARY AND CONCLUSIONS

The functional link between the brain and gastrointestinal motor function has been established experimentally since the beginning of this century. During the last decade, a resurgence of interest in the elucidation of brain pathways and neurochemical coding of brain–gut interaction resulted from the use of electrophysiological, retrograde and anterograde tracing techniques, and the characterization of biologically active peptides in the brain and gut.

Using electrical lesions and stimulation and more recently chemical stimulation, the hypothalamus including the lateral, ventromedial, and medial, and paraventricular parts, the dorsal vagal complex, the nucleus ambiguus, and the periaqueductal gray matter were demonstrated to influence gastrointestinal motor function. New findings with potentially important physiological implications came from the demonstration that the brain and the spinal cord are target sites of action for peptides to alter gut transit and motor activity.

4.1. Brain Peptides and CNS Modulation of Gastrointestinal Transit

The central action of petides to influence gastrointestinal transit in experimental animal is summarized in Table I. TRH is thus far the only peptide stimulating simultaneously gastric, intestinal, and colonic transit[35] whereas opioid peptides acting on μ brain receptors exert an opposite effect and inhibit concomitantly gastric, intestinal, and colonic transit.[102] Bombesin and CRF were found to act centrally to inhibit gastric and intestinal transit whereas they stimulated colonic transit.[66,126] The antitransit effect of calcitonin and CGRP is limited to the stomach and small intestine.[139] Nothing is known about brain sites through which these peptides act to alter gastric emptying and colonic transit. The lateral and medial hypothalamus and medial septum are responsive sites of action for TRH-induced stimulation of intestinal transit in the rat,[11] and the periaqueductal gray matter is a responsive site for μ receptor agonist- and neurotensin-induced inhibition of intestinal transit.[111,113] Further studies on the identification of brain sites of action for these peptides will generate important information on the brain structures regulating gut transit. The central action of peptides to stimulate or inhibit gastrointestinal transit is vagally mediated.[36,39,67,68,108,111,126,139] It is not known whether the vagally mediated inhibition of gastrointestinal transit by these peptides results from a decrease in the activity of vagal preganglionic fibers synapsing with excitatory myenteric neurons or an activation of vagal preganglionic neurons synapsing with inhibitory myenteric neurons. Although the lack of specific antagonists for these peptides has hampered the assessment of their physiological role in the control of gastrointestinal transit, the use of the recently developed CRF antagonist indicates that central CRF may be involved in mediating restraint-induced inhibition of gastric emptying and increase in colonic transit.[70,101] Moreover, neuropharmacological and neuroanatomical evidence substantiates a role of TRH in the dorsal vagal complex in the centrally mediated vagal stimulation of gastrointestinal transit.

4.2. Brain Peptides and Modulation of Gastrointestinal Motility

The same peptides influencing gastrointestinal transit are exerting a CNS action to alter the pattern of gastrointestinal motility. TRH produced a marked stimulation of gastric, intestinal, and colonic motor activity.[28,42–44,47] The delay in gastrointestinal transit elicited by the central action of peptides is associated with the inhibition of gastrointestinal motility for most of the peptides except central bombesin, which increases gastrointestinal motility.[132,133] A number of peptides including μ opioid peptides,[117,120] calcitonin,[145] CGRP,[145] neurotensin,[143] and NPY[154] act centrally to induce the fasted MMC pattern of motility in fed animals. The dorsal vagal complex (nucleus tractus solitarius and/or dorsal motor nucleus of the vagus) are sites of action for TRH and bombesin-induced stimulation of gastric contractility,[14,18,19,23,132] and for CCK-, oxytocin-, and substance P-induced decrease in gastric contractions or intraluminal pressure.[14,143,151] The mechanism through which TRH, bombesin, calcitonin, neurotensin, CCK, and oxytocin alter gastrointestinal motility is vagally dependent.

4.3. Conclusions

Peptides have emerged as new probes to gain insight on brain sites and neural pathways involved in the central regulation of gut motor function. Further studies will be needed to evaluate whether they are involved in modulating autonomic efferent neurons in response to gastrointestinal afferent vagal and splanchnic input to the brain and whether they play a physiological role in the extrinsic regulation of gut motility in response to neural stimuli. Preliminary evidence in experimental animals suggests that CRF may have physiological relevance in the gastrointestinal response to stress and TRH in the central control exerted by the vagus on lower peripheral circuitry involved in the regulation of gastrointestinal motor function.

ACKNOWLEDGMENTS. The author thanks M. David Claus for helping in the preparation of the manuscript. Supported by the national Institute of Mental Health, Grant MH-00663, and the National Institute of Arthritis, Metabolism and Digestive Diseases, Grants DK-33061 and DK-30110.

REFERENCES

1. Cabanis PJG: Introduction: On the relations between the physical and moral aspects of man, in Mora G, Saidi MD (eds):, Baltimore, Johns Hopkins University Press, 1981, p 650
2. Beaumont W: in Osler W (ed): Experiments and Observations on the Gastric Juice and the Physiology of Digestion. New York, Dover Publications, 1833, p 1
3. Cannon WB: Bodily Changes in Pain, Hunger, Fear and Rage. New York, Appleton, 1929
4. Roman C, Gonella J: Extrinsic control of digestive tract motility, in Johnson LR (ed): Physiology of the Gastrointestinal tract, ed 2. New York, Raven Press, 1987, p 507
5. Rostad H: Colonic motility in cat. 3. Influence of hypothalamic and mesencephalic stimulation. Acta Physiol Scand 89:104–115, 1973
6. Folkow B, Rubinstein EH: Behavioural and autonomic patterns evoked by stimulation of the lateral hypothalamic area in the cat. Acta Physiol Scand 65:292–299, 1965
7. Lee ZL: Effects of stimulation of the satiety and feeding centers on gastric, cecal and rectal motility in the rat. Acta Med Okayama 36:213–222, 1982
8. Takeda M: Studies on the motility of the gastrointestinal tract by the electrical stimulation in the hypothalamus of rabbits. Med J Osaka Univ 2:335–355, 1950
9. Feng HS, Brobeck RJ, Brooks FP: Lateral hypothalamic sites in cats for stimulation of gastric antral contractions. Clin Invest Med 10:140–144, 1987
10. Costall B, Gunning SJ, Naylor RJ: An analysis of the hypothalamic sites at which substituted benzamide drugs act to facilitate gastric emptying in the guinea-pig. Neuropharmacology 24:869–875, 1985
11. Carino MA, Horita A: Localization of TRH-sensitive sites in the rat brain mediating intestinal transit. Life Sci 41:2663–2667, 1988
12. Wood KL, Addae JI, Andrews PL, et al: Injection of baclofen into the ventromedial hypothalamus stimulates gastric motility in the rat. Neuropharmacology 26:1191–1194, 1987
13. Duggan JP, Booth DA: Obesity, overeating, and rapid gastric emptying in rats with ventromedial hypothalamic lesions. Science 231:609–611, 1986
14. Rogers RC, Hermann GE: Oxytocin, oxytocin antagonist, TRH, and hypothalamic paraventricular nucleus stimulation effects on gastric motility. Peptides 8:505–513, 1987
15. Pagani FD, Norman WP, Kasbekar DK, et al: Localization of sites within dorsal motor nucleus of vagus that affect gastric motility. Am J Physiol 249:G73–G84, 1985
16. Norman WP, Pagani FD, Ormsbee HS 3d, et al: Use of horseradish peroxidase to identify hindbrain sites that influence gastric motility in the cat. Gastroenterology 88:701–705, 1985
17. Brooks, FP, Feng YS, Brobeck JR: Efferent nervous control of gastric acid secretion and phasic antral contractions in the anesthetized cat. Gastroenterology 86:1036, 1984 (abstr)
18. Rossiter CD, Pineo SV, Norman WP, et al: Effects of microinjections of thyrotropin releasing hormone into the dorsal motor nucleus of the vagus on gastrointestinal motility, blood pressure and heart rate in the cat. Gastroenterology 94:A622, 1988 (abstr)
19. Raybould HE, Jackobsen LJ, Novin D, et al: TRH stimulation and L-glutamic inhibition of proximal gastric motor activity in the rat dorsal vagal complex. Brain Res. 1989 (in press) gastric motility by picomole quantities of glutamic acid and TRH in the dorsal complex (DVC) in rats. Soc Neurosci Abstr 13:736, 1987
20. Lynn RB, Han J, Feng H-S, et al: TRH injection into the dorsal motor nucleus of the vagus (DMV) increases gastric acid output and the force of gastric contractions in anesthetized cats. Gastroenterology 94:A274, 1988 (abstr)
21. Pagani FD, Norman WP, Kasbekar DK, et al: Effects of stimulation of nucleus ambiguus complex on gastroduodenal function. Am J Physiol 246:G253–G262, 1984
22. Williford DJ, Ormsbee HS 3d, Norman W, et al: Hindbrain GABA receptors influence parasympathetic outflow to the stomach. Science 214:193–194, 1981
23. Garrick T, Stephens R, Ishikawa T, et al: TRH-analogue, RX 77368, microinjected into the dorsal vagal complex and nucleus ambiguus stimulates gastric contractility in the rat. Am J Physiol 1989 (in press)

24. Krieger DT: Brain peptides: What, where and why? Science 222:975–985, 1983
25. Diz DI, Barnes KL, Ferrario CM: Functional characteristics of neuropeptides in the dorsal medulla oblongata and vagus nerve. Fed Proc 46:30–35, 1987
26. Leslie RA: Neuroactive substances in the dorsal vagal complex of the medulla oblongata: Nucleus of the tractus solitarius, area postrema, and dorsal motor nucleus of the vagus. Neurochem Int 7:191–211, 1985
27. Swanson LW, Sawchenko PE: Hypothalamic integration: Organization of the paraventricular and supraoptic nuclei. Annu Rev Neurosci 6:269–324, 1983
28. Smith JR, LaHann TR, Chesnut RM, et al: Thyrotropin-releasing hormone: Stimulation of colonic activity following intracerebroventricular administration. Science 196:660–661, 1977
29. Burks TF: Central sites of action of gastrointestinal drugs [editorial]. Gastroenterology 74:322–324, 1978
30. Bueno L, Ferre JP: Central regulation of intestinal motility by somatostatin and cholecystokinin octapeptide. Science 216:1427–1429, 1982
31. Passaro E Jr, Debas H, Oldendorf W, et al: Rapid appearance of intraventricularly administered neuropeptides in the peripheral circulation. Brain Res 241:335–340, 1982
32. Tannenbaum GS, Patel YC: On the fate of centrally administered somatostatin in the rat: Massive hypersomatostatinemia resulting from leakage into the peripheral circulation has effects on growth hormone secretion and glucoregulation. Endocrinology 118:2137–2143, 1986
33. Morimito T, Okamoto M, Nakamuta H, et al: Intracerebroventricular injection of 125I-salmon calcitonin in rats: Fate, anorexia and hypocalcemia. Jpn J Pharmacol 37:21–29, 1985
34. Yarbrough GG: On the neuropharmacology of thyrotropin releasing hormone (TRH). Prog Neurobiol 12:291–312, 1979
35. Taché Y, Stephens RL, Ishikawa T: Central nervous system action of TRH to influence gastrointestinal function and ulceration. Ann NY Acad Sci 553: 269–285 (1989)
36. Maeda-Hagiwara M, Taché Y: Central nervous system action of TRH to stimulate gastric emptying in rats. Regul Pept 17:199–207, 1987
37. Parolaro D, Sala M, Patrini G, et al: Further investigations on neurotensin as central modulator of intestinal motility in rats. Regul Pept 17:111–117, 1987
38. Bhargava HN, Pillai NP: Studies on the mechanism of thyrotropin releasing hormone induced inhibition of gastrointestinal transit. Peptides 6:185–187, 1984
39. Horita A, Carino MA: Centrally administered thyrotropin-releasing hormone (TRH) stimulates colonic transit and diarrhea production by a vagally mediated serotonergic mechanism in the rabbit. J Pharmacol Exp Ther 222:367–371, 1982
40. Horita A, Carino MA, Pae Y-S: Blockade by naloxone and naltrexone of the TRH-induced stimulation of colonic transit in the rabbit. Eur J Pharmacol 108:289–293, 1985
41. Beleslin DB, Jovanovic Micic D, Samardzic R, et al: Studies of thyrotropin-releasing hormone (TRH)-induced defecation in cats. Pharmacol Biochem Behav 26:639–641, 1987
42. Garrick T, Buack S, Veiseh A, et al: Thyrotropin-releasing hormone (TRH) acts centrally to stimulate gastric contractility in rats. Life Sci 40:649–657, 1987
43. Ruckebusch Y, Malbert CH: Stimulation and inhibition of food intake in sheep by centrally-administered hypothalamic releasing factors. Life Sci 38:929–934, 1986
44. LaHann TR, Horita A: Thyrotropin releasing hormone: Centrally mediated effects on gastrointestinal motor activity. J Pharmacol Exp Ther 222:66–70, 1982
45. Somiya H, Tonoue T: Neuropeptides as central integrators of autonomic nerve activity: Effects of TRH, SRIF, VIP and bombesin on gastric and adrenal nerves. Regul Pept 9:47–52, 1984
46. Taché Y, Goto Y, Hamel D, et al: Mechanisms underlying intracisternal TRH-induced stimulation of gastric acid secretion in rats. Regul Pept 13:21–30, 1985
47. Tonoue T, Nomoto T: Effect of intracerebroventricular administration of thyrotropin-releasing hormone upon the electroenteromyogram of rat duodenum. Eur J Pharmacol 58:369–377, 1979
48. Kubek MJ, Rea MA, Hodes ZI, et al: Quantitation and characterization of thyrotropin-releasing hormone in vagal nuclei and other regions of the medulla oblongata of the rat. J Neurochem 40:1307–1313, 1983
49. Palkovits M, Mezey E, Eskay RL, et al: Innervation of the nucleus of the solitary tract and the dorsal vagal nucleus by thyrotropin-releasing hormone-containing raphe neurons. Brain Res 373:246–251, 1986.
50. Mantyh PW, Hunt SP: Thyrotropin-releasing hormone (TRH) receptors. Localization by light microscopic autoradiography in rat brain using [3H][3-Me-His2]TRH as the radioligand. J Neurosci 5:551–561, 1985
51. Manaker S, Winokur A, Rostene WH, et al: Autoradiographic localization of thyrotropin-releasing hormone receptors in the rat central nervous system. J Neurosci 5:167–174, 1985

52. Neuhuber WL, Sandoz PA: Vagal primary afferent terminals in the dorsal motor nucleus of the rat: Are they making monosynaptic contacts on preganglionic efferent neurons? Neurosci Lett 69:126–130, 1986

53. Shapiro RE, Miselis RR: The central organization of the vagus nerve innervating the stomach of the rat. J Comp Neurol 238:473–488, 1985

54. Gwyn DG, Leslie RA, Hopkins DA: Observations on the afferent and efferent organization of the vagus nerve and the innervation of the stomach in the squirrel monkey. J Comp Neurol 239:163–175, 1985

55. Arancibia S, Tapia-Arancibia L, Assenmacher I, et al: Direct evidence of short-term cold-induced TRH release in the median eminence of unanesthetized rats. Neuroendocrinology 37:225–228, 1983

56. Arancibia S, Assenmacher I: Sécrétion de TRH dans le troisième ventricle cérébral lors de l'exposition aigue au froid chez le rat non anesthésie. Effect des drogues α-adrénergiques. C R Soc Biol 181:323–331, 1987

57. Yano S, Akahane M, Harada M: Role of gastric motility in development of stress-induced gastric lesions of rats. Jnp J Pharmacol 28:607–615, 1978

58. Koo MWL, Cho CH, Ogle CW: Effect of cold-restraint stress on gastric ulceration and motility in rats. Pharmacol Biochem Behav 25:775–779, 1986

59. Garrick T, Buack S, Bass P: Gastric motility is a major factor in cold restraint-induced lesion formation in rats. Am J Physiol 250:G191–G199, 1986

60. Yano S, Matsukura H, Shibata M, et al: Stress procedures lowering body temperature augment gastric motility by increasing the sensitivity to acetylcholine in rats. J Pharmacobiodyn 5:582–592, 1982

61. Taché Y, Ishikawa T, Stephens R, et al: Stressor specific alterations of gastric function in rats: Role of brain TRH and CRF. Gastroenterology 94:A452, 1988 (abstr)

62. Koo MWL, Ogle CW, Cho CH: The effect of cold-restraint stress on gastric emptying in rats. Pharmacol Biochem Behav 23:969–972, 1985

63. Barone FC, Deegan JF, Fowler PJ, et al: Stress-induced diarrhea is not associated with abnormal gut secretion. Gastroenterology 90:1337, 1986 (abstr)

64. Williams CL, Villar RG, Peterson JM, et al: Stress-induced changes in intestinal transit in the rat: A model for irritable bowel syndrome. Gastroenterology 94:611–621, 1988

65. Rivier CL, Plotsky PM: Mediation by corticotropin releasing factor (CRF) of adenohypophysial hormone secretion. Annu Rev Physiol 48:475–494, 1986

66. Taché Y, Gunion MM, Stephens R: CRF: Central nervous system action to influence gastrointestinal function and role in the gastrointestinal response to stress, in De Souza EB, Nemeroff CB (eds): Corticotropin-Releasing Factor: Basic and Clinical Studies of a Neuropeptide. Boca Raton, FL. CRC Press, 1989.

67. Taché Y, Maeda-Hagiwara M, Turkelson CM: Central nervous system action of corticotropin-releasing factor to inhibit gastric emptying in rats. Am J Physiol 253:G241–G245, 1987

68. Lenz HJ, Burlace M, Raedler A, et al: Central nervous system effects of corticotropin-releasing factor on gastrointestinal transit in the rat. Gastroenterology 94:598–602, 1988

69. Broccardo M, Improta G, Melchiorri P: Effect of sauvagine on gastric emptying in conscious rats. Eur J Pharmacol 85:111–114, 1982

70. Williams CL, Peterson JM, Villar RG, et al: Corticotropin-releasing factor directly mediates colonic responses to stress. Am J Physiol 253:G582–G586, 1987

71. Lenz HJ: Brain regulation of gastric secretion, emptying and blood flow by neuropeptides in conscious dogs. Gastroenterology 92:1500, 1987 (Abstract)

72. Pappas TN, Welton M, Taché Y, et al: Corticotropin-releasing factor inhibits gastric emptying in dogs: Studies on its mechanism of action. Peptides 8:1011–1014, 1988

73. Gue M, Fioramonti J, Bueno L: Comparative influences of acoustic and cold stress on gastrointestinal transit in mice. Am J Physiol 253:G124–G128, 1987

74. Bueno L, Gue M: Evidence for the involvement of corticortropin-releasing factor in the gastrointestinal disturbances induced by acoustic and cold stress in mice. Brain Res 441:1–4, 1988

75. Garrick T, Veiseh A, Sierra A, et al: Corticotropin-releasing factor acts centrally to suppress stimulated gastric contractility in the rat. Regul Pept 21:173–181, 1988

76. Bueno L, Fioramonti J: Effects of corticotropin-releasing factor, corticotropin and cortisol on gastrointestinal motility in dogs. Peptides 7:73–77, 1986

77. Bueno L, Fargeas MJ, Gue M, et al: Effects of corticotropin-releasing factor on plasma motilin and somatostatin levels and gastrointestinal motility in dogs. Gastroenterology 91:884–889, 1986

78. Brown MR, Gray TS, Fisher LA: Corticotropin-releasing factor receptor antagonist: Effects on the autonomic nervous system and cardiovascular function. Regul Pept 16:321–329, 1986

79. Tazi A, Dantzer R, Le Moal M, et al: Corticotropin-releasing factor antagonist blocks stress-induced fighting in rats. Regul Pept 18:37–42, 1987

80. Lenz HJ, Raedler A, Greten H, et al: CRF initiates biological actions within the brain that are observed in response to stress. Am J Physiol 252:R34–R39, 1987

81. Swanson LW, Sawchenko PE, Rivier J, et al: Organization of ovine corticotropin-releasing factor immunoreactive cells and fibers in the rat brain: An immunohistochemical study. Neuroendocrinology 36:165–186, 1983

82. Merchenthaler I: Corticotropin releasing factor (CRF)-like immunoreactivity in the rat central nervous system. Extrahypothalamic distribution Peptides 5(suppl 1):53–69, 1984

83. De Souza EB: Corticotropin-releasing factor receptors in the rat central nervous system: Characterization and regional distribution. J Neurosci 7:88–100, 1987

84. Fioramonti J, Bueno L: Gastrointestinal myoelectric activity disturbances in gastric ulcer disease in rats and dogs. Dig Dis Sci 25:575–580, 1980

85. Gue M, Bueno L: Diazepam and muscimol blockade of the gastrointestinal motor disturbances induced by acoustic stress in dogs. Eur J Pharmacol 131:123–127, 1986

86. Dorval ED, Mueller GP, Eng RR, et al: Effect of ionizing radiation on gastric motility in monkeys. Gastroenterology 89:374–380, 1985

87. Taché Y, Stephens RL, Ishikawa T: Stress-induced alterations of gastrointestinal function: Involvement of brain CRF and TRH, in Weiner H, Florin I, Hellhammer D, et al (eds): IV. New Frontiers of Stress Research. Bern, Huber, 1988, p 1.

88. Gue M, Fioramonti J, Frexinos J, et al: Influence of acoustic stress by noise on gastrointestinal motility in dogs. Dig Dis Sci 32:1411–1417, 1987

89. Williams CL, Burks TF: Stress, opioids, and gastrointestinal transit, in Taché Y, Morley JE, Brown MR (eds): Hans Selye Symposia: Neuropeptides and Stress. Berlin, Springer-Verlag 1989, pp 175–187

90. Enck P, Wienbeck M, Merlin V, et al: Panic induced changes of gastrointestinal transit in the rat. Gastroenterology 94:A115, 1988 (abstr)

91. Valori RM, Kumar D, Wingate DL: Effects of different types of stress and of "prokinetic" drugs on the control of the fasting motor complex in humans. Gastroenterology 90:1890–1900, 1986

92. Mcrae S, Younger K, Thompson DG, et al: Sustained mental stress alters human jejunal motor activity. Gut 23:404–409, 1982

93. Stanghellini V, Malagelada J-R, Zinsmeister AR, et al: Stress-induced gastroduodenal motor disturbances in humans: Possible humoral mechanisms. Gastroenterology 85:83–91, 1983

94. Thompson DG, Richelson E, Malagelada J-R: Perturbation of gastric emptying and duodenal motility through the central nervous system. Gastroenterology 83:1200–1206, 1982

95. Simpson KH, Stakes AF: Effect of anxiety on gastric emptying in preoperative patients. Br J Anaesth 59:540–544, 1987

96. Thompson DG, Richelson E, Malagelada J-R: Perturbation of upper gastrointestinal function by cold stress. Gut 24:277–283, 1983

97. Cann PA, Read NW, Cammack J, et al: Psychological stress and the passage of a standard meal through the stomach and small intestine in man. Gut 24:236–240, 1983

98. Welgan P, Meshkinpour H, Hoehler F: The effect of stress on colon motor and electrical activity in irritable bowel syndrome. Psychosom Med 47:139–149, 1985

99. Narducci F, Snape WJ, Battle WM Jr, et al: Increased colonic motility during exposure to a stressful situation. Dig Dis Sci 30:40–44, 1985

100. O'Brien JD, Thompson DG, Burnham WR, et al: Action of centrally mediated autonomic stimulation on human upper gastrointestinal transit: A comparative study of two stimuli. Gut 28:960–969, 1987

101. Lenz HJ, Raeder A, Greten H, et al: Stress-induced gastrointestinal secretory and motor responses in rats are mediated by endogenous corticotropin-releasing factor. Gastroenterology 95:1510–1517, 1988

102. Porreca F, Galligan JJ, Burks TF: Central opioid receptor involvement in gastrointestinal motility. Trends Pharmacol Sci 7:104–107, 1986

103. Manara L, Bianchetti A: The central and peripheral influences of opioids on gastrointestinal propulsion. Annu Rev Pharmacol Toxicol 25:249–273, 1985

104. Ewart WR, Wingate DL: Central representation and opioid modulation of gastric mechanoreceptor activity in the rat. Am J Physiol 244:27–32, 1983

105. Porreca F, Cowan A, Raffa RB, et al: Ketazocines and morphine: Effects on gastrointestinal transit after central and peripheral administration. Life Sci 32:1785–1790, 1983

106. Ward SJ, Takemori AE: Relative involvement of receptor subtypes in opioid-induced inhibition of gastrointestinal transit in mice. J Pharmacol Exp Ther 224:359–363, 1983

107. Porreca F, Mosberg HI, Hurst R, et al: Roles of mu, delta and kappa opioid receptors in spinal and supraspinal mediation of gastrointestinal transit effects and hot-plate analgesia in the mouse. J Pharmacol Exp Ther 230:341–348, 1984

108. Stewart JJ, Weisbrodt NW, Burks TF: Central and peripheral actions of morphine on intestinal transit. J Pharmacol Exp Ther 205:547–555, 1978

109. Broccardo M: Pituitary–adrenal mediation of dermorphin-induced inhibition of gastric emptying in rats. Eur J Pharmacol 142:151–154, 1987

110. Galligan JJ, Burks TF: Inhibition of gastric and intestinal motility by centrally and peripherally administered morphine. Proc West Pharmacol Soc 25:307–311, 1982

111. Parolaro D, Sala M, Crema G, et al: Effect on intestinal transit of neurotensin administered intracerebroventricularly to rats. Life Sci 33:485–488, 1983

112. Galligan JJ, Burks TF: Centrally mediated inhibition of small intestinal transit and motility by morphine in the rat. J Pharmacol Exp Ther 226:356–361, 1983

113. Parolaro D, Crema G, Sala M, et al: Intestinal effect and analgesia: Evidence for different involvement of opioid receptor subtypes in periaqueductal gray matter. Eur J Pharmacol 120:95–99, 1986

114. Porreca F, Filla A, Burks TF: Spinal cord-mediated opiate effects on gastrointestinal transit in mice. Eur J Pharmacol 86:135–136, 1982

115. Koslo RJ, Vaught JL, Cowan A, et al: Intrathecal morphine slows gastrointestinal transit in rats. Eur J Pharmacol 119:243–246, 1985

116. Vaught JL, Cowan A, Gmerek DE: A species difference in the slowing effect of intrathecal morphine on gastrointestinal transit. Eur J Pharmacol 94:181–184, 1983

117. Ruckebusch Y, Ferre JP, Du C: In vivo modulation of intestinal motility and sites of opioid effects in the rat. Regul Pept 9:109–117, 1984

118. Ferre JP, Du C, Soldani G, et al: Peripheral versus central components of the effects of dermorphin on intestinal motility in the fed rat. Regul Pept 13:109–117, 1986

119. Ruckebusch Y: Ruminoreticular functions: A pharmacological approach, in Milligan LP, Grovum WL, Dobson A (eds): Control of Digestion and Metabolism in Ruminants. Englewood Cliffs, NJ, Prentice–Hall, 1986, p 60

120. Bueno L, Fioramonti J, Honde C, et al: Central and peripheral control of gastrointestinal and colonic motility by endogenous opiates in conscious dogs. Gastroenterology 88:549–556, 1985

121. Ruckebusch Y, Ferre J-P, Bardon T: Opioid control of colonic motility in different species, in Lewin MJM, Bonfils S (eds): Regulatory Peptides in Digestive, Nervous and Endocrine Systems. Amsterdam, Elsevier, 1985, p 335

122. Khachaturian H, Lewis ME, Schafer MK-H, et al: Anatomy of the CNS opioid systems. Trends Neurosci 8:111–119, 1985

123. Kaufman PN, Krevsky B, Malmud LS, et al: Role of opiate receptors in the regulation of colonic transit. Gastroenterology 94:1351–1356, 1988

124. Primi MP, Bueno L: Effects of centrally administered naloxone on gastrointestinal myoelectrical activity in morphine-dependent rats. J Pharmacol Exp Ther 240:320–326, 1987

125. Taché Y, Vale W, Rivier J, et al: Brain regulation of gastric secretion: Influence of neuropeptides. Proc Natl Acad Sci USA 77:5515–5519, 1980

126. Porreca F, Burks TF: Centrally administered bombesin affects gastric emptying and small and large bowel transit in the rat. Gastroenterology 85:313–317, 1983

127. Moody TW, O'Donohue TL, Jacobowitz DM: Biochemical localization and characterization of bombesin-like peptides in discrete regions of rat brain. Peptides 2:75–79, 1981

128. Zarbin MA, Kuhar MJ, O'Donohue TL, et al: Autoradiographic localization of (125I-Tyr4) bombesin-binding sites in rat brain. J Neurosci 5:429–437, 1985

129. Gmerek DE, Cowan A: Pituitary–adrenal mediation of bombesin-induced inhibition of gastrointestinal transit in rats. Regul Pept 9:299–304, 1984

130. Koslo RJ, Gmerek DE, Cowan A, et al: Intrathecal bombesin-induced inhibition of gastrointestinal transit: Requirement for an intact pituitary–adrenal axis. Regul Pept 14:237–242, 1986

131. Koslo RJ, Burks TF, Porreca F: Centrally administered bombesin affects gastrointestinal transit and colonic bead expulsion through supraspinal mechanisms. J Pharmacol Exp Ther 238:62–67, 1986
132. Spencer SE, Talman WT: Centrally administered bombesin modulates gastric motility. Peptides 8:887–891, 1987
133. Porreca F, Burks TF, Koslo RJ: Centrally-mediated bombesin effects on gastrointestinal motility. Life Sci 37:125–134, 1985
134. Porreca F, Fulginiti JT, Burks TF: Bombesin stimulates small intestinal motility after intracerebroventricular administration to rats. Eur J Pharmacol 114:167–173, 1985
135. Goltzman D, Mitchell J: Interaction of calcitonin and calcitonin gene-related peptide at receptor sites in target tissues. Science 227:1343–1346, 1985
136. Rosenfeld MG, Mermod J-J, Amara SG, et al: Production of a novel neuropeptide encoded by the calcitonin gene via tissue-specific RNA processing. Nature 304:129–135, 1983
137. Taché Y: Central regulation of gastric acid secretion, in Johnson LR, Christensen J, Jackson M, et al (eds): Physiology of the Gastrointestinal tract, ed 2. New York, Raven Press, 1987, p 911
138. Taché Y, Kolve E, Maeda-Hagiwara M, et al: CNS action of calcitonin to alter experimental gastric ulcers in rats. Gastroenterology 41:651–655, 1987
139. Lenz HJ: Calcitonin and CGRP inhibit gastrointestinal transit via distinct neuronal pathways. Am J Physiol 254:G920–G924, 1988
140. Bueno L, Fargeas MJ, Julie P: Effects of calcitonin and CGRP alone or in combination on food intake and forestomch (reticulum) motility in sheep. Physiol Behav 36:907–911, 1986
141. Bueno L, Fargeas MJ, Fioramonti J, et al: Central control of intestinal motility by prostaglandins: A mediator of the actions of several peptides in rats and dogs. Gastroenterology 88:1888–1894, 1985
142. Bueno L, Fioramonti J, Ferre JP: Calcitonin–CNS action to control the pattern of intestinal motility in rats. Peptides 4:63–66, 1983
143. Bueno L, Ferre JP, Fioramonti J, et al: Effects of intracerebroventricular administration of neurotensin, substance P and calcitonin on gastrointestinal motility in normal and vagotomized rats. Regul Pept 6:197–205, 1983
144. Fargeas MJ, Fioramonti J, Bueno L: Central action of calcitonin on body temperature and intestinal motility in rats: Evidence for different mediations. Regul Pept 11:95–103, 1985
145. Fargeas MJ, Fioramonti J, Bueno L: Calcitonin gene-related peptide: Brain and spinal action on intestinal motility. Peptides 6:1167–1171, 1985
146. Fargeas MJ, Fioramonti J, Bueno L: Protaglandin E2: A neuromodulator in the central control of gastrointestinal motility and feeding behavior by calcitonin. Science 225:1050–1052, 1984
147. Amara SG, Arriza JL, Leff SE, et al: Expression in brain of a messenger RNA encoding a novel neuropeptide homologous to calcitonin gene-related peptide. Science 229:1094–1097, 1985
148. Raybould HE, Kolve E, Taché Y: Central nervous sytem action of calcitonin-gene related peptide to inhibit gastric emptying in the conscious rat. Peptides 9:735–737, 1988
149. Bueno L, Fioramonti J, Fargeas MJ, et al: Neurotensin: A central neuromodulator of gastrointestinal motility in the dog. Am J Physiol 248:G15–G19, 1985
150. Minty FM, Tepperman BL, Evered MD: The effect of intracranial injections of gastrin-like peptides on gastric motor activity in the rat. Gastroenterology 82:1132, 1988 (abstr)
151. Talman WT, Andreasen K: Centrally administered CCK changes gastric pressure and contractile rhythmicity. FASEB J 2:A438, 1988 (abstr)
152. Della Fera MA, Baile CA: CCK-octapeptide injected in CSF and changes in feed intake and rumen motility. Physiol Behav 24:943–950, 1980
153. Bueno L, Duranton A, Ruckebusch Y: Antagonistic effects of naloxone on CCK-octapeptide induced satiety and rumino-reticular hypomotiity in sheep. Life Sci 32:855–863, 1983
154. Nitecki S, Szurszewski JH: The effect of central and peripheral administration of NPY on gastrointestinal myoelectrical activity in the dog. Gastroenterology 94:A325, 1988 (abstr)
155. Hashmonai M, Go VL, Yaksh T, et al: Effect of central administration of motilin on migrating complexes in the dog. Am J Physiol 252:G195–G199, 1987
156. Spencer SE, Talman WT: Central modulation of gastric pressure by substance P: A comparison with glutamate and acetylcholine. Brain Res 385:371–374, 1986

5

Effect of Diet on Intestinal Function and Dysfunction

Kenneth W. Heaton

1. INTRODUCTION

This chapter is an attempt to make some sense out of the effects of diet and eating habits on the intestine with special reference to functional disorder of the intestine, commonly called irritable bowel syndrome (IBS). The chapter does not cover the role of diet in causing and treating organic gastrointestinal disease nor the effects on the gut of under-nutrition including specific deficiencies.

There are many complexities in this area that at times make it difficult to reach scientifically valid conclusions about published work:

1. Physical factors may be as important as chemical ones in determining the reaction of the gut to foods. These factors include the temperature of the food or drink, its osmolality, its histological integrity, its consistency, and its particle size. All of these factors are affected by cooking and other types of food processing.
2. Psychological factors can be crucial. A meal may be handled quite differently by the gut when a person is angry, anxious, tense, or unhappy compared to when the person is relaxed.
3. Interactions occur such that the effect of one food component is modified by the presence of another.
4. Events in one part of the gut can modify events in another part. The best known example is the colonic response to eating, especially in the morning. In addition, entry of fat into the ileum can slow down gastric emptying, and distension of the rectum can do the same. Thus, the function of the stomach can depend on what was eaten hours or even days ago.
5. Food and bacteria interact in important ways before the food is eaten, and when

Kenneth W. Heaton • University Department of Medicine, Bristol Royal Infirmary, Bristol BS2 8HW, England.

its undigested residues enter the colon. Infected food is beyond the scope of this chapter but it is, of course, responsible for much bowel dysfunction. Fermentation of food residues in the colon is crucial and will be discussed later.

2. EFFECTS OF EATING ON THE COLON

The symptoms of IBS are often brought on or exacerbated by eating. Thus, patients' pain and bloated feelings, which are clearly from the colon because they are lower abdominal and are eased by defecation, are often precipitated or worsened by food. The urgent calls to stool that dominate some patients' lives are often precipitated by eating or drinking. The patient may be forced to give up eating away from home, which can ruin social activities.

The physiology of the colonic response to eating is still poorly understood. It is wrong to call it the gastrocolic reflex since it is independent of the stomach and still occurs in the gastrectomized patient.[1] It is also not a reflex in the sense of requiring extrinsic innervation since it remains in the vagotomized patient. It does, however, depend to some extent on cholinergic stimulation since it can be reduced by an anticholinergic drug[2] and such drugs are generally accepted as liable to cause constipation. All the same, a hormonal element may exist. Certainly, intravenous infusions of cholecystokinin and gastrin lead to increased colonic motor activity[3] and cholecystokinin release associated with magnesium sulfate administration can evoke the pain of IBS.[4]

Meal Composition and the Gastrocolonic Response

Surprisingly few studies have been done on how the colonic response to eating varies with different types of meal and different food components. The size of the meal is probably important since a 350-kcal meal has much less effect on myoelectrical and motor activity in the left colon than a 1000-kcal meal.[3] In addition, the fat content of the meal may be crucial. The colonic effect of a 1000-kcal mixed meal can be reproduced simply by drinking 70 ml olive oil (providing 600-kcal).[5] An isocaloric drink of glucose has no effect while an amino acid drink either has no effect or even inhibits the colon.[5,6] These findings may explain the Greek tradition of starting the day with a glass of olive oil. In France, constipated women have been reported to eat, on average, 24% less fat than matched controls with normal bowel habit.[7] More data are needed on the effects of dietary fats and, especially, fats taken at breakfast time, on colonic function and bowel habit.

In some patients with IBS the pain is small intestinal in origin[8-10] and can be reproduced by infusing cholecystokinin octapeptide at physiological rates.[11] One study of liquid and solid meals suggested that the motility of the ileum increases after a liquid meal (containing amino acids, glucose polymers, and corn oil) as much as after a normal solid one,[6] but more data are needed on meals of different composition.

3. CARBOHYDRATE

The effects of carbohydrate on the gut are extremely variable depending on the nature of the carbohydrate, whether it is simple or complex, digestible or indigestible, processed or unprocessed. Indeed, in their effects on the body, carbohydrates vary as much as vitamins and it is as important as with vitamins to consider separately each carbohydrate or groups of similar carbohydrates. Generalizations about carbohydrate are meaningless.

3.1. Simple Sugars

For practical purposes, simple sugars are the mono- and disaccharides. Henceforth I call these sugars. Virtually all naturally occurring sugars are absorbed and metabolized by healthy people, the only common exception being lactose in people who have lost the enzyme lactase from their small intestinal brush border. Some artificial sugars and sugar alcohols are not absorbed or are absorbed slowly, e.g., lactulose, lactitol, mannitol, xylitol and sorbitol. These must be considered separately. They are increasingly used as therapeutic agents and sucrose substitutes, especially by diabetics.

3.1.1. Absorbable Sugars

The main absorbable sugars in our diet are the monosaccharides glucose and fructose and the disaccharide sucrose. Beer drinkers ingest maltose and consumers of dairy products (especially milk) consume lactose. The average intake of sugars other than lactose in the United States is 80 g/day[12] and the average intake of sucrose and glucose in the United Kingdom is 120 g/day[13] but there is wide individual variation. An appreciable number of young people consume over 200 g of sugars daily. Most of the sugars consumed today are in the form of refined or fiber-depleted sugars. These are often called added sugars but are best described as extracted or extracellular sugars. The majority consists of sucrose which has been extracted from sugar cane and sugar beet but also included are corn syrup (a hydrolyzate of maize starch which contains maltose and other oligosaccharides), other syrups, and honey. The sugars in fruit juices are also in the category of extracellular sugars.

The important differences between extracellular sugars and the naturally occurring sugars in fruits and vegetables are as follows: (1) they are consumed in larger amounts because they do not have to be chewed (indeed, they can often be drunk) or because they are in concentrated form; (2) they are absorbed more rapidly and also, probably, more proximally in the small intestine; (3) they are unaccompanied by dietary fiber.

To illustrate these points, the world's biggest selling candy bar contains nearly 40 g of extracellular sugars and some people eat two or three such bars in a day. The world's biggest selling soft drink contains 38 g of sugars in a can and, again, it is not unusual for a person to drink several cans in a day. Consuming such candy or soft drink leads to higher insulin responses and a greater postabsorptive swing of plasma glucose than eating whole food containing the same amount of sugars in intracellular form, implying that the sugars are being absorbed more rapidly.[14]

Relevance to Bowel Disease. There is a dearth of good studies on the effects of absorbable sugars on intestinal function. It is widely assumed that, because they are absorbed, their effects must be negligible. This may not be true. In one study, published so far only in abstract form, the addition of 120 g/day refined sugar to a defined diet for 2 weeks had the following significant effects: mean whole-gut transit time lengthened from 57 to 64 hr, fecal concentration of secondary bile acids rose by 29% from 5.6 to 7.2 mg/g and, after an oral load of lactulose, there was increased excretion of hydrogen in the breath implying greater fermentation of carbohydrate.[15] Clearly further studies are needed but, in the judgment of this author, it would be unwise to ignore the possible role of sugars in future research on gut function, if only because of suggestive links between sugar consumption and Crohn's disease[16] and because even refined sucrose is not 100% absorbed.[17]

3.1.2. Unabsorbable Sugars and Sugar Alcohols

These differ radically from ordinary sugars in their effect on the gut. Since they exert osmotic effects in the lower small intestine and, like dietary fiber, provide substrate for colonic bacteria, they speed up intestinal transit, and increase the bulk and softness of the stools. Lactulose is the prototype and is of course much used as a laxative but other artificial sugars and sugar alcohols (namely, lactitol, mannitol, and xylitol) have the same effect. The same may well apply to stachyose, a tetrasaccharide present in beans, and to raffinose, a trisaccharide of glucose, fructose, and galactose present in beans and molasses, since these oligosaccharides are often blamed for flatulence after eating beans. However, systematic studies are lacking. Sorbitol is a slowly absorbed sugar alcohol that is widely used as a sweetener of diabetic foods. Occasionally, patients who eat a large amount of such foods experience diarrhea and urgency of defecation, which may lead the unwary physician to diagnose IBS.

3.1.3. Lactose Intolerance and Hypolactasia

Unabsorbed lactose is equivalent in its physiological effects to lactulose and people with intestinal hypolactasia are liable to notice a laxative effect from drinking milk (half a pint or 227 ml cow's milk contains 10–15 g lactose). However, this does not necessarily amount to symptomatic diarrhea and, if it does, the subject is usually aware of the connection and avoids drinking milk. It was suggested in the 1960s that some cases of IBS are caused by hypolactasia[18,19] and since that time many thousands of patients with IBS have undergone tests for hypolactasia and have been prescribed lactose-free diets. However, few gastroenterologists now consider hypolactasia to be a common cause of chronic diarrhea or other symptoms that lead to the diagnosis of IBS. No one has confirmed a Danish report that 13% of IBS patients were cured by a lactose-free diet[20] and this could well have been a nonspecific placebo response. In a series of 16 Scottish patients there was not a single case of lactose intolerance.[21] Newcomer and McGill[22] found 5 cases of hypolactasia among 80 white non-Jewish patients with IBS. However, only one of them showed sustained improvement on a lactose-free diet. Even in this case one cannot be sure of the significance without blind challenges of lactose and placebo. People who do get IBS symptoms from lactose-containing foods are probably supersensitive to unabsorbed carbohydrate[23] as well as having hypolactasia and may be regarded as predisposed to IBS. It is now believed that most people with hypolactasia do not get abdominal symptoms after a glass of milk.[24]

3.2. Starch

Standard physiological teaching until recently had been that dietary starch is fully digested and absorbed provided it is adequately cooked. Despite this, medical textbooks up until the 1950s described patients who experienced abdominal discomfort, bloating, borborygmi, and sometimes acid diarrhea when they ate starchy foods, a syndrome that was quaintly called "intestinal carbohydrate dyspepsia."[25] The syndrome was blamed on rapid small bowel transit, often as the result of emotional distress, and diagnosis rested on finding iodine-positive starch granules in fresh stool. Treatment was a low-starch diet with, sometimes, the addition of a sedative. For 30 years this syndrome has been discredited and largely forgotten but it may be due for a renaissance since, with improved methodology, we now know that even normal people digest cooked starch imperfectly and that there is wide variation, perhaps from 2 to 20%, in the percent of starch that is malabsorbed and enters the colon, even after a standard meal.[26,27] The reason for this starch malabsorption is unclear, as is the reason for the wide person-to-person variation. Small bowel transit time seems not to be the limiting factor[27,28] although artificially speeding up small bowel transit can increase the fraction escaping absorption.[29] Exclusion of wheat and corn products alleviates the symptoms in some IBS patients.[30]

3.2.1. Effect of Unabsorbed Starch on the Colon

Scientific work on the interaction between unabsorbed starch and the colon is in its infancy. In vitro and in vivo, starch is readily fermented by intestinal bacteria[31] and the end products are the same as with the fermentation of nonstarch polysaccharide (the major component of dietary fiber), namely, short-chain fatty acids and gases (H_2, CO_2, CH_4). Therefore, insofar as the effects of dietary fiber are exerted via its fermentation products, or by the multiplication of bacteria that fermentation allows, the effects of unabsorbed starch should be similar to those of fiber. However, if the starch is fermented very rapidly there may be gaseous distension of the right colon, which could cause pain and bloated feelings and, if peristalsis is provoked, diarrhea. In one study,[32] addition of 100 g corn starch daily to the diet of young Indian men caused 24-hr fecal weight to increase from 187 to 246 g. No data are given on symptoms. Similar studies are needed using different sources of starch, using subjects who are more and less efficient at digesting starch and using subjects who have faster and slower colonic transit. It may be that dietary starch has laxative properties only in people with intrinsically poor starch-digesting capacity and/or fairly rapid colon transit (note that the subjects in the cornstarch study already had bulky stools by Western standards). People who get symptoms from dietary starch may be those whose cecal flora is especially active at fermenting starch.

In a French study,[33] 50 g wheat starch was instilled into the terminal ileum over 4 hr. All five volunteers experienced bloating and two had pain, proving that starch in the colon can cause IBS-type symptoms. The starch in this study was raw, which may have slowed down its fermentation and limited cecal distension by gases. The volatile fatty acids produced must have been completely absorbed because there was no rise in fecal VFA concentration.

3.2.2. Factors Affecting the Digestibility of Starch

Englyst and Cummings[34] have worked extensively on the digestibility of starch in vitro and in vivo and their findings have led them to propose three categories of starch: readily digestible, partially resistant, and resistant (Table I). Several plausible hypotheses arise from this classification: (1) foods rich in inaccessible, crystalline or retrograded starch have laxative properties; (2) in predisposed individuals the same foods produce IBS

Table I. Classification of Dietary Starch According to
Its Digestibility[a]

Readily digestible starch (RDS)	
RDS1	Fully gelatinized starch, as in freshly cooked food
RDS2	Type A crystalline starch, as in raw cereals (slowly but completely digested)
Partially resistant starch (PRS)	
PRS1	Physically inaccessible starch, as in whole or coarsely milled cereals and pulses
PRS2	Type B or C crystalline starch, as in intact starch granules of raw potato and unripe banana
PRS3	Retrograded amylopectin, as in cooked, then cooled potato
Resistant starch (RS)	
Mainly retrograded amylose, as in cooked, then cooled potato	

[a]After Englyst and Cummings.[34]

symptoms; (3) in other predisposed individuals consumption of starch only in readily digestible form contributes to the development of constipation. There is already experimental evidence that, when people eat bread made from coarsely milled rather than conventional finely ground flour, the starch is digested more slowly,[35] more starch escapes from the ileum[35a] and the feces are bulkier.[36,37]

3.2.3. Starch-Digesting Capacity and Colonic Dysfunction

Diverticular disease of the colon is generally believed to be the result of colonic dysfunction in the form of high intraluminal pressures and, in the clinic, symptomatic diverticular disease is indistinguishable from IBS.[38] It is of interest therefore that, as judged by their generation of hydrogen and its excretion in the breath after a test meal, eight patients with symptomatic diverticular disease were three or four times more efficient at digesting potato starch than matched controls.[39] These important findings need to be confirmed and to be extended to asymptomatic cases of diverticular disease and to patients with IBS and a normal barium enema. We need to know whether superefficient starch digestion is a feature of diverticulosis or of a subtype of IBS.

4. DIETARY FIBER

Despite 20 years of research and discussion there are still problems in the definition and classification of dietary fiber,[40] controversy about how best to measure it, ignorance as to the physiological meaning of measured food values,[41] and uncertainty about recommending daily intakes. For a full discussion of these questions the reader is referred to recent multiauthor books on dietary fiber.[42-46] Progress in understanding the role of fiber in health and disease has been hampered by the protean nature of fiber components, by the crucial role of physical factors such as histological integrity and particle size, and by the varying reaction of different individuals to fiber.

Table II. Relationship between Plant Cell
Wall and Dietary Fiber as Usually
Defined—Overlap, Not Identity

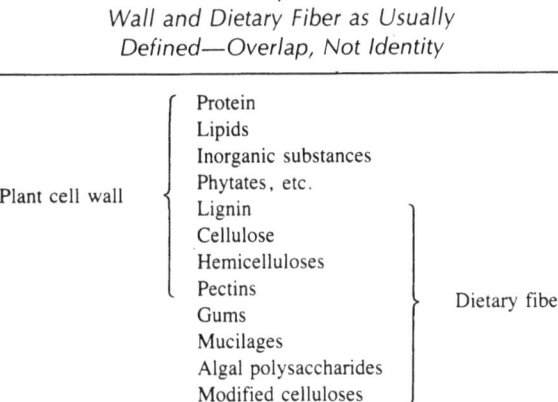

4.1. Definition and Classification

An attractively simple working definition is nonstarch polysaccharides and lignin. The justification for combining these two very different classes of polymer is that they occur together in plant cell walls. However, there are anomalies. The plant cell wall contains protein, lipids, and inorganic constituents that are inextricably combined with the nonstarch polysaccharides and lignin but are not usually classed as dietary fiber while, on the other hand, the term nonstarch polysaccharides is used to include non-cell wall materials like gums and mucilages and even artificial derivatives like methyl cellulose. Indeed the most widely prescribed pharmaceutical fiber preparations, the ispaghula husk preparations, consist chiefly of intracellular mucilages (those of the seeds of *Plantago* species). Thus, the plant cell wall is far from synonymous with dietary fiber (Table II).

The original unifying concept of dietary fiber was nondigestibility by mammalian enzymes.[47] However, there are anomalies with this idea too. We now know that in the average Westerner's diet at least half the undigested polysaccharide entering the colon is starch. There are also other undigested polymers in the diet like amylose–lipid complexes and Maillard products, not to mention nondigestible sugars and sugar alcohols. Thus, dietary fiber is far from synonymous with nondigestible food matter. There is even a small fraction of fiber, perhaps 5–8%, that is hydrolyzed in the stomach.[48]

Nondigestibility is a useful concept only if it predicts physiological effects. Unfortunately, it does not. Nondigestible might be expected to imply nonnutritious but it does not; most of the noncellulosic polysaccharides are extensively fermented in the colon and the fermentation products are efficiently absorbed. Nondigestible might be expected to imply laxative, or stool-bulking. Again, it does not necessarily do so. In tolerable doses, pectin, the gums, and lignin have little if no laxative action (lignin may even be constipating).

Thus dietary fiber is an imprecise and misleading term. It has served a useful purpose in focusing scientific and medical attention on neglected areas of nutrition, food science, and physiology but perhaps it should now be avoided in original scientific publications and replaced with more precise terms, such as cellulose, guar gum, pectin, powdered ispaghula, and of course wheat bran, corn bran, rice bran, and so forth. A naturally fiber-rich diet is best described as a diet rich in whole plant foods.

Table III. Demonstrated Changes
in Human Large Bowel Function with Addition
of Wheat Bran or Ispaghula to the Diet[54,58]

Transit time shortened (unless already < 48 hr)
Intraluminal pressure lowered (in sigmoid)
Volatile fatty acid production increased
pH lowered
Bacterial turnover increased
Bacterial metabolism decreased, e.g., of bile acids
Stool made bulkier and softer
Defecation made easier (and more frequent)

Most of the recent work on the effects of dietary fiber on colonic function and dysfunction has been done with wheat bran and ispaghula husk. There is inadequate physiological and therapeutic information on the other fiber-rich preparations and isolated fiber components. This chapter will therefore deal only with bran and ispaghula.

4.2. Actions of Wheat Bran and Ispaghula on the Colon

Probably every single function of the colon is altered by a change in the amount of solid matter that enters it, particularly if that matter is fermentable or has water-holding properties. However, even the ingestion of 15 g daily of small plastic particles has appreciable effects on stool weight and intestinal transit time.[49]

The demonstrated changes in large bowel function when bran or ispaghula is added to the diet are listed in Table III. There is appealing simplicity in the statement that bran and ispaghula produce a larger, softer stool that contains more water and moves faster. However, the mechanisms that produce these changes are complex and imperfectly understood. It is usually assumed that the bulkier stool stimulates colonic peristalsis, but if colonic peristalsis is stimulated chemically (by senna laxative) the results mimic those of fiber; the stool becomes bulkier, bacterial excretion increases, and bacterial metabolism is reduced.[50,51] Fiber could stimulate peristalsis in several ways—by direct mechanical stimulation, by distending the colon with gases (H_2, CO_2, CH_4), by acid inhibition of salt and water absorption, and by carrying bile acids into the colon. Much experimental work is needed to sort out these possible mechanisms.

4.2.1. Stool Bulk and Composition

The increased stool bulk with added fiber is generally believed to have two main mechanisms—water-holding and fermentation leading to increased bacterial mass.[52] Fermentation cannot be the main or only mechanism because pectin is almost entirely fermented and has little fecal bulking effect. On the other hand, the relationship between the in vitro water-holding capacity of a fiber preparation and its in vivo fecal bulking capacity is opposite to what one would expect.[53] This paradox may be because the fibers with the greatest water-holding capacity in vitro, namely the gums and pectin, are also, being soluble, the fibers which are most easily and completely fermented. Once a fiber has been fermented it can no longer contribute to fecal bulk except by the bulk of the bacteria which have fed on it. Bran and ispaghula may owe their effectiveness to the fact that they combine reasonable water-holding capacity (3 g water is held by 1 g bran on average but this varies with cooking and particle size and the method used for measuring water-holding[54]) with relative resistance to bacterial attack, only a quarter to a half of bran fiber being lost during passage through the gut.[55]

Dose–response studies in normal subjects have shown a straight-line relationship between the amount of bran or wholemeal bread eaten and the weight of the stools per 24 hr.[55–57] The increment of stool weight per gram of wheat fiber has varied from 2.7 to 7.5 g. This variation may be due to differences in particle size, cooking technique, strain of wheat, or characteristics of the subjects. There are some data to suggest that the fecal bulking effect of bran is less in subjects with diverticular disease[58] and in subjects with low initial stool-weights[59] but the evidence is not conclusive.

With ispaghula there are few data on dose–response[60] and these are derived from Indian men who began with relatively bulky stools by Western standards. When direct comparison has been made between ispaghula and bran in fiber-equivalent amounts, ispaghula has had a greater effect on stool bulk in normal subjects[61] and probably in patients with diverticular disease[62] and with constipation.[63]

Corn bran seems to be less effective than wheat bran. In four published studies the mean increase in fecal output per gram of corn fiber was 3.3 g compared with 5.7 g in 31 studies with wheat fiber.[58] The equivalent figure for soya fiber was 2.8. Bran made from soft white wheat is less effective than bran from hard red spring wheat.[64]

The percentage of water in the stool in increased by bran in some studies but not in others. This inconsistent situation may relate to the fact that bacteria have similar water content to formed stools, namely 80%. On the other hand, the superior bulking action of ispaghula is explicable by its ability to increase the water content of the stool.[61]

Softening of the stool with addition of fiber to the diet is commonly ascribed in part to increased gas content. This is a plausible idea but there are no good data to support or refute it. It has not even been shown that stools are more likely to float in water on a high-fiber diet.

Data on stool composition are patchy but generally show little or no change with added fiber. Absolute excretion of fat, nitrogen, and minerals tends to increase pro rata with stool weight. Studies of fecal flora have also been disappointing in the main, pointing up the stability of the flora in an individual and the methodological difficulties of this field.[54,65] In any event, examination of stools tells us little or nothing about events in the right colon.

4.2.2. Colonic Transit Time

Most studies report whole-gut transit time but all but 5 or 6 hr of this consists of colonic transit time and there is little scope for changes in gastric and small bowel transit. Therefore, changes in whole-gut transit time are practically synonymous with changes in colonic transit time.

Transit time is related inversely in a curvilinear fashion to fecal output, the shape of the curve being such that there are substantial changes in transit time with changes in the lower range of fecal weights as found in most normal Westerners.[66–69] Beyond a fecal

Table IV. Stool Form Scale Used in Bristol
to Assess Intestinal Transit Time

Type 1—Separate hard lumps, like nuts
Type 2—Sausage shaped but lumpy
Type 3—Like a sausage or snake but with cracks on its
surface
Type 4—Like a sausage or snake, smooth and soft
Type 5—Soft blobs with clear-cut edges
Type 6—Fluffy pieces with ragged edges, a mushy stool
Type 7—Watery, no solid pieces

weight of 160–200 g/day, transit time is nearly always less than 2 days[69] and it does not consistently shorten as fecal output increases further.

When transit time is initially slow, addition of bran to the diet almost invariably speeds it up.[70,71] The effect is distinctly less with finely particulate bran than with coarse bran.[72–74] The greater efficacy of coarse bran could be due to greater water-holding capacity,[54] to more mechanical stimulation of the colon, or to reduced fermentability. Acceleration in transit is not always associated with more frequent bowel motions.[71,75–77]

Some workers have noted that initially fast transit is slowed down to about 48 hr when bran is added to the diet, suggesting a normalizing effect on colonic function.[70,71] For many physicians this has provided the rationale for treating IBS with bran. Skeptics doubt the reality of the finding and it must be admitted that the studies cited lacked a placebo control.

In the outpatient clinic or office it is not feasible for the physician to measure transit time in every patient with bowel dysfunction. But the patient's symptoms can be misleading. The patient may complain of frequent defecations and urgency yet, on close inquiry, the stools are of normal or even hard consistency. This pseudodiarrhea or tachychezia can be easily distinguished from true diarrhea by the use of a stool form scale (Table IV). Stool type on this 1 to 7 scale correlates well with mean transit time whereas stool frequency does not correlate at all.[78] Patients with IBS seem to be quite reliable at recording their stool type when asked to do so by the physician in the clinic. Whether they can reliably report their usual stool form without keeping a record remains to be seen.

4.2.3. Intraluminal Pressures

In several studies, mainly from Edinburgh, administration of wheat bran of the coarse variety has been shown to lower the rectosigmoid pressures of patients with symptomatic diverticular disease.[62,67,72,79–81] The same effect has been reported in IBS.[80,82] Methyl cellulose has also been reported to lower intracolonic pressure in diverticular disease.[83] Paradoxically, an ispaghula preparation was found to raise intracolonic pressure at the same time as it increased fecal weight and relieved symptoms[62]—an odd finding that needs to be confirmed as it makes no sense.

In a controlled double-blind study, psyllium hydrocolloid (which is the same as ispaghula) failed to lower sigmoid pressures any more than placebo in patients with diverticular disease.[84] In a similar study in IBS patients there was no difference in rectosigmoid pressures after 6 weeks on placebo and after 6 weeks on a dose of bran which raised stool weight substantially.[77] This raises the awkward question whether the reduced pressures noted in earlier uncontrolled studies were all placebo effects—an idea which is in line with the well-known fact that sigmoid motility increases under stress[85] and with the fact that the colon is less reactive when the subject is familiarized with the laboratory.[86] On the other hand, careful studies in monkeys with graded fiber intakes from 0 to 20 g daily showed that intrasigmoid pressures decreased as the fiber intake increased.[87] This is what one would expect from Laplace's law, which states that the tension in the walls of a tube is proportional to the pressure exerted multiplied by the radius; assuming that the tension in the walls of the colon does not change, an increased radius due to bulkier stools should entail fall in pressure.[88] But the colon is not a simple tube.

If bran and other fiber sources affect colonic motility, it is not necessarily through their bulking effect. The products of bacterial fermentation and metabolism might have spasmogenic or antispasmodic effects and physiologically active substances in the lumen might be adsorbed or bound by fibrous residues. For example, deoxycholic acid can stimulate colonic motility[89]; it is also bound hydrophobically by dietary fiber[90] and its formation from cholic acid and/or its absorption are reduced by bran.[91]

4.3. Effects of Bran and Ispaghula on Symptoms of Irritable Bowel

Since the early 1970s wheat bran has probably been the most widely prescribed treatment for IBS but, in Britain at least, its use is now waning. Ispaghula or psyllium hydrocolloid has always been popular and continues to be so. It is interesting to consider the reasons for the rise and fall of bran and the continued success of ispaghula.

Enthusiasm for bran came as part of the wave of interest in dietary fiber. Its use in IBS seemed logical for several reasons: (1) IBS was becoming recognized as a condition in which pain can be associated with a rise in intraluminal pressures and reports were published that bran lowers such pressures; (2) IBS was postulated to be one of the diseases of Western civilization[92]; (3) bran was reported to normalize colonic transit whether it was fast or slow[70] and IBS is characterized by alternating diarrhea and constipation; (4) the therapeutic value of ispaghula preparations was generally accepted and, in a wheat-eating population, bran seemed a more natural way of providing undigestible material to bulk the stools.

At that time the size of the placebo response in IBS was poorly appreciated and the role of psychological factors in the genesis of IBS had not been explored scientifically. The favorable results of uncontrolled trials of bran in IBS[93] and symptomatic diverticular disease[94] were accepted uncritically. When a controlled trial was published concluding that bran was no better than placebo,[95] it was criticized as using an inactive form of bran and, within a few months, it was contradicted by a controlled trial which reported reduced pain frequency and severity, improved bowel habit, and reduced passage of mucus on a bran-rich diet compared with a diet avoiding whole-grain products; there was also a fall in fasting sigmoid motility on the bran-rich diet.[82] Several years passed before any more controlled trials were published. However, since 1984 four such trials have been published and all four have failed to demonstrate any superiority of bran over placebo[77,96–98] (Table V).

Table V. Controlled Trials of Wheat Bran in Irritable Bowel Syndrome: Synopsis of All Six Studies Which Have Been Published in Full[a]

Authors (city)	Design of study and No. of subjects	Type and dose of bran	Nature of placebo	Assessments	Findings
Søltoft et al.[95] (Hellerup)	Randomized: 32 to bran, 27 to placebo, for 6 weeks	Fine bran baked into biscuits 10 g × 3 daily	Wheat biscuits	Diary records of pain, distention, borborygmi, stools, laxative use	No difference in overall assessment, days with pain or bloating, number or consistency of stools, laxative use
Manning et al.[82] (Bristol)	Randomized: 14 to bran, 12 to placebo for 6 weeks	Fine bran 20 g or four slices wholemeal bread daily	Diet sheet avoiding whole-grain products	Diary records of pains, stools. Questionnaire on pain, bowels, mucus. Sigmoid motility	Frequency and severity of pain reduced (but not constantly) on bran. Bowel habit improved. Mucus and fasting motility reduced
Cann et al.[96] (Sheffield)	Crossover. Bran first openly 4 weeks, then placebo (as part of drug trial) 5 weeks; 28 patients	Coarse bran 9–38 g daily (median 20) increasing as desired	Tablets	Diary records of pain, distention, urgency, stools, flatus, borborygmi. Stool weight, transit time	Of all symptoms, only constipation improved with bran more than placebo. Bran responders tended to start constipated. Pain and diarrhea worse with bran
Arffmann et al.[77] (Copenhagen)	Double-blind, crossover, 18 patients, 6 weeks	Coarse bran 30 g daily	Bread crumbs of similar appearance	Diary records of pain, distention, rumbling, stools. Stool weight, transit time, rectosigmoid motility	No difference in symptoms or motility indices. Stools heavier and transit faster on bran
Kruis et al.[97] (Munich)	Randomized: 40 to bran, 40 to placebo, 40 to mebeverine	"53% cellulose fibers" 15 g daily	Tablets	Monthly report on change in pain, distension, bowel irregularity	Bran overall superior to placebo and mebeverine at 8 and 12 weeks but not at 16 weeks
Lucey et al.[98] (London)	Double-blind, crossover. 28 patients 12 weeks	Bran biscuits 12 daily (12.8 g dietary fiber)	Low-fiber biscuits	Monthly questionnaire on pain, straining, incomplete evacuation, bloating, flatus, stools. Stool weight	No overall difference in pain, bowel symptoms, or stool weight. Bowel score worsened in 14 going from bran to placebo

[a]Of the controlled trials published only in abstract form, most show no advantage of bran over placebo.

A high-fiber diet is a more natural way to increase fiber intake than raw bran and the one controlled trial that found bran to be useful supplied it largely in the form of whole-meal bread.[82] However, a trial of a high-fiber diet versus "routine instruction and treatment" found no overall benefit, though colicky pain was reduced.[99] Two gastroenterologists who routinely prescribe a high-fiber diet reevaluated a large number of their patients several years later and found the great majority to be improved.[100,101] However, a third gastroenterologist did not find this[102] and, in a prospective assessment of 14 patients who had been carefully instructed in a high-fiber diet 2 years previously, there was no change in their symptom score.[103] Thus, the value of bran or a high-fiber diet remains unproven.

This conclusion is disappointing but not unexpected in the light of recent advances in understanding the psychological aspects of IBS.[104] Even in normal subjects psychological factors account for as much variance in stool weight as dietary fiber intake[64] and the same must be true of other aspects of colonic function.

Some patients with IBS have slow transit and a low stool output and it is still appropriate to treat them with bran or a high-fiber diet and the Sheffield trial suggests they are likely to benefit.[96] The symptoms of IBS can be produced in healthy volunteers by inducing constipation pharmacologically[105] and it is reasonable to suppose that they can also be produced by diet-induced constipation. Indeed, in the author's experience, women sometimes develop IBS when they go on a slimming diet and become constipated. It must, of course, be conceded that constipation can have nondietary causes, including psychological ones, and some constipated IBS sufferers can be expected not to respond to bran, especially those in whom the primary problem is in anorectal function.

The continued use of ispaghula in IBS is justified by the results of placebo-controlled trials. Three such trials have shown ispaghula to have the advantage over placebo.[106-108] One trial has found no significant difference[109] but in this study no less than 71% of patients felt better on placebo (77% on psyllium). In a dose–response study using 10, 20, or 30 g of ispaghula daily the fall in symptom score correlated with the rise in stool weight,[60] which raises the possibility that bran might be more effective if given in larger than usual doses. However, compliance is likely to be a problem especially in those patients whose symptoms worsen initially on bran.

The published results of treating symptomatic diverticular disease with bran and ispaghula are similar to the results with IBS[110] and will not be considered further.

5. OTHER DIETARY FACTORS

Food poisoning is beyond the scope of this chapter but some consideration must be given to food allergy and intolerance. In the mind of the general public they are a common and important problem.

5.1. Food Allergy and Intolerance

True food allergy, that is, an abnormal immunological reaction to food, is indeed an important problem but it is a rare one.[111-113] Proof of the diagnosis requires a positive skin-test reaction to the food or a positive radioallergosorbent test for IgE antibodies.[114]

Table VI. Conditions and Syndromes
That Are Confirmed as Sometimes Being
Caused by IgE-Mediated Food Allergy[a]

Acute, generalized
Angioedema, anaphylaxis
Gastrointestinal
Lip, mouth, and throat tingling, itching, swelling
Epigastric pain, vomiting
Abdominal pain, bloating, diarrhea
Malabsorption
Respiratory
Sneezing, rhinorrhea, nasal stuffiness
Asthma
Skin
Urticaria
(Eczema; pathophysiology uncertain)

[a] After Pearson.[115]

Manifestations of confirmed food allergy (Table VI), include a number of gastrointestinal symptoms—epigastric pain, vomiting, abdominal pain, bloating, diarrhea, and malabsorption. The pattern of response depends on the level of IgE-sensitization of the different organ systems and on the dose of food ingested.[115] Different foods can give different patterns of response in the same patient. Symptoms tend to multiply as larger amounts of food are eaten. With low levels of sensitivity or small amounts of the provocative food, reactions are usually confined to the gastrointestinal tract. Established examples of "pure" intestinal food allergy include celiac disease (gluten enteropathy) and cow's milk protein-induced colitis in children.

These facts and the great commonness of unexplained gastrointestinal symptoms in the general population provide the foundations for the myth that food allergy is a common cause of gastrointestinal symptoms. The patients who believe this or worry about it are invariably adults. But the facts are that, though food allergy is quite common in infancy, it becomes increasingly uncommon with advancing age. IgE-mediated hypersensitivity to food developing for the first time after childhood has never been demonstrated.[115] The range of foods which are known to cause it is very limited (particularly milk, eggs, fish, and legume seeds including soya and peanuts).

There are many other causes for adverse reactions to food besides true allergy (Table VII) and the commonest reason for failing to tolerate a specific food is psychological.[115] True organic food intolerance other than allergy does occur but it can be proved to exist only by double-blind feeding tests. These are tedious and impractical in day-to-day clinical practice but they are essential in any scientific investigation of the role of food intolerance.

Unfortunately, there are few published reports in which double-blind feeding tests have been used in adult patients with IBS (and even fewer in functional or nonulcer dyspepsia). Hunter and his colleagues[30] reported that 14 out of 21 IBS patients lost their symptoms after 1 week on a diet of a single meat, a single fruit, and distilled or spring

Table VII. Adverse Reactions to Food—
An Etiological Classification[a]

Usual or expected
  Toxins, pharmacologically active agents, etc.
Unusual—intolerance of usually nontoxic substances
  Organic (true food intolerance)
    Allergic (immunologic)
      IgE mediated
      ? nonreaginic (unproven)
    Idiosyncratic (nonimmunologic)
      Metabolic, e.g., alactasia
      Pharmacologic, e.g., salicylic acid sensitivity
      Autonomic, e.g., sulfur dixoide effects
    Idiopathic
  Psychogenic
    Food aversion (distaste, phobias)
    Pseudo-food allergy syndrome
    Munchausen's syndrome

---

[a]After Pearson.[115]

water and that, when foods were introduced one by one, all 14 patients could identify foods that reproduced their symptoms. Six of the fourteen were subjected to blind testing. They could distinguish a provocative food from a control food in 21 out of 24 blind testings when it was given via a nasogastric tube. However, Bentley et al.[116] found only 3 patients out of a group of 27 in whom blind provocation tests established a food item as causing their IBS symptoms. In 2 of the 3 patients the item concerned was milk and the patients already knew that milk upset them (though they were not lactose intolerant). Similarly, Farah et al.[117] considered 49 IBS patients as possible cases of food intolerance. After 2 weeks on a "hypoallergic" diet, 13 had remission of their symptoms, of whom 8 identified a reintroduced food as provoking their symptoms. However, only 3 of them reacted to this food more than to placebo when both were fed as capsules for a week and then stayed well when the food was excluded (the offending items being eggs, peas, and coffee). In a third study, McKee et al.[118] treated 40 consecutive IBS patients with lamb, pears, and spring water for 1 week. Six patients (15%) had a marked reduction in two or more symptoms and could then identify a provocative food (eggs, milk, potatoes, or wheat) on open challenge but no blind testing was done. All 6 had diarrhea at least part of the time on their original diet.

It does appear therefore that a tiny minority of IBS patients, perhaps 5–10%, have an important element of food intolerance and that for the physician this is worth considering when diarrhea is a prominent symptom. But in practice there are problems. Exclusion diets are demanding and time-consuming for patient, dietitian, and physician; a non-specific placebo response is likely to occur in a large proportion; in some patients the results are inconclusive or confusing; and, in faddy or hypochondriacal patients, there is a risk that they will end up avoiding so many foods that they become socially crippled and possibly even nutritionally depleted. In the author's opinion, elimination diets should be reserved for the occasional, intelligent, well-motivated patient, and then only if physician and dietitian can work in close liaison and are prepared to see the patient at frequent intervals.

The dietary items which are most commonly blamed for causing IBS symptoms are wheat, corn (maize), dairy products, coffee, tea, and citrus fruits. However, many other items have been blamed, including tap water, and patients often have multiple intolerances.

Pseudo-Food Allergy

Pseudo-food allergy has been well described by Pearson.[115] Out of 24 women with this condition (it is rare in men), 9 had irritable bowel symptoms, the others having chronic hyperventilation syndrome or somatic features of depression. Women with pseudo-food allergy tended to be 35–45 years old, middle-class, articulate, and under-employed for their level of intelligence. All were polysymptomatic but were adamant that their symptoms were not "psychological," claiming rather that food was responsible for panic attacks, agarophobia, irritability, mood swings, uncontrolled weeping, and even suicidal thoughts. On formal analysis these patients suffer from the same spectrum of psychiatric disorder as unselected new referrals to a psychiatric outpatient department.

There can of course be overlap between organic and psychosomatic disease so that one reinforces the other. Just as an asthmatic who is genuinely allergic to roses can develop bronchospasm upon seeing artificial roses, so patients with organic food intolerance may "overreact" to foods to which they have a genuine physical reaction.

A major problem with the scientific acceptance of organic food-intolerant gastrointestinal symptoms is the unavailability of a simple test for altered gastrointestinal function comparable with the peak flow meter in asthma. However, this should not be used as an excuse for total rejection of the idea. There are sufficient data from double-blind food tests to prove that these reactions do occur, albeit rarely. A second problem is the lack of a proven mechanism for these reactions but this may simply reflect the neural and hormonal complexity of the gastrointestinal tract, its relative inaccessibility for investigation, and the failure of major gastrointestinal research centers to address this problem.

5.2. Protein and Fat

There are few good scientific studies of the physiological effects on the gut of protein and fat at different levels of intake or in different forms. The usual assumption is that fat and protein are fully digested and absorbed in the small intestine but this is not necessarily the case. Solid food must be broken down into small particles before digestive enzymes can work to maximum effect. If lumps of food are swallowed without chewing, recognizable remnants can be recovered from the feces. This applies to 1-g lumps of cooked pork, bacon, beef, and lamb as well as to boiled potatoes, carrots, and, especially, peas.[119] Similarly, clinical steatorrhea can be produced by eating peanuts in large quantities.[120] Whether this unabsorbed protein and fat causes symptoms is unknown. In healthy people a high intake of meat protein (136 g/day) and a high intake of animal fat (152 g/day) make no difference in fecal weight, intestinal transit time, or bowel frequency.[121,122] On the other hand, unabsorbed fat reaching the ileum may result in slowing of gastric emptying and feelings of epigastric fullness—the so-called ileal brake effect.[123]

6. CONCLUSIONS

The effect of diet on the intestine is a poorly researched area with the partial exception of dietary fiber. Understanding is hindered by the many variables in food and food preparation as well as in the intestinal response to food. Nevertheless, this is an important subject and a rewarding area for research. Patients with functional gut symptoms expect dietary advice and in some it is crucial. The role of wheat bran in IBS must be questioned but that of ispaghula (psyllium) seems more secure. Food intolerance of the nonallergic kind is occasionally the cause of IBS but double-blind challenges are essential to prove it. Hypolactasia rarely causes IBS, at least in people of northern European origin.

REFERENCES

1. Holdstock DJ, Misiewicz G: Factors controlling colonic motility: Colonic pressures and transit time after meals in patients with total gastrectomy, pernicious anaemia or duodenal ulcer. Gut 11:100–110, 1970
2. Snape WJ, Wright SH, Battle WM, et al: The gastrocolic response: Evidence for a neural mechanism. Gastroenterology 77:1235–1240, 1979
3. Snape WJ, Matarazzo SA, Cohen S: Effect of eating and gastrointestinal hormones on human colonic myoelectrical and motor activity. Gastroenterology 75:373–378, 1978
4. Harvey RF, Read AE: Effects of oral magnesium sulphate on colonic motility in patients with the irritable bowel syndrome. Gut 14:983–987, 1973
5. Wright SH, Snape WJ, Battle W, et al: Effect of dietary components on gastrocolonic response. Am J Physiol 238:G228–232, 1980
6. Kerlin P, Zinsmeister A, Phillips S: Motor responses to food of the ileum, proximal colon and distal colon of healthy humans. Gastroenterology 84:762–770, 1983
7. Meyer F, Le Quintrec Y: Rapport entre fibres alimentaires et constipation. Nouv Presse Med 10:2479–2481, 1981
8. Moriarty KJ, Dawson AM: Functional abdominal pain: Further evidence that whole gut is affected. Br Med J 284:1670–1672, 1982
9. Kingham JGC, Dawson AM: Origin of chronic right upper quadrant pain. Gut 26:783–788, 1985
10. Kellow JE, Phillips SF: Altered small bowel motility in irritable bowel syndrome is correlated with symptoms. Gastroenterology 92:1885–1893, 1987
11. Kellow JE, Zinsmeister AR, Phillips SF: Ileal dysmotility and abdominal symptoms provoked by stimuli in irritable bowel syndrome. Gastroenterology 90:1489, 1986
12. Glinsmann WH, Irausquin H, Park YK: Evaluation of health aspects of sugars contained in carbohydrate sweeteners. Report from FDA's Sugars Task Force. J Nutr 116(suppl 11S):S1–216, 1986
13. BNF Task Force on Sugars and Syrups: Sugars and Syrups. London, British Nutrition Foundation, 1987
14. Oettlé GJ, Emmett PM, Heaton KW: Glucose and insulin responses to manufactured and whole-food snacks. Am J Clin Nutr 45:86–91, 1987
15. Kruis W, Forstmaier G, Sheurlen C, et al: Influence of diets high and low in refined sugar on stool qualities, gastrointestinal transit time and fecal bile acid excretion. Gastroenterology 92:1483, 1987 (abstr)
16. Heaton KW: Dietary sugar and Crohn's disease. Can J Gastroenterol 2:41–44, 1988
17. Bond JH, Currier BE, Buchwald H, et al: Colonic conservation of malabsorbed carbohydrate. Gastroenterology 78:444–447, 1980
18. McMichael HB, Webb J, Dawson AM: Lactase deficiency in adults: Cause of "functional" diarrhoea. Lancet 1:717–720, 1965
19. Weser EW, Rubin W, Ross L, et al: Lactase deficiency in patients with the "irritable-colon syndrome." N Engl J Med 273:1070–1075, 1965
20. Gudmand-Hoyer E, Riis P, Wulff HR: The significance of lactose malabsorption in the irritable colon syndrome. Scand J Gastroenterol 8:273–278, 1973
21. Eastwood MA, Walton BA, Brydon WG, et al: Faecal weight, constituents, colonic motility, and lactose tolerance in the irritable bowel syndrome. Digestion 30:7–12, 1984

22. Newcomer AD, McGill DB: Irritable bowel syndrome. Role of lactase deficiency. Mayo Clin Proc 58:339–341, 1983

23. Sciarretta G, Giacobazzi G, Verri A, et al: Hydrogen breath test quantification and clinical correlation of lactose malabsorption in adult irritable bowel syndrome and ulcerative colitis. Dig Dis Sci 29:1098–1104, 1984

24. Dawson AM: Discussion statement, in Read NW (ed): Irritable Bowel Syndrome. New York, Grune & Stratton, 1985, p 50

25. Hunt TC: Intestinal carbohydrate dyspepsia, in Hunter D (ed): Price's Textbook of the Practice of Medicine, ed 9. London, Oxford University Press, 1956, pp 629–631

26. Anderson IH, Levine AS, Levitt MD: Incomplete absorption of the carbohydrate in all-purpose wheat flour. N Engl J Med 304:891–892, 1981

27. Stephen AM, Haddad AC, Phillips SF: Passage of carbohydrate into the colon. Direct measurements in humans. Gastroenterology 85:589–595, 1983

28. Thornton JR, Dryden A, Kelleher J, et al: Super-efficient starch absorption. A risk factor for colonic neoplasia? Dig Dis Sci 32:1088–1091, 1987

29. Chapman RW, Sillery JK, Graham MM, et al: Absorption of starch by healthy ileostomates: Effect of transit time and of carbohydrate load. Am J Clin Nutr 41:1244–1248, 1985

30. Jones VA, McLaughlan P, Shorthouse M, et al: Food intolerance: A major factor in the pathogenesis of irritable bowel syndrome. Lancet 2:1115–1117, 1982

31. Flourié B, Florent C, Etanchaud F, et al: Starch absorption by healthy man evaluated by lactulose hydrogen breath test. Am J Clin Nutr 47:61–66, 1988

32. Shetty PS, Kurpad AV: Increased starch intake in the human diet increases fecal bulking. Am J Clin Nutr 43:210–212, 1986

33. Flourié B, Florent C, Jouany J-P, et al: Colonic metabolism of wheat starch in healthy humans. Effects on fecal outputs and clinical symptoms. Gastroenterology 90:111–119, 1986

34. Englyst HN, Cummings JH: Digestion of polysaccharides of potato in the small intestine of man. Am J Clin Nutr 45:423–431, 1987

35. Heaton KW, Marcus SN, Emmett PM, et al: Particle size of wheat, maize and oats test meals: Effects on plasma glucose and insulin responses and on the rate of starch digestion in vitro. Am J Clin Nutr 47:675–682, 1988

35a. O'Donnell LJD, Emmett PM, Heaton KW: Size of flour particles and its relation to glycaemia, insulinaemia and colonic disease. Br Med J (in press)

36. Macrae TF, Hutchinson JCD, Irwin JO, et al: Comparative digestibility of wholemeal and white breads and the effect of the degree of fineness of grinding on the former. J Hyg 42:423–435, 1942

37. Wisker E, Krumm U, Feldheim W: Einfluss der Partikelgrösse von Getreideprodukten auf das Stuhlgewicht von jungen Frauen. Akt Ernährungsmed 11:208–211, 1986

38. Thompson, WG, Patel DG, Tao H, et al: Does uncomplicated diverticular disease cause symptoms? Dig Dis Sci 27:605–608, 1982

39. Thornton JR, Dryden A, Kelleher J, et al: Does superefficient starch absorption promote diverticular disease? Br Med J 292:1708–1710, 1986

40. Asp N-G: Definition and analysis of dietary fibre. Scand J Gastroenterol 22(suppl 129):16–20, 1987

41. Eastwood MA: What does the measurement of dietary fibre mean? Lancet 1:1487–1488, 1986

42. Trowell H, Burkitt D, Heaton K: Dietary Fibre, Fibre-depleted Foods and Disease. New York, Academic Press, 1985

43. Vahouny GV, Kritchevsky D (eds): Dietary Fiber: Basic and Clinical Aspects. New York, Plenum Press, 1986

44. Spiller GA (ed): CRC Handbook of Dietary Fiber in Human Nutrition. Boca Raton, CRC Press, 1986

45. Pilch SM (ed): Physiological Effects and Health Consequences of Dietary Fiber. A Report Prepared for Center for Food Safety and Applied Nutrition, Food and Drug Administration, Dept. of Health and Human Services, Washington, DC. Bethesda, Life Sciences Research Office, FASEB, 1987

46. Holmgren L (ed): Symposium on dietary fibre with clinical aspects, Helsingør, Denmark, 11–13 June 1986. Scand J Gastroenterol 22(suppl 129):1–295, 1987

47. Trowell HC: Crude fibre, dietary fibre and atherosclerosis. Atherosclerosis 16:138–140, 1972

48. Andersen JR, Bukhave K, Højgaard L, et al: Decomposition of wheat bran and ispaghula husk in the stomach and small intestine of healthy men. J Nutr 118:326–331, 1988

49. Tomlin J, Read NW: The effect of inert plastic particles on colonic function in human volunteers. Gastroenterology 94:A463, 1988

50. Stephen AM, Wiggins HS, Cummings JH: Effect of changing transit time on colonic microbial metabolism in man. Gut 28:601–609, 1987

51. Marcus SN, Heaton KW: Intestinal transit, deoxycholic acid and the cholesterol saturation of bile—Three inter-related factors. Gut 27:550–558, 1986

52. Stephen AM, Cummings JH: Mechanism of action of dietary fibre in the human colon. Nature 284:283–284, 1980

53. Stephen AM, Cummings JH: Water-holding by dietary fibre in vitro and its relationship to faecal output in man. Gut 20:722–729, 1979

54. Eastwood MA, Brydon WG: Physiological effects of dietary fibre on the alimentary tract, in Trowell H, Burkitt D, Heaton K (eds): Dietary Fibre, Fibre-depleted Foods and Disease. New York, Academic Press, 1985, pp 105–131

55. Stephen AM, Wiggins HS, Englyst HN, et al: The effect of age, sex and level of intake of dietary fibre from wheat on large-bowel function in thirty healthy subjects. Br J Nutr 56:349–361, 1986

56. Spiller GA, Story JA, Wong LG, et al: Effect of increasing levels of hard wheat fiber on fecal weight, minerals and steroids and gastrointestinal transit time in healthy young women. J Nutr 116:778–785, 1986

57. Jenkins DJA, Peterson RD, Thorne MJ, et al: Wheat fiber and laxation: Dose response and equilibration time. Am J Gastroenterol 82:1259–1263, 1987

58. Cummings JH: The effect of dietary fiber on fecal weight and composition, in Spiller GA (ed): CRC Handbook of Dietary Fiber in Human Nutrition. Boca Raton, CRC Press, 1986, pp 211–280

59. Müller-Lissner SA: Effect of wheat bran on weight of stool and gastrointestinal transit time: A meta analysis. Br Med J 296:615–617, 1988

60. Kumar A, Kumar N, Vij JC, et al: Optimum dosage of ispaghula husk in patients with irritable bowel syndrome: Correlation of symptom relief with whole gut transit time and stool weight. Gut 28:150–155, 1987

61. Stevens J, Van Soest PJ, Robertson JB, et al: Comparison of the effects of psyllium and wheat bran on gastrointestinal transit time and stool characteristics. J Am Diet Assoc 88:323–326, 1988

62. Eastwood MA, Smith AN, Brydon WG, et al: Comparison of bran, ispaghula and lactulose on colon function in diverticular disease. Gut 19:1144–1147, 1978

63. Smith RG, Rowe MJ, Smith AN, et al: A study of bulking agents in elderly people. Age Ageing 9:267–271, 1980

64. Tucker DM, Sandstead HH, Logan GM, et al: Dietary fiber and personality factors as determinants of stool output. Gastroenterology 81:879–883, 1981

65. Woods MN, Gorbach SL: Influences of fiber on the ecology of the intestinal flora, in Spiller GA (ed): CRC Handbook of Dietary Fiber in Human Nutrition. Boca Raton, CRC Press, 1986, pp 289–291

66. Burkitt DP, Walker ARP, Painter NS: Effect of dietary fibre on stools and transit-times, and its role in the causation of disease. Lancet 2:1408–1412, 1972

67. Findlay JM, Smith AN, Mitchell WD, et al: Effects of unprocessed bran on colon function in normal subjects and in diverticular disease. Lancet 1:146–149, 1974

68. Stasse-Wolthuis M, Katan MB, Hautvast JGAJ: Fecal weight, transit time, and recommendations for dietary fiber intake. Am J Clin Nutr 32:909–910, 1979

69. Spiller GA: Suggestions for a basis on which to determine a desirable intake of dietary fiber in Spiller GA (ed): CRC Handbook of Dietary Fiber in Human Nutrition. Boca Raton, CRC Press, 1986, pp 281–283

70. Harvey RF, Pomare EW, Heaton KW: Effects of increased dietary fibre on intestinal transit. Lancet 1:1278–1280, 1973

71. Payler DK, Pomare EW, Heaton KW, et al: The effect of wheat bran on intestinal transit. Gut 16:209–213, 1975

72. Smith AN, Drummond E, Eastwood MA: The effect of coarse and fine Canadian Red Spring Wheat and French Soft Wheat bran on colonic motility in patients with diverticular disease. Am J Clin Nutr 34:2460–2463, 1981

73. van Dokkum W, Pikaar NA, Thissen JTNM: Physiological effects of fibre-rich types of bread. 2. Dietary fibre from bread: Digestion by the intestinal microflora and water-holding capacity in the colon of human subject. Br J Nutr 50:61–74, 1983

74. Wrick KL, Robertson JB, van Soest PJ, et al: The influence of dietary fiber on human intestinal transit and stool output. J Nutr 113:1464–1479, 1983

75. Wyman JB, Heaton KW, Manning AP, et al: The effect on intestinal transit and the feces of raw and cooked bran in different doses. Am J Clin Nutr 29:1474–1479, 1976

76. Heller SN, Hackler LR, Rivers JM, et al: Dietary fiber: The effect of particle size of wheat bran on colonic function in young adult men. Am J Clin Nutr 33:1734–1744, 1980

77. Arffmann S, Andersen JR, Henghoj J, et al: The effect of coarse wheat bran in the irritable bowel syndrome. A double-blind cross-over study. Scand J Gastroenterol 20:295–298, 1985

78. O'Donnell LJD, Heaton KW: Pseudo-diarrhoea in the irritable bowel syndrome: Patients' records of stool form reflect transit time while stool frequency does not. Gut 29:A1455 (abstr)

79. Kirwan WO, Smith AN, McConnell AA, et al: Action of different bran preparations on colonic function. Br Med J 4:187–189, 1974

80. Kirwan WO, Smith A: Colonic propulsion in diverticular disease, idiopathic constipation, and the irritable colon syndrome. Scand J Gastroenterol 12:331–336, 1977

81. Brodribb AJM, Humphreys DM: Diverticular disease: Three studies. Br Med J 1:424–430, 1976

82. Manning AP, Heaton KW, Harvey RF, et al: Wheat fibre and irritable bowel syndrome. A controlled trial. Lancet 2:417–418, 1977

83. Hodgson J: Effect of methylcellulose on rectal and colonic pressures in treatment of diverticular disease. Br Med J 3:729–731, 1972

84. Howell DA, Crow HC, Almy TP, et al: A controlled double-blind study of sigmoid motility using psyllium mucilloid in diverticular disease. Gastroenterology 74:1046, 1978 (abstr)

85. Almy TP, Kern F, Tulin M: Alterations in colonic function in man under stress. II Experimental production of sigmoid spasm in healthy persons. Gastroenterology 12:425–436, 1949

86. Narducci T, Snape WJ, Battle WM, et al: Increased colonic motility during exposure to a stressful situation. Dig Dis Sci 30:40–44, 1985

87. Brodribb J, Condon RE, Cowles V et al: Influence of dietary fiber on transit time, fecal composition, and myoelectrical activity of the primate right colon. Dig Dis Sci 25:260–266, 1980

88. Almy TP: Diverticular disease of the colon—The new look. Gastroenterology 49:109–112, 1965

89. Kirwan WO, Smith AN, Mitchell WD, et al: Bile acids and colonic motility in the rabbit and the human. Gut 16:894–902, 1975

90. Eastwood MA, Hamilton D: Studies on the adsorption of bile salts to nonabsorbed components of diet. Biochim Biophys Acta 152:165–173, 1968

91. Pomare EW, Heaton KW: Alteration of bile salt metabolism by dietary fibre (bran). Br Med J 4:262–264, 1973

92. Painter NS: Irritable or irritated bowel. Br Med J 2:46, 1972

93. Piepmeyer JL: Use of unprocessed bran in treatment of irritable bowel syndrome. Am J Clin Nutr 27:106–107, 1974

94. Painter NS, Almeida AZ, Colebourne KW: Unprocessed bran in treatment of diverticular disease of the colon. Br Med J 2:137–140, 1972

95. Søltoft J, Gudmand-Høyer E, Krag B, et al: A double-blind trial of the effect of wheat bran on symptoms of irritable bowel syndrome. Lancet 1:270–272, 1976

96. Cann PA, Read NW, Holdsworth CD: What is the benefit of coarse wheat bran in patients with the irritable bowel syndrome? Gut 25:168–173, 1984

97. Kruis, W, Weinsierl M, Schüssler P, et al: Comparison of the therapeutic effect of wheat bran, mebeverine and placebo in patients with the irritable bowel syndrome. Digestion 34:196–201, 1986

98. Lucey MR, Clark ML, Lowndes J, et al: Is bran efficacious in irritable bowel syndrome? A double blind placebo controlled crossover study. Gut 28:221–225, 1987

99. Rasmussen SN, Bondesen S, Edmund C, et al: Behandling af colon irritabile med kostfiberrig diaet. En kontrolleret klinisk undersøgelse. Ugeskr Laeg 144:2415–2417, 1982

100. Sullivan SN: Management of the irritable bowel syndrome: A personal view. J Clin Gastroenterol 5:499–502, 1983

101. Harvey RF, Mauad EC, Brown AM: Prognosis in the irritable bowel syndrome: A 5-year prospective study. Lancet 1:963–965, 1987

102. Nyhlin H, Eastwood MA: Comparison of various treatments for irritable bowel syndrome. Br Med J 282:74–75, 1981

103. Hillman LC, Stace NH, Pomare EW: Irritable bowel patients and their long-term response to a high fiber diet. Am J Gastroenterol 79:1–7, 1984

104. Creed F, Guthrie E: Psychological factors in the irritable bowel. Gut 28:1307–1318, 1987

105. Marcus SN, Heaton KW: Irritable bowel type symptoms in spontaneous and induced constipation. Gut 28: 156–159, 1987

106. Ritchie JA, Truelove SC: Treatment of irritable bowel syndrome with lorazepam, hyoscine butylbromide, and ispaghula husk. Br Med J 1:376–378, 1979

107. Ritchie JA, Truelove SC: Comparison of various treatments for irritable bowel syndrome. Br Med J 281:1317–1319, 1980

108. Prior A, Whorwell PJ: Double blind study of ispaghula in irritable bowel syndrome. Gut 28:1510–1513, 1987

109. Longstreth GF, Fox DD, Youkeles L, et al: Psyllium therapy in the irritable bowel syndrome. Ann Intern Med 95:53–56, 1981

110. Heaton KW: Role of dietary fibre in irritable bowel syndrome, in Read NW (ed): Irritable Bowel Syndrome. New York, Academic Press, 1985, pp 203–218

111. Lessof MH (ed): Clinical Reactions to Food. New York, Wiley, 1983

112. Brostoff J, Challacombe SJ (eds): Food Allergy and Intolerance. London, Ballière Tindall, 1987

113. Joint Committee of the Royal College of Physicians and the British Nutrition Foundation: Food intolerance and food aversion. J R Coll Physicians London 18:83–123, 1984

114. Lessof MH: Clinical reactions to food. Br J Hosp Med, February 1988, pp 138–142

115. Pearson DJ: Food allergy, hypersensitivity and intolerance. J R Coll Physicians London 19:154–162, 1985

116. Bentley SJ, Pearson DJ, Rix KJB: Food hypersensitivity in irritable bowel syndrome. Lancet 2:295–297, 1983

117. Farah DA, Calder I, Benson L, et al: Specific food intolerance: Its place as a cause of gastrointestinal symptoms. Gut 26:164–168, 1985

118. McKee AM, Prior A, Whorwell PJ: Exclusion diets in irritable bowel syndrome: Are they worthwhile? J Clin Gastroenterol 9:526–528, 1987

119. Farrell JH: The effect of mastication on the digestion of food. Br Dent J 100:149–155, 1956

120. Levine AS, Silvis SE: Absorption of whole peanuts, peanut oil, and peanut butter. N Engl J Med 303:917–918, 1980

121. Cummings JH, Wiggins HS, Jenkins DJA et al: The influence of diets high and low in animal fat on bowel habit, gastrointestinal transit time, faecal microflora, bile acid and fat excretion. J Clin Invest 61:953–963, 1978

122. Cummings JH, Hill MJ, Jivray T, et al: The effect of meat protein and dietary fiber on colonic function and metabolism. I. Changes in bowel habit, bile acid excretion and calcium absorption. Am J Clin Nutr 32:2086–2093, 1979

123. Welch IM, Sepple CP, Read NW: Comparisons of the effects on satiety and eating behaviour of infusion of lipid into the different regions of the small intestine. Gut 29:306–311, 1988

6

Disorders of Intestinal Motility Resulting from Drug Therapy

M. A. K. Khalil and W. G. Thompson

1. INTRODUCTION

The approach to a patient with gastrointestinal symptoms must include a careful drug history. Perusal of drug formularies and pharmacopoeias reveals that few drugs do not have potential gut side effects. Much suffering might be avoided if the constipated patient with low back pain would discontinue codeine, or the diarrhea patient with peptic ulcers cease magnesium-containing antacids. Such undesirable effects are so ubiquitous that, on principle, any drug the gut complainant takes should be suspect.

It is clearly not possible to catalogue all the possible side effects that are known or suspected, or that are understood or not understood. Therefore, this chapter will concentrate on those classes of drugs that have known receptors in the gut, and that have known pharmacologic effects on gut motility in vitro or in vivo (Table I). In the interest of a more complete explanation of drug effects, drugs within these classes used for gastrointestinal complaints will be included as examples. An understanding of these should help the reader predict undesirable effects of these classes of drugs. Laxatives and drugs with laxative action such as antacids are discussed elsewhere.[1] Discussion of many drugs that are said without authority to cause gut symptoms will be omitted.

2. CHOLINERGIC AGENTS

Acetylcholine is excitatory to enteric nerves and gut smooth muscle. The synapse with the smooth muscle is muscarinic and the pre- and postganglionic synapses are nicotinic.[2] There are two types of muscarinic receptors, M_1 and M_2, mediating different effects in different tissues.

M. A. K. Khalil and W. G. Thompson • Digestive Diseases Research Group, Division of Gastroenterology, University of Ottawa, Ottawa Civic Hospital, Ottawa, Ontario K1Y 4E9, Canada

Table I. Summary of Those Classes of Drugs with Known Receptors in the Gut

Class	Receptor	Action	Example	Effect
Cholinergic	Nicotinic Muscarinic	Agonist	Bethanechol	Increase contraction, motility
	(Nonselective)	Antagonist	Atropine	Delay GI transit, reduce contractions
	M_1 selective	Antagonist	Pirenzepine	Enhance GI transit, reduce segmental colonic contraction
Adrenergic	α_1	Antagonist	Dihydroergotamine Phentolamine	Enhance GI transit
	α_2	Agonist	Clonidine	Delay GI transit
	β_1	Antagonist	Metaprolol	Increase motility index in sigmoid colon
	β_2	Agonist	Terbutaline	Reduce contractions in esophagus and colon
	β_1 and β_2	Antagonist	Propranolol	Increase motility index in sigmoid colon
				Increase esophagus and stomach contractions
Dopamine	D_1 and D_2	Agonist	Dopamine	Delay gastric emptying
			Levodopa	Increase sigmoid colon contraction
	D_2	Antagonist	Domperidone	Enhance gastric emptying, reduce sigmoid colon contraction
Opiate	μ, δ, and κ	Agonist	Codeine	Delay gastric emptying, slow gut transit
		Antagonist	Naloxone	Increase fecal weight, frequency
Calcium channel		Antagonist	Nifedipine	Reduce colon contraction
Prostaglandin		PGE	Misoprostil	Cause longitudinal muscle contraction, circular muscle relaxation
				Enhance GI transit

Parasympathetic cholinergic nerves enhance intestinal smooth muscle tone and motility, relax sphincters and thereby ease the passage of chyme through the gut. Both methacholine (Rx Mecholyl) and bethanechol (Rx Urecholine) are potent, muscarinic cholinergic receptor agonists, moderately selective for smooth muscle. The latter is used to treat nonobstructive urinary retention due to neurogenic atony. Bethanechol is more selective for the gut than other tissues, and is almost completely resistant to inactivation by acetylcholinesterase.[2] It causes both small bowel and colonic contractions, which are disordered. These produce colicky abdominal pain, nausea, and diarrhea.[2] Perforation has occurred when bethanechol was used to treat paralytic ileus. Some patients with gastroesophageal reflux improve on these drugs, which augment peristalsis and increase lower esophageal sphincter tone.[2,3]

Cholinesterase inhibitors increase acetylcholine at the muscarinic receptor, thus prolonging cholinergic effects. Preparations clinically used for myasthenia gravis include neostigmine (Rx Prostigmin), endrophonium (Rx Tensilon), and pyridostigmine bromide (Rx Mestinon). Nausea, vomiting, cramps, and diarrhea may occur with their use. In fact, the ability of endrophonium to cause gut smooth muscle contraction has led to its use for provocation of esophageal spasm during motility studies in the differential diagnosis of noncardiac chest pain. Oral neostigmine has occasionally benefited patients with idiopathic megacolon.[4]

Aside from its role in motility, the parasympathetic system is involved in secretion and absorption. Cholinergic drugs induce net secretion by reducing water and chloride absorption. These effects are inhibited by atropine.[5]

Atropine is an antagonist at both M_1 and M_2 receptors, with anticholinergic effects on the small and large bowel. The clinical importance of these effects on the colon is controversial. Christensen believes the inhibitory effects of atropine on the colon to be minor, and has found no effect of atropine on electromyograms.[6] Others have shown in normals, and in patients with gastrointestinal disease, that atropine produces prolonged inhibitory effects on the motor activity of the stomach, duodenum, jejunum, ileum, and colon—characterized by a decrease in tone, amplitude, and frequency of contractions.[2] Snape et al. have demonstrated that anticholinergic drugs inhibit the meal-induced gastrocolonic response: i.e., increased colon myoelectric and motor activity.[7] Therefore, there appears to be a cholinergically mediated gastrocolonic response.

Phenothiazines and tricyclic antidepressants demonstrate anticholinergic properties. Gastrointestinal complaints, especially constipation, occur frequently as undesirable effects of these drugs. The combination of phenothiazines with antidepressants or antiparkinsonian drugs may further enhance the anticholinergic effect. Several cases of fatal adynamic ileus resulting in perforation, peritonitis, and septicemia have been reported due to phenothiazines[8,9] and the tricyclic antidepressant nortriptyline.[10]

In an extensive review of the literature, Ivey failed to find a well-controlled study of the efficacy of nonselective anticholinergics such as propantheline (Rx Pro-banthine) in the treatment of irritable bowel syndrome.[11] However, he did conclude there was a suggestion of benefit in patients in whom pain and/or constipation was a major feature.

Pirenzepine (Rx Gastrozepin) is a selective muscarinic blocker of the M_1 subtype, which is used to treat peptic ulcer disease. In contrast to conventional, nonselective antimuscarinics, it seems to increase bowel activity in volunteers and patients and may produce diarrhea.[12] Atropine and L-hyoscyamine produce a prolonged reduction in rectosigmoid motility index (RSMI), but pirenzepine does so only transiently.[12] L-Hyoscyamine prolongs gastrointestinal transit time but pirenzepine actually reduces it below control values.[12] Pirenzepine seems to coordinate intestinal migrating motor complexes, which are interrupted and rarefied by atropine.[13] These differences are present at equivalent acid-suppressing doses. Pirenzepine inhibits segmental contractions of the colon but does not inhibit propulsive action, the net result being diarrhea.[12,14]

Thus, the muscarinic cholinergic drugs through stimulation of gut activity cause nausea, vomiting, diarrhea, and abdominal cramps. Anticholinergics have variable effects on the colon, apparently depending on the receptor involved. Nonspecific anticholinergics constipate by blocking M_1 and M_2 receptors, while pirenzepine through M_1 blockade causes diarrhea (Table II).

Table II. Summary of Gut Side Effects of Some Classes of Drugs

	Nausea, vomiting	Diarrhea	Constipation	Abdominal pain
Cholinergics				
Cholinergic (bethanechol, Tensilon, Mestinon)	+	+		+
Anticholinergic (tricyclics, phenothiazines— M₁, M₂ pirenzepine)		+	+	
Adrenergics				
α₂ agonist (clonidine, lidamidine)			+	
α₁ antagonist (phentolamine)	+	+		+
β₁, β₂ antagonist (propranolol)	+	+		+
Dopamine				
D₁ and D₂ agonist (L-Dopa bromocriptine)	+ +		+ +	+
Opiates			+	
Ca²⁺ channel blockers			+	
PGE₂		+		+
Erythromycin	+			+

3. ADRENERGIC AGENTS

The sympathetic nervous system has important regulatory activities on many organ systems including the gastrointestinal tract. Sympathetic stimulation is mediated by norepinephrine. Drugs that partly or completely mimic epinephrine or norepinephrine should also be expected to have effects on the gut.[15]

The development of more specific adrenergic agents has led to greater understanding of adrenergic effects on gastrointestinal motility. The postganglionic sympathetic nerves appear to act by regulating cholinergic enteric nerves. They also terminate in intramural ganglia, blood vessels, and gastrointestinal smooth muscle, so that the contractile state of the gut can be modified by adrenergic agents.[2]

Four types of adrenergic receptors are identified by pharmacological means. α_1 receptors are found postsynaptically and mediate effects on nerves, glands, and smooth muscles. α_2-Adrenergic receptors are located presynaptically and modulate feedback inhibition of norepinephrine release. β-Adrenergic receptors are found postsynaptically on neurons, glands, and smooth muscle.

α and β receptor stimulation relaxes isolated human colon preparations in vitro.[16] Sympathetic (adrenergic) nervous activity has been demonstrated to suppress gastrointestinal motility after abdominal surgery, at least partly, modulated by β-adrenoreceptor stimulation. In a study of 20 patients undergoing abdominal surgery randomized to receive the nonselective β blocker propranolol (Rx Inderal) or placebo, the treatment group passed flatus and first stool significantly sooner than the placebo group.[17] Similar studies have shown a reduction in postoperative ileus with the use of an α_1-adrenergic blocker. In a group of cholecystectomy patients, dihydroergotamine (an α_1 blocker) produced first bowel movement significantly sooner than placebo.[18]

Clonidine (Rx Catapress) is a selective agonist at the presynaptic α_2 adrenergic receptor, and modulates feedback inhibition of norepinephrine release. Clonidine also acts as an agonist at postsynaptic α_2 receptors and thus possesses some sympathetic activity.[2] It delays gastrointestinal transit and may produce constipation at doses used to treat hypertension. Some of clonidine's constipating effect is due to stimulation of α_2 receptors on mucosa promoting net water absorption. Clonidine reduces the cramps and diarrhea associated with narcotic withdrawal.[19] Lidamidine, an experimental α_2 agonist, has been used as an antidiarrheal with limited success.[19]

β_2 receptor stimulation with terbutaline (Px Bricanyl) given intravenously causes a decrease in wave amplitude in the esophagus and reduces the motility index (amplitude times duration of contraction) in the sigmoid colon. β_1 receptor agonists cause relaxation in the esophagus but have no effect in the distal colon.[20] Propranolol increases peristaltic mean amplitude and wave duration in human distal esophagus and lower esophageal sphincter.[21] β blockade also shortens gastric emptying time.[22] Theoretically, it may help heartburn and worsen esophageal spasm. Both the α_1 antagonist phentolamine (Rx Regitine) and the nonselective β antagonist propranolol increase basal electrical rhythm and spike activity in the stomach.[21]

The β_1 blocker metaprolol (Rx Lopressor) causes an increase in the colon motility index in healthy volunteers at plasma levels similar to those seen when the drug is used for hypertension or angina.[22] Propranolol 5 mg given intravenously increased the contractile activity in 9 out of 10 patients with irritable bowel syndrome. These patients had colonic pressure waves with longer duration and higher amplitude compared to baseline. The drug produced symptoms in two of these patients.[23]

β blockers may also influence gut peptide release and the secretion and absorption of water, which secondarily affect motility.

In summary, α_2 agonists (e.g., clonidine) may cause constipation. α_1 antagonists (e.g., phentolamine) may cause nausea, vomiting, diarrhea, and cramps. β blockers are commonly used drugs and their effect on gastrointestinal motility may also cause nausea, vomiting, cramps, and diarrhea. In a survey of reports to the manufacturer, nausea occurred in 1% of 1500 patients and diarrhea in 0.5%.[24] In one report gut disturbances were the most common adverse reactions, occurring in 11.2% of 797 patients.[25]

4. DOPAMINERGIC AGENTS

The role of dopamine in gastrointestinal motility is just beginning to be understood. There are distinct dopamine receptors on nerves and smooth muscle. At high dosages, dopamine can act on α_1-adrenergic and cardiac β_1-adrenergic receptors. Two types of dopaminergic receptors have been identified, D_1 and D_2.

Dopamine inhibits contraction of human gastric muscle strips in vitro. Dopamine also reduces phasic contractile activity and blocks antroduodenal coordination in guinea pigs.[26] Domperidone (Rx Motillium), a selective D_2 antagonist, reverses these effects.[27] In humans with diabetic gastroparesis, domperidone[28] and metoclopramide (Rx Maxeran)[29] improve solid- and liquid-phase gastric emptying. Some of the effects of metoclopramide may be blocked by atropine, suggesting that its mechanism of action is not entirely by dopaminergic receptor antagonism.

About 80% of patients receiving levodopa (Rx L-Dopa), a dopaminergic used in Parkinson's disease, experience anorexia, nausea, vomiting, or epigastric discomfort, at least early in the course of treatment.[30] These effects are partially caused by stimulation of the medullary emetic center, but some may be due to impaired gastroduodenal motility. Another drug used in Parkinson's disease is bromocriptine (Rx Parlodel), which at high doses exerts adverse effects on the gastrointestinal tract mainly by its dopaminergic activity. Nausea and vomiting are noted with onset of treatment and constipation with long-term use.[30] Many of these dopaminergic side effects may be alleviated by the D_2 antagonist domperidone without reducing the antiparkinsonian activity.[31] The antiemetic effect of dopamine antagonists is believed to be mediated through the chemoreceptor trigger zone of the area postrema in the brain.[30] Domperidone may be used with levodopa and bromocriptine to permit more rapid increases in dosage of the antiparkinsonism drugs with fewer side effects.[32]

The importance of dopamine receptors in the lower gastrointestinal tract is less well studied. Dopamine infused intravenously at 5 μg/kg per min increased the colon motility index. This effect was unaltered by α- and β-adrenergic antagonists, suggesting specific dopamine receptors in the sigmoid colon.[33] In another study, dopamine increased contractility, which was inhibited by domperidone, but not by atropine, phentolamine, and propranolol.[34] The increased motility is nonpropulsive and may explain the constipation that occurs with antiparkinsonism drugs.

Domperidone has not been shown to produce any change in basal motor activity in the sigmoid colon in a group of patients with irritable bowel syndrome.[35] However, it did antagonize the effects of intravenously administered dopamine.[35] Thus, the dopaminergic drugs levodopa and bromocriptine cause nausea, vomiting, and constipation, which may be prevented by the D_2 antagonist domperidone.[36,37]

5. OPIATES

Morphine's use for diarrhea predates its use as an analgesic. Opiate receptors are present in the central nervous system, peripheral nerves, and throughout the gastrointestinal tract. In the gut they are located presynaptically on cholinergic motor nerves and on smooth muscle. There are three major types of receptors: μ, δ, and κ. The relative importance of these receptors is uncertain. The effects of specific opioid alkaloids and peptides on motility depend on the receptor selectivity of the opiate, the species, and the particular tissue.[2]

Morphine given intravenously lowers LES pressure and delays gastric emptying of both solids and liquids.[2] However, the morphine antagonist naloxone (Rx Narcan) does not appear to increase gastric emptying.[38]

Electromyographic studies in the opossum small bowel demonstrate that morphine increased phase II activity and reduced phase III activity resulting in segmental nonpropulsive contractions.[39,*] These changes were shown to be more intense with morphine

*Phase I: no spike activity, intestine quiescent; phase II: spike activity begins, irregular, nonpropulsive; phase III: intense spike activity on every slow wave, propulsive; phase IV: short, decreasing spike activity.

than with meperidine (Rx Demerol) or pentazocine (Rx Talwin).[39] However, most work shows reduced phase II activity but also decreased transit.[40] The site and phase of activity at which narcotics have their constipating effect are in dispute. Some have shown the main effects in the jejunum with little contribution from the ileum or colon. However, everyone agrees that opiates prolong total bowel transit time by increasing intestinal tone, and disorganizing contractions; effects that impair propulsion. The constipating effect of morphine is probably due to the following: delayed gastric emptying, reduced small bowel transit, reduced large bowel transit, increased anal sphincter tone, and inattention to sensory stimuli for the defecation reflex.[41,45]

The mechanisms by which other opiates produce constipation may be similar in nature but different in degree. Both pentazocine and meperidine produce less constipation than morphine at equivalent analgesic doses. With continuous use, some tolerance develops to opiates.

The effects of opiates on gastrointestinal motility are mediated directly and via the brain and spinal cord. Opiates that do not cross the blood–brain barrier exert their influence peripherally. One opiate, etorphine, acts mainly at the central level, methadone (Rx Amidom) acts centrally and peripherally, and morphine acts mainly at the peripheral level. It requires less morphine to affect gut motility than to produce analgesia.[2]

A recent review outlines the possible role of endogenous opiates on motility. The small intestine contains an abundance of enkephalins, mainly in the myenteric ganglia and smooth muscle layers.[42] A randomized clinical trial of the opiate antagonist naloxone in elderly patients with constipation demonstrated increased fecal weight and frequency.[43] Since naloxone is poorly absorbed it must exert its effects directly on the gut. This study implies a possible role for endogenous opiates in gastrointestinal motility and may, in the future, explain some drug effects.

Some of the antidiarrheal effect of narcotics is probably through inhibition of secretion,[44] although many investigators have been unable to document a change in absorption by the mucosa.

Loperamide (Rx Imodium), diphenoxylate (Rx Lomotil), and codeine act peripherally and are used as antidiarrheal agents. Loperamide is the most selective antidiarrheal opiate due to its inability to penetrate the central nervous system. Although the precise role of the various opiate receptors is unknown, delayed gastric emptying, slowed gut transit, and perhaps reduced gut secretion mediated centrally and peripherally cause nausea, vomiting, anorexia, and constipation.

6. CALCIUM CHANNEL BLOCKERS

The influx of extracellular calcium into the smooth muscle cell is necessary to generate an electrical spike potential and corresponding muscle contraction. This influx occurs through calcium channels, located on cell membranes. The calcium channel blockers are a class of drugs used mainly for cardiac disorders. They also relax arteriolar smooth muscle in Raynaud's phenomenon, hypertension, and esophageal smooth muscle in the "nutcracker" esophagus.

In vitro studies of circular muscle strips from dog and monkey colons show that calcium channel blockers reduce contractile activity in response to a number of colonic stimulants such as acetylcholine, substance P, and electrical field stimulation.[46] Thus, intracellular movement of calcium (Ca^{2+}) has a role in the mediation of colonic motility. At least part of the antidiarrheal effects of loperamide may be mediated through calcium channel antagonism.[47] Calcium channel blockers used in coronary artery disease [especially verapamil (Rx Isoptin)] cause constipation. Intravenous calcium chloride may relieve constipation and fecal impaction secondary to verapamil.[48]

Calcium channel blockers have no effect on gastric emptying,[49] but reduce colonic electrical activity and contractions after a meal.[50] In IBS patients, sublingual nifedipine (Rx Adalat) reduces the postprandial increase in colon spike potential activity and motility index[50] (gastrocolonic response). Intravenous nicardipine causes a reduction in number and amplitude of colon contractions after a meal in IBS patients.[51] However, the above studies fail to address symptoms. Considering the poor correlation between gut symptoms and gut motor and electrical activity, little can be said about the possible use of calcium channel blockers in IBS. Nonetheless, these drugs may be expected to cause constipation when used for nongut disorders.

7. PROSTAGLANDINS

Prostaglandins are distributed widely in the mucosa and muscle of the gastrointestinal tract. Prostaglandins (PG) of the E and F series affect the tone of isolated intestinal smooth muscle strips of all species studied.[52] As well as direct effects on smooth muscle, they act via neural receptors. Prostaglandins may inhibit norepinephrine release and maintain release of acetylcholine.[53]

The effects of exogenous prostaglandins on intestinal motility in vitro show considerable variability that depends on the type of prostaglandin, its concentration, the species and even the muscle layer studied.[54]

Prostaglandins of the E and F series alter gastrointestinal tract secretions by inhibiting Na^+ absorption and increasing Cl^- secretion in the small bowel.[55] The relative importance of this mechanism in producing diarrhea is uncertain since 16,16-dimethyl PGE_2 produced diarrhea in rats even after their ileocecal junctions were tied. This suggests increased colonic transit is an important mechanism of this diarrhea.[56]

In a group of patients with diarrhea as a manifestation of their IBS, 10 out of 17 showed elevated PGE_2 levels in jejunal fluid when compared to healthy volunteers or alcoholics with diarrhea. Furthermore, in 6 of these patients, indomethacin (Rx Indocid), a prostaglandin inhibitor, reduced volume and frequency of stools.[57] However, diarrhea and not constipation is a side effect of Indocid use.

Prostaglandins (Rx Prostin E_2) used therapeutically to induce or maintain uterine contractions are frequently associated with diarrhea. Misoprostil (Rx Cytotec), currently available in Canada for treatment of peptic ulcer disease, often induces diarrhea. The effect of many laxatives such as ricinoleic acid (castor oil), oleic acid, bisacodyl, and phenolphthalein may at least partially be due to their ability to stimulate colonic PGE synthesis.[58]

Responses to prostaglandins, in vitro and in vivo, vary greatly depending on the segment, type of muscle, concentration of drug, and particular prostaglandin. Currently used prostaglandins of the E group cause diarrhea and cramps, as well as nausea and vomiting.[59]

8. ANTIBIOTICS

The effects of some antibiotics on neuromuscular transmission in skeletal muscle are well documented, but little work has been done on their effects on smooth muscle. Of course, antibiotic-associated diarrhea may be caused by several mechanisms. Diarrhea that commonly occurs with ampicillin may be due to altered colonic flora. Pseudomembranous colitis is due to overgrowth of *Clostridium difficile* producing a cytotoxin. Since patients chronically using laxatives or antidiarrheal drugs are predisposed to pseudomembranous colitis, perhaps impaired motility of the gastrointestinal tract predisposes a person to proliferation of *C. difficile*.[60,61] The antibiotics ampicillin, doxycycline, mecillinan, and metronidazole at concentrations that include the therapeutic range had no in vitro effect on gut motility. However, clindamycin, gentamicin, kanamycin, pivmecillinam, and trimethoprim all inhibited evoked reflex responses in guinea pig ileum. This inhibition occurred at doses often higher than the therapeutic range,[62] so the importance of this effect is uncertain.

Erythromycin commonly causes abdominal pain, nausea, and vomiting. It affects the small bowel migrating motor complex. Given orally or intravenously in dogs, erythromycin induces immediate strong contractions in the stomach, duodenum, and jejunum, which are initially uncoordinated. Vomiting occurs during the initial phase. The motor activity induced by erythromycin is suppressed by atropine, suggesting a cholinergic pathway.[63] In humans the interval between migrating motor complexes is shortened and phase III is prolonged.[64] To what extent these changes in motility contribute to symptoms is uncertain, but erythromycin commonly causes abdominal pain, nausea, and vomiting. Antibiotic-associated diarrhea has several mechanisms, and a direct effect on gut motility may be one.

9. MISCELLANEOUS

The diarrheagenic effects of some antacid preparations are due to the osmotic effect of magnesium hydroxide. The constipating effect of calcium carbonate and aluminum hydroxide is not understood. Digitalis preparations cause nausea and vomiting, oral colchicine causes diarrhea, intravenous vasopressin causes diarrhea, and sucralfate causes constipation. The list of unwanted gut effects of drugs is seemingly endless, and the mechanisms are often unknown. The physician inquiring about a gut symptom must suspect any drug that the patient is currently taking.

On the other hand, many putative gut side effects of drugs are not clearly established. Placebo-controlled trials have taught us that placebos can induce gut symptoms. Thus, minor gut complaints of a patient on essential drugs must be evaluated carefully.

10. SUMMARY

Recognition of specific receptors in the enteric nervous system has permitted us to understand the effects of some drugs on the gut. Such knowledge will increasingly help us predict how various classes of drugs may affect the gut. Although we have concentrated here on agonists and antagonists of the cholinergic, adrenergic, dopaminergic, opiate, prostaglandin, and calcium channel receptors, it is likely that new receptors and drugs that affect them will be recognized. For the present, the physician would be wise to suspect any drug a patient has taken as the cause of a new gut symptom. In the absence of a logical explanation, he or she should critically evaluate the new symptom in the light of known pharmacology, and the imponderable side effects due to placebo.

REFERENCES

1. Thompson WG: Laxatives: Clinical pharmacology and rational use. Drugs 19:49–58, 1980
2. Burks TF: Actions of drugs on gastrointestinal motility, in Johnson LR (ed): Physiology of the gastrointestinal tract, ed 2. New York, Raven Press, 1987, pp 723–743
3. Farrar JT: The effects of drugs on intestinal motility. Clin Gastroenterol 11(3):673–681, 1982
4. Connell AM: Colonic motility in megacolon. Proc R Soc Med 54:1040–1043, 1961
5. Morris AI, Turnberg LA: The influences of a parasympathetic agonist and antagonist on human intestinal transport in vivo. Gastroenterology 79:861–866, 1980
6. Christensen J: Motility of the colon, in Johnson LR (ed): Physology of the Gastrointestinal Tract, ed 2. New York, Raven Press, 1987, pp 665–692
7. Sun EA, Snape WJ, Cohen S, et al: The role of opiate receptors and cholinergic neurons in the gastrocolonic response. Gastroenterology 82:689–693, 1982
8. Warnes H, Lehman HE: Adynamic ileus during psychoactive medication: A report of three fatal and five severe cases. Can Med Assoc J 96:1112–1113, 1967
9. Giordano J, Huang A, Canter JW: Fatal paralytic ileus complicating phenothiazine therapy. South Med J 68(13):351–353, 1975
10. Milner G, Hill NF: Adynamic ileus and nortriptyline. Br Med J 1:841–842, 1966
11. Ivey KJ: Are anticholinergics of use in the irritable colon syndrome? Gastroenterology 68:1300–1307, 1975
12. Jay BH, Abrahamsson H, Stockbruegger RW, et al: Effect of selective and non-selective antimuscarinics on rectosigmoid motility and gastrointestinal transit. Scand J Gastroenterol 20:1101–1109, 1985
13. Lederer PC, Thiemann R, Femppel J, et al: Influence of atropine, pirenzepine and cimetidine on nocturnal gastrointestinal motility and gastric acid secretion. Scand J Gastroenterol 17(suppl 72):131–137, 1982
14. Kleist OV, Janisch HD, Bauer FE: Proceedings of the XII International Congress of Gastroenterology, Lisbon, 1984 (abstr)
15. Hoffman BB: Adrenergic receptor-activating drugs, in Katzung BG (ed): Basic and Clinical Pharmacology, ed 2. Lange Medical Publications, Los Altos, Calif, 1984, pp 86–106
16. Bucknel A, Whitney B: A preliminary investigation of the pharmacology of the human isolated toenia coli prep. Br J Pharmacol 23:164–175, 1964
17. Glise H, Hallerback B: Effects of propranolol on post-op ileus after colonic surgery. Gastroenterology 84:1169, 1983
18. Altaparmakov IA, Erckenbrecht JF, Wienbeck M: Modulation of adrenergic system in the treatment of post-op bowel atonia. Scand J Gastroenterol 1104–1106, 1984
19. Weiner N: Drugs that inhibit adrenergic nerves and block adrenergic receptors, in Gilman AG, Goodman LS, Rall TW (eds): The Pharmacological Basis of Therapeutics, ed 7. New York, Macmillan Co, 1985, p 203
20. Jaffe, JH: Drug addiction and drug abuse, in Gilman AG, Goodman LS, Rall TW (eds): The Pharmacological Basis of Therapeutics, ed 7. New York, Macmillan Co, 1985, p 569
21. Thorpe JAC: Effect of propranolol on lower esophageal sphincter in man. Curr Med Res Opinion 7:91–95, 1980
22. Lyrenas E: Beta adrenergic influence on esophageal and colonic motility in man. Scand J Gastroenterol Suppl 116:1–48, 1985
23. Abrahamsson H, Dotevall G: Effects of propranolol on colonic pressure in patients with irritable bowel syndrome. Scand J Gastroenterol 16:1021–1024, 1981
24. Zacharias FJ: Patient acceptability of propranolol and the occurrence of side effects. Postgrad Med J 52(suppl 4):87–89, 1976

25. Greenblatt DJ, Koch-Weser J: Adverse reactions to β-adrenergic receptor blocking drugs: A report from the Boston collaborative drug surveillance program. Drugs 7:118–129, 1974
26. VanNueten JM, Schuurkes JAJ: Studies on the role of dopamine and dopamine blockers in gastroduodenal motility. Scand J Gastroenterol Suppl 96:90–99, 1984
27. Schuurkes JAJ, VanNueten JM: Is dopamine an inhibitory modulator of gastrointestinal motility? Scand J Gastroenterol 16(suppl 67):33–36, 1981
28. Horowitz M, Harding PE, Chatterton BE, et al: Acute and chronic effects of domperidone on gastric emptying in diabetic autonomic neuropathy. Dig Dis Sci 30(1):1–9, 1985
29. Schade RR, Dugas MC, Lhotsky DM, et al: Effect of metoclopramide on gastric liquid emptying in patients with diabetic gastroparesis. Dig Dis Sci 30(1):10–15, 1985
30. Bianchine JR: Drugs for Parkinson's disease, spasticity and acute muscle spasm, in Gilman AG, Goodman LS, Rall TW (eds): The Pharmacological Basis of Therapeutics, ed 7. New York, Macmillan Co, 1985, pp 473–490
31. Schindler JS, Finnerty GJ, Towlson K, et al: Domperidone and levodopa in Parkinson's disease. Br J Clin Pharmacol 18:959–962, 1984
32. Quinn N, Illas A, Lhermitte F, et al: Bromocriptine and domperidone in the treatment of Parkinson's disease. Neurology 31:662–667, 1981
33. LanFranchi GA, Marzio L, Cortini C, et al: Motor effect of dopamine on human sigmoid colon. Am J Dig Dis 23(3):257–263, 1978
34. Wiley J, Owyang C: Dopaminergic modulation of rectosigmoid motility: Action of domperidone. Pharmacol Exp Ther 242(2):548–551, 1987
35. LanFranchi GA, Bazzocchi G, Fois F, et al: Effect of domperidone and dopamine on colonic motor activity in patients with irritable bowel syndrome. Eur J Clin Pharmacol 29:307–310, 1985
36. Cann PA, Read NW, Holdsworth CD: Oral domperidone: Double blind comparison with placebo in IBS. Gut 24:1135–1140, 1983
37. Fielding JF: Domperidone treatment in IBS. Digestion 23:125–127, 1982
38. Shea-Donahue PT, Adams N, Arnold J, et al: Effects of met-enkephalin and naloxone on gastric emptying and secretion in rhesus monkeys. Am J Physiol 245:G196–G200, 1983
39. Coelho JCU, Runkel N, Herfarth C, et al: Effect of analgesic drugs on electromyographic activity of the gastrointestinal tract and sphincter of Oddi and on biliary pressure. Ann Surg 204(1):53–58, 1984
40. Wingate DL, Malagelada JR, Read NW, et al: General discussion—phase activity. Scan J Gastroenterol Suppl 96:157–158, 1984
41. Jaffe JH, Martin WR: Opioid analgesics and antagonists, in Gilman AG, Goodman LS, Rall TW (eds): The Pharmacological Basis of Therapeutics, ed 7. New York, Macmillan Co, pp 491–531, 1985
42. Diamant N: Enkephalinergic control of gastrointestinal motility: From "gut brain" to trimebutine. Can J Gastroenterol 1(1):41–43, 1987
43. Kreek MJ, Shaefer RA, Elliot FH: Naloxone, a specific opioid antagonist, reverses chronic idiopathic constipation. Lancet 1:261–262, 1983
44. Kachur JF, Miller RJ, Field M: Control of guinea pig intestinal electrolyte secretion by delta receptors. Proc Natl Acad Sci USA 77:2753–2756, 1980
45. Manara L, Bianchetti A: The central and peripheral influences of opioids on gastrointestinal propulsion. Annu Rev Pharmacol Toxicol 25:249–273, 1985
46. Barone FC, White RF, Ormsbee HS, et al: Effects of calcium channel entry blockers, nifedipine and nilvadipine on colonic motor activity. Pharmacol Exp Ther 237(1):99–106, 1986
47. Reynolds IJ, Gould RJ, Snyder HS: Loperamide: Blockade of calcium channels as a mechanism for anti-diarrheal effect. Pharmacol Exp Ther 231:628–632, 1984
48. Ward DJ, Ward JW, Griffo W, et al: Intravenous Ca^{2+} for fecal impaction secondary to verapamil. N Engl J Med 307(27):1709, 1982
49. Traube M, Lange RC, McAllister RG, et al: Effect of nifedipine on gastric emptying in normal subjects. Dig Dis Sci 30(8):710–712, 1985
50. Narducci F, Bassotti G, Gaburri M, et al: Nifedipine reduces the colonic motor response to eating in patients with the irritable colon syndrome. Am J Gastroenterol 80(5):317–319, 1985
51. Prior A, Harris SR, Whorwell PJ: Reduction of colonic motility by intravenous nicardipine in irritable bowel syndrome. Gut 28:1609–1612, 1987
52. Bennett A, Eley KG, Scholes GB: Effect of PGE_1 and E_2 on human, guinea pig and rat isolated small intestine. Br J Pharmacol 34:630–638, 1968

53. Bennett A, Eley KG, Stockley A: Inhibition of peristalsis in guinea pig isolated ileum and colon by drugs that block prostaglandin synthesis. Br J Pharmacol 57:335–340, 1976
54. Thor P, Konturek JW, Konturek SJ: Role of prostaglandins in control of intestinal motility. Am J Physiol 248:G353–G359, 1985
55. Horton EW, Main IHM, Thompson LJ, et al: The effect of orally administered prostaglandin E on gastric secretion and gastrointestinal motility in man. Gut 9:655–658, 1968
56. Rush RD, Ruwart MJ: The role of accelerated colonic transit in prostaglandin induced diarrhea and its inhibition by prostacyclin. Br J Pharmacol 83:157–159, 1984
57. Bukhave K, Rask-Madsen J: Prostaglandin E in jejunal fluids and its potential diagnostic value for selecting patients with indomethacin sensitive diarrhea. Eur J Clin Invest 11:191–197, 1981
58. Beubler E, Jaun H: Effect of ricinoleic acid and other laxatives on net water flux and prostaglandin E release by rat colon. J Pharm Pharmacol 31:681–685, 1979
59. Moncada S, Flower RJ, Vane JR: Prostaglandins, prostacyclin, thromboxane A_2 and leukotrienes, in Gilman AG, Goodman LS, Rall TW, et al (eds): The Pharmacological Basis of Therapeutics, ed 7. New York, Macmillan Co, 1985, p 667
60. Pittman FE: Antibiotic associated colitis: An update. Adverse Drug Reaction Bull. 75:268–271, 1979
61. Shulze-Delrieu K: Pseudomembraneous colitis and the neuromuscular actions of antibiotics. Gastroenterology 85(5):1221–1222, 1983
62. Lees GM, Percy WH: Antibiotic associated colitis: An in-vitro investigation of the effects of antibiotics on intestinal motility. Br J Pharmacol 73:553–557, 1981
63. Itoh Z, Suzuki T, Nakaya M, et al: Gastrointestinal motor stimulating activity of macrolide antibiotics and analysis of their side effects on canine gut. Antimicrob Agents Chemother 26(6):863–869, 1984
64. Tomomasa T, Kuroume T, Arai H, et al: Erythromycin induces migrating motor complex in human GI tract. Dig Dis Sci 31(2):157–161, 1986

7

Functional Diseases of the Esophagus

Joel E. Richter

1. INTRODUCTION

Although recognized as early as the 17th century, functional disorders of the esophagus attracted only sporadic interest until the mid 20th century. The awareness that esophageal abnormalities are frequently found in patients with noncardiac chest pain has led to a resurgence of interest in esophageal motility disorders (EMDs). Improvement in manometric instrumentation as well as increased frequency of manometric evaluations in patients with noncardiac chest pain have provided more specific characterizations of EMDs. "New" disorders such as high-amplitude peristalsis (nutcracker esophagus) and hypertensive lower esophageal sphincter (LES) have been defined and associated with chest pain syndromes and dysphagia. "Older" disorders such as achalasia and diffuse esophageal spasm have been further characterized and attempts made to correlate the motility disorders with symptomatic complaints of chest pain and dysphagia.

In this chapter, I will review the current "state of the art" relevant to the definitions, diagnosis, and treatment of EMDs. Specific attention will be directed to abnormalities of the upper esophageal sphincter (UES), primary EMDs (achalasia, diffuse esophageal spasm, nutcracker esophagus, hypertensive LES), and secondary EMDs resulting from systemic diseases. There continues to be many sphinxlike qualities to the functional derangements of the esophagus. These gaps in our knowledge and controversies also will be pointed out.

2. CLINICAL PRESENTATION

The hallmark of functional disorders of the esophagus is dysphagia. Dysphagia is divided into two distinct syndromes: that produced by abnormalities affecting the finely

Joel E. Richter • Section on Gastroenterology, Department of Medicine, The Bowman Gray School of Medicine, Wake Forest University, Winston-Salem, North Carolina 27103.

tuned neuromuscular mechanism of the pharynx and UES (oropharyngeal dysphagia) and that due to any one of a variety of disorders affecting the esophagus itself (esophageal dysphagia).

Oropharyngeal dysphagia is usually described as an inability to initiate the act of swallowing. It is a "transfer" problem, due to the impaired ability to transfer food from mouth to upper esophagus. These patients present with a variety of complaints including food sticking in the throat, difficulty initiating a swallow, nasal regurgitation, and coughing during swallowing. They may also complain of dysarthria or display nasal speech because of associated muscle weaknesses.

Three major functions occur in the pharynx during the process of deglutition: (1) the propulsion of food into the esophagus (buccal phase); (2) the closure of the entrances into the nasal pharynx and larynx (pharyngeal phase); and (3) the opening of the UES (cricopharyngeal phase). Abnormal function of any one of these processes can lead to dysphagia. However, many of the diseases associated with oropharyngeal dysphagia affect multiple aspects of deglutition.

The esophageal dysphagia associated with motility disorders is usually slowly progressive, present with liquids and solids, and may be associated with weight loss. It is often relieved by repeated swallowing, a Valsalva maneuver, or by throwing the arms over the head. In contrast, patients with obstructive lesions usually have dysphagia only for solid foods which is extremely difficult to relieve with the above-mentioned maneuvers. The site at which the patient localizes the symptom is of limited value. While symptoms in the substernal area frequently correspond to the site of obstruction, dysphagia localized to the neck is often referred from below. Dysphagia associated with heartburn should suggest gastroesophageal reflux and its related complications. Occasionally, patients also will complain of odynophagia but if this is a prominent symptom, an infectious or caustic cause should be sought.

The symptom of dysphagia results from interference in the orderly "transport" of liquids or solids down the esophagus into the stomach. Radiographic studies have shown that during primary peristalsis the esophageal lumen is obliterated by the contraction wave, imparting an inverted V configuration to the tail of the barium column.[1] The point of the tail corresponds precisely to the upstroke of the peristaltic complex as recorded by simultaneous esophageal manometry. Subsequent studies[2,3] have shown that peristaltic pressure complexes elict normal bolus transport, regardless of the number of repetitive waves or the duration of the complex. Wave amplitude must be sufficient to seal the esophageal lumen, but otherwise does not correlate with the efficacy of bolus transport. Therefore, only motility disturbances characterized by simultaneous contractions, nonconducted swallows, or low-amplitude waves that do not seal the esophageal lumen, should be associated with dysphagia. However, these nonpropulsive contractions do not consistently produce this symptom, suggesting that other factors (luminal distension, bolus size) may contribute to dysphagia. Dysfunction of the LES, particularly incomplete relaxation or elevated basal pressures, also has been associated with dysphagia. In achalasia, incomplete relaxation leaves a residual pressure gradient between the nadir of LES relaxation and intragastric pressure that acts as a functional obstruction. Pneumatic dilatation or surgical myotomy reduces this pressure gradient, thereby improving the dysphagia. Patients with a hypertensive LES frequently complain of dysphagia. However, it is unclear how this otherwise normally functioning valve should produce this symptom unless there is some subtle delay in esophageal emptying.

It has been stated that dysphagia always indicates the presence of esophageal dysfunction. It is important, therefore, that one not confuse dysphagia with "globus hystericus," the sensation of a "lump in the throat." This is a more constant symptom that usually does not interfere with swallowing and may be relieved during deglutition. Although poorly documented, this symptom has been associated with a hypertensive UES,[4] gastroesophageal reflux disease,[5] and personality disorders.[6]

In recent years we have become increasingly aware that patients with EMDs may present with unexplained chest pain. Pain arising from the esophagus may produce a retrosternal chest discomfort not unlike that secondary to coronary insufficiency. Therefore, it frequently is necessary to rule out a cardiac etiology of these patients' chest pain. Some features suggesting esophageal rather than cardiac pain[7] include pain that is nonexertional and continues for hours; pain without lateral radiation; pain that interrupts sleep or is meal related; pain relieved with antacids; or the presence of associated esophageal symptoms including heartburn, dysphagia, or regurgitation. Unfortunately, as many as 50% of patients with cardiac pain may have one or more symptoms of esophageal pain.[7]

The specific mechanisms by which abnormalities of esophageal function produce chest pain are not well understood (Fig. 1). The acid sensitivity observed during intraesophageal acid perfusion or esophageal pH monitoring suggests that this pain is secondary to stimulation of acid-sensitive chemoreceptors in the esophageal mucosa. EMDs occasionally may be evoked by acid perfusion,[8] but acid-induced pain usually is not associated with a dysmotility problem.[9] In addition, esophageal acid stimulation may induce ischemic EKG changes and increased myocardial work load in patients with concomitant heart disease and gastroesophageal reflux.[10] It has been suggested that

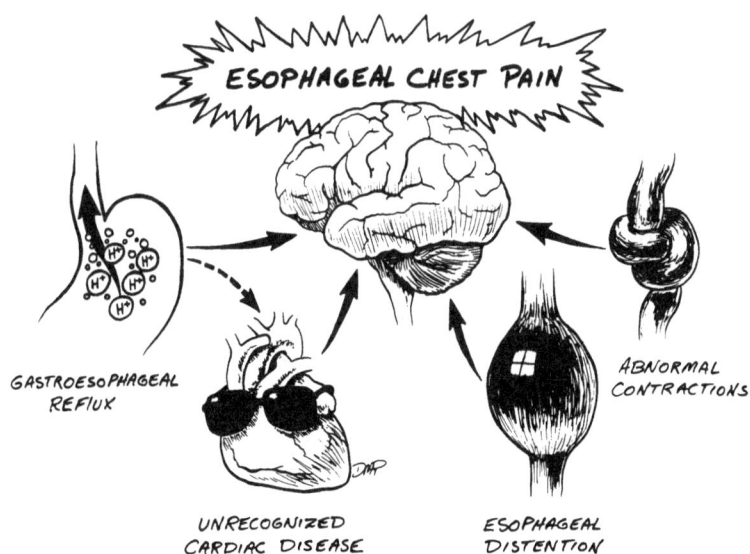

Figure 1. Potential mechanisms for esophageal chest pain. These stimuli reach the brain via the afferent sensory fibers of the vagus nerve. The perception and verbal report of chest pain is an interaction between these internal stimuli and psychologic factors such as anxiety, depression, individual cultural values, and environmental events.

EMDs may produce chest pain as the result of high intramural esophageal tension inhibiting blood flow at critical time periods, i.e., myoischemia.[11] However, the arterial blood supply of the esophagus is extensive and comes from five separate tributaries including the thoracic aorta and bronchial arteries. Therefore, it is unlikely that esophageal blood flow could be critically compromised by local esophageal contractions. Furthermore, if we are to attribute esophageal chest pain to high-amplitude or simultaneous contractions, then why are these patients usually asymptomatic when these contraction abnormalities are identified? Possibly these contractions are a marker for more severe EMDs present during chest pain.[12] However, prolonged ambulatory esophageal motility studies suggest this is infrequently the case.[13,14] In addition, chest pain improvement has not predictably correlated with amplitude reduction produced by either calcium channel blockers[15] or surgical myotomy.[16] Other potential causes of esophageal chest pain include excitation of temperature receptors or acute luminal distension. Very cold liquids may produce severe esophageal chest pain which is associated with aperistalsis and dilatation rather than esophageal spasm.[17] It is possible that the chest pain experienced by patients with EMDs is due to proximal distension of the esophageal body by an abnormal distal contraction or by a lack of coordination between LES relaxation and the esophageal contraction advancing toward it.[18] However, the absolute degree of esophageal distension may not be the only factor in these patients' chest pains. We recently have shown that patients with suspected esophageal chest pain frequently note replication of their pain with smaller volumes of esophageal balloon distension than those required to produce pain in asymptomatic control subjects.[19] Thus, lower pain thresholds may also contribute to these patients' interpretation of pain.

3. CLASSIFICATION OF EMDs

3.1. Disorders of the UES

Abnormal UES function may be one of altered resting tone or abnormal relaxation. It may be an isolated defect in deglutition, but more commonly is part of diffuse neuromuscular diseases affecting several aspects of the swallowing mechanism (Table I).

3.1.1. Hypertensive UES

High UES pressures have been described in so-called "spasm" of the cricopharyngeus and in globus hystericus. Some authors have measured higher than normal pressures in the presence of esophagitis.[20] Recent studies using modern manometric techniques have shown that UES resting pressure increases significantly in response to both saline and acid perfusion of the esophagus.[21] Early reports suggested that globus sensation may be caused by significantly higher than normal resting UES pressures but there have been no more recent studies to confirm or refute this observation.[4]

3.1.2. Hypotensive UES

Lower than normal UES pressures have been reported in patients with esophagopharyngeal reflux.[22] Not only was UES pressure low in these patients, but the sphincter

Table I. Neuromuscular Diseases as the Cause
of Oropharyngeal Dysphagia

Central nervous system
  Cerebral vascular accidents
  Parkinson's disease
  Multiple sclerosis
  Amyotrophic lateral sclerosis
  Syringobulbia
  Stiff man syndrome
  Brain stem tumor
  Tabes dorsalis
  Bulbar poliomyelitis
  Congenital Riley–Day syndrome
Peripheral nervous system
  Mononeuritis multiplex
  Diabetic neuropathy
  Miscellaneous (diphtheria, tetanus, botulism)
Motor endplate
  Myasthenia gravis
Muscle
  Dystrophia myotonica
  Oculopharyngeal muscular dystrophy
  Polymyositis and dermatomyositis
  Metabolic myopathies

appeared to have lost the ability to increase pressure in response to intraesophageal acid. In this situation, UES hypotension may be secondary to esophageal damage with interruption of a protective reflex mechanism. UES hypotension is found after cricopharyngeal myotomy and after laryngectomy, yet these patients do not necessarily suffer from esophagopharyngeal reflux. Hypotension may also occur secondary to some neuromuscular disorders including amyotrophic lateral sclerosis, myasthenia gravis, oculopharyngeal muscular dystrophy, and dystrophia myotonica.[23]

3.1.3. Abnormalities of UES Relaxation

Three types of abnormalities in UES relaxation have been described: incomplete relaxation, delayed relaxation, and premature closure.[24] The term *cricopharyngeal achalasia* has been used to refer to all these abnormalities, but is perhaps better reserved specifically for the disorder of incomplete relaxation. UES resting pressure normally falls to within 5 mm Hg of intraesophageal pressure, as the swallow is initiated, and does not return to baseline resting pressure until the bolus has passed. Patients with cricopharyngeal achalasia should show incomplete UES relaxation after the majority of swallows. It has been described as an isolated phenomenon in children[25] and in adults, usually secondary to underlying neuromuscular diseases such as cerebral vascular accidents affecting the brain stem, bulbar poliomyelitis, and thyrotoxic myopathies.[26] Although radiography may show functional delay of barium at the level of the cricopharyngus, the correlation with manometric studies identifying incomplete relaxation is poor. Patients with familial

Table II. Manometric Criteria for Primary Esophageal Motility Disorders[a,b]

Motility diagnosis	Required criteria	Patient may have
Achalasia	Aperistalsis of esophageal body	Incomplete LES relaxation Elevated LES pressure (> 45 mm Hg) Elevated intraesophageal pressure
Diffuse esophageal spasm	Simultaneous contractions (> 10% wet swallows) Intermittent normal peristalsis	Repetitive contractions (> two peaks) Increased duration Increased amplitude Spontaneous contractions Incomplete relaxation
Nutcracker esophagus	Normal peristalsis Increased distal amplitude (> 180 mm Hg)	Increased duration (> 6 sec)
Hypertensive LES	Elevated LES pressure (> 45 mm Hg) Normal LES relaxation Normal peristalsis	
Nonspecific esophageal motility disorder	Any combination of criteria at right	Increased nontransmitted waves (> 20%) Increased duration Triple-peaked contractions Retrograde contractions Low-amplitude peristalsis (< 30 mm Hg)

[a]Based on studies of 95 healthy subjects ranging in age from 22 to 79 years.
[b]All values in parentheses $> x \pm 2$ S.D.

dysautonomia (Riley–Day syndrome) may develop a number of disturbances related to autonomic function including sucking and swallowing difficulties. Radiologic studies have shown delayed opening in the cricopharyngus with normal pharyngeal motor activity.[27] Manometric studies of the UES have not been reported in these patients. It has been reported that premature closure of the UES is an important factor in the pathogenesis of Zenker's diverticulum. Manometric studies have not resolved this issue so far, since groups of patients have been reported where all,[28] some,[29] and none[30] showed premature UES closure.

3.2. Primary EMDs

The development of precise infusion systems to allow accurate pressure recordings brought studies of esophageal motility into the modern age. This new technology has allowed us to establish criteria for normals based on large numbers of healthy adults.[31,32] At the same time, a variety of new esophageal motility "disorders" have been recognized, particularly in patients with noncardiac chest pain syndromes. Specific manometric characteristics of these abnormalities have recently been defined (Table II). Whether these newer abnormal motility patterns represent important disturbances of esophageal function or simply "curious" manometric findings is a controversial issue. One authority[33] recently has suggested the following general criteria to define a manometric finding as an important esophageal disease: (1) the motility event must be a major "alteration" of esophageal physiology, (2) motility change must be associated temporally with symptoms of esophageal disease, (3) the abnormality of esophageal function must be demonstrated by other independent measures, and (4) the symptoms or signs of esophageal abnormality must be improved as the esophageal disorder is corrected. These may be worthwhile criteria, but on closer scrutiny would permit only achalasia to be defined as a true clinical EMD. Further studies are required to understand the clinical significance and complex neurophysiologic and possibly psychophysiologic interactions contributing to the other primary EMDs.

3.2.1. Achalasia

The best known and characterized primary EMD is achalasia. First described by Willis in the 17th century, its manometric hallmarks are aperistalsis in the esophageal body, failure of complete relaxation of the LES, and increased LES pressure (Fig. 2). In addition, elevated intraesophageal pressures relative to intragastric pressures are occasionally found. Achalasia may present at any age and is equally common in males and females. The most common symptom is slowly progressive dysphagia for both liquids and solids, often accompanied by weight loss. Nocturnal cough and regurgitation in the absence of heartburn should suggest achalasia. Chest x-ray may show a widened mediastinum secondary to esophageal dilatation and absence of the gastric air bubble. Barium studies usually reveal a dilated esophagus with tapering or "beaking" at the distal end and often the presence of an air–fluid level. Liquid radionuclide transit studies show a markedly prolonged transit time with an adynamic pattern whereas solid upright radionuclide studies reveal delayed esophageal emptying.

Several variations of the classic achalasia pattern have been reported. There is a subset of patients with complete absence of peristalsis and the other manometric features of achalasia, who exhibit higher-amplitude (> 60 mm Hg) simultaneous, repetitive contractions in response to swallows. This manometric pattern has been called "vigorous" achalasia.[34] These patients differ from those with classic achalasia in that they have a greater incidence of severe chest pain and less esophageal dilatation on x-ray. A second group with all the clinical and radiologic hallmarks of achalasia have manometric evidence of absent peristalsis but apparently normal LES relaxation.[35] They usually have less weight loss, dysphagia of shorter duration, and less esophageal dilatation than patients with classical achalasia. Esophageal manometry, even with the Dent sleeve, has demonstrated relaxation of the LES to the gastric baseline. However, the duration of relaxation [7.2 ± 0.6 sec (± S.E.)] is significantly shorter than healthy controls (11.7 ± 0.6 sec). We believe this LES relaxation is artifactual and related to the relatively small diameter of the motility catheter and the degree of opening of the esophageal lumen. These patients may represent an early stage of achalasia as we have seen several patients progress from aperistalsis and complete LES relaxation to incomplete LES relaxation over a period of several years. Achalasia secondary to a carcinoma has been reported in association with pancreatic, bronchogenic, gastric, and prostate cancers as well as lymphomas. The manometric features are identical to those of idiopathic achalasia but patients are usually older (mean age 65 years), have rapidly progressive dysphagia, and weight loss is prominent.[36] The mechanism of this form of achalasia is uncertain. Tumors of the esophageal wall can destroy the myenteric plexus, induce a peripheral neuropathy, or produce distal obstruction with aperistalsis as a nonspecific reaction. Peristalsis may return after successful treatment or removal of the tumor.

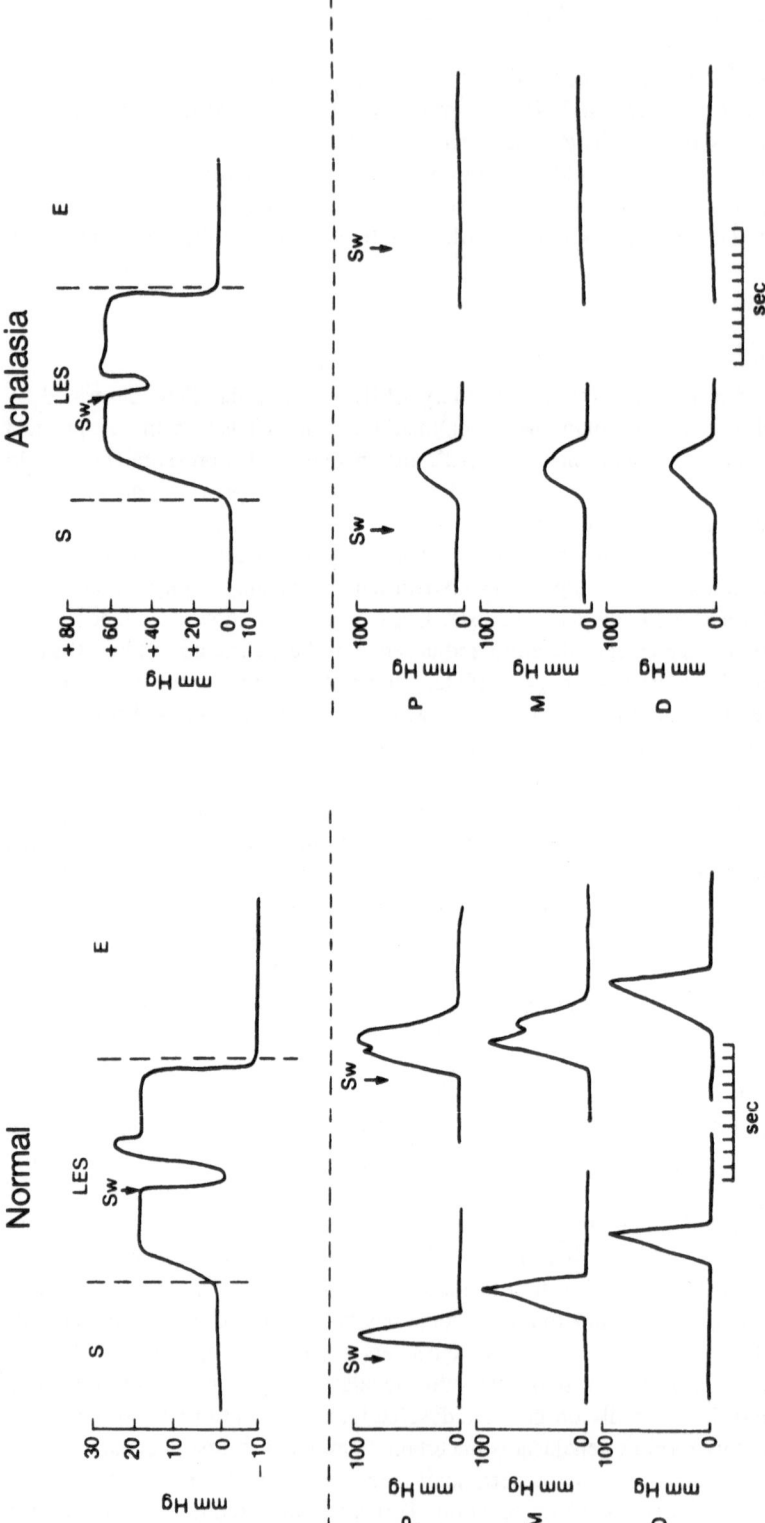

Figure 2. Diagrammatic examples of esophageal manometric tracings in normal subject (left) and patient with achalasia (right). Upper portion: pull-through of catheter from stomach (S), across lower esophageal sphincter (LES), to esophagus (E). Relaxation of LES evaluated during a swallow (Sw). Lower portion: catheter placed in distal esophagus with openings 5 cm apart from proximal (P), middle (M), and distal (D) recording sites. Response to two wet swallows (Sw) is shown. Left: Example of normal LES with complete relaxation after a swallow. Contractions in the body of the esophagus are peristaltic with an average amplitude of 100 mm Hg. Double-peaked waves are a variation of normal. Right: In achalasia, LES pressure is usually increased with incomplete relaxation after a swallow. Activity in the esophageal body reveals either low-amplitude simultaneous waves of the complete lack of esophageal contractions.

The etiology of achalasia has not been completely determined, but several pathologic findings may help explain the characteristic manometric findings. Degenerated or absent myenteric ganglion cells have been described in the distal smooth muscle segment of the esophagus and LES.[37] However, these findings best correlate with the duration of the disease and are likely not to reflect the primary lesion.[38] In contrast, lesions of the vagus nerve can be found in even early cases of achalasia and reportedly resemble Wallerian degeneration. Thus, it is currently thought that a degenerative lesion in the dorsal motor nucleus of the vagus or in the peripheral nerve itself is responsible for idiopathic achalasia.[39]

3.2.2. Diffuse Esophageal Spasm (DES)

This syndrome is characterized by intermittent chest pain and/or dysphagia that is usually not progressive or associated with weight loss. The pain may mimic angina pectoris and frequently is triggered by the ingestion of either very hot or cold liquids. In severe cases, the barium esophagram reveals diffuse, incoordinated contractions of the lower esophagus with barium propelled both retrogradely and into the stomach. These contractions distort the esophagus, resulting in graphic descriptions such as the "corkscrew" or "rosary-bead" esophagus. More commonly, however, the esophagram will show marginal serrations of the barium column—"tertiary contractions." Caution must be used in interpreting these tertiary contractions as they are occasionally seen in normals, particularly the elderly, and are seldom associated with chest pain. Radionuclide studies often show chaotic, to-and-fro bolus transit but overall emptying in the upright position is not significantly delayed.

There is controversy over the manometric criteria for the diagnosis of DES. A recent literature review[40] has indicated that the manometric hallmarks of this disease are simultaneous contractions intermixed with normal peristaltic sequences. In our laboratory, we require two manometric findings to make the diagnosis of DES: (1) simultaneous contractions occurring after greater than 10% of transmitted wet swallows and (2) some normal peristaltic waves (Fig. 3). Others have proposed a minimum of 30% simultaneous contractions after dry swallows for such a diagnosis.[41] However, we do not believe dry swallows should be used to define EMDs because simultaneous contractions may be seen after 80% and even 100% of dry swallows in healthy adults.[32] Repetitive contractions (> two peaks), spontaneous contractions, increased amplitude or duration of contractions, increased LES pressure, and incomplete LES relaxation may be seen in DES but are not absolutely required for the diagnosis.[40] Using these criteria, DES accounts for about 10% of EMDs diagnosed in patients with noncardiac chest pain referred to our laboratory.[42]

Although simultaneous contractions represent a major alteration in esophageal function, their pathologic cause is not understood. Some DES patients will develop classic achalasia suggesting an evolving neuropathic disorder.[38] The occasional finding of poor LES relaxation in DES patients has suggested that simultaneous contractions may simply be a response to distal obstruction.[25,41] However, a more diffuse lesion seems likely since abnormal contraction waves are always observed, yet failed LES relaxation is noted in less than one-third of patients. Recent electromyographic studies in DES patients have demonstrated spike-independent contractions of the esophageal body and increased excit-

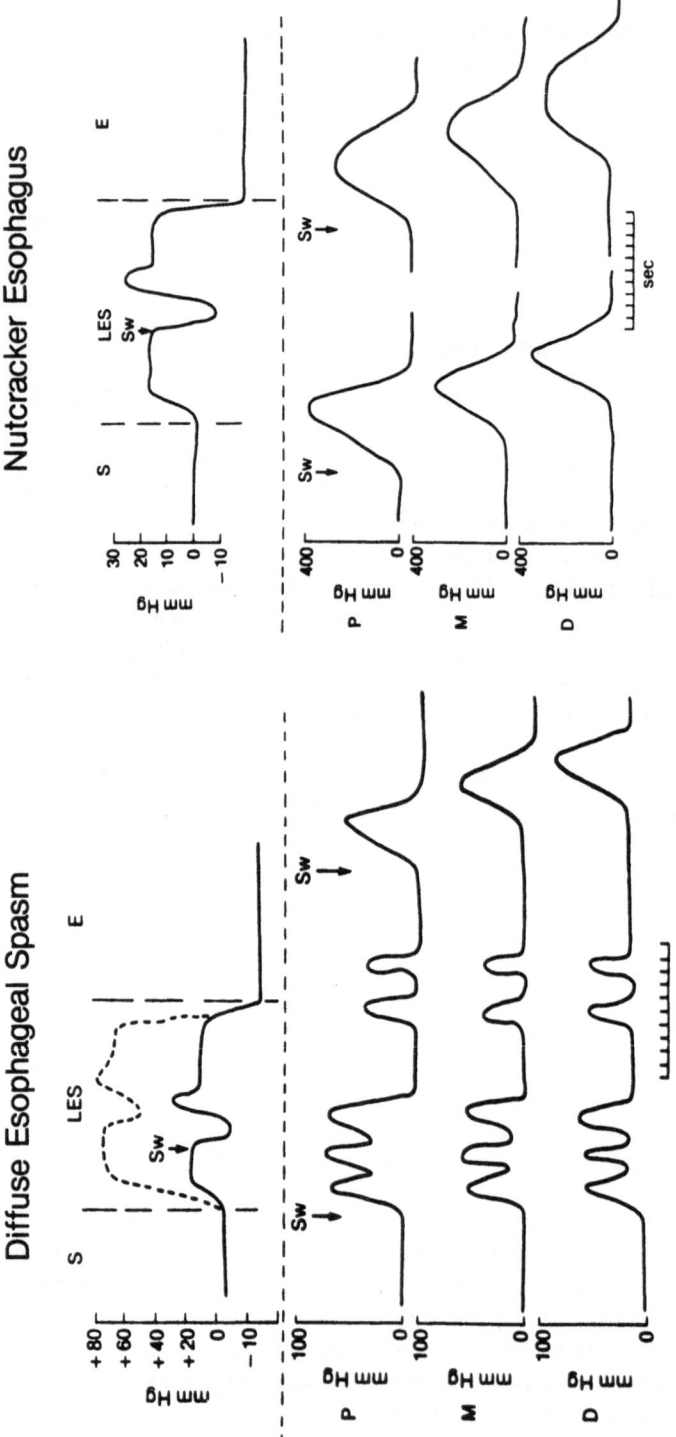

Figure 3. Diagrammatic examples of esophageal manometric tracings in patient with diffuse esophageal spasm (left) and nutcracker esophagus (right). Similar arrangement of LES and esophageal body contractions as in Fig. 2. Left: LES pressure and relaxation are usually normal in diffuse esophageal spasm. However, a third of patients may have a hypertensive LES with incomplete relaxation. Contractions in the body of the esophagus are a mixture of normal peristaltic waves and simultaneous contractions. Simultaneous contractions may be multipeaked, spontaneous (not associated with a swallow), or associated with high-amplitude or long-duration wave forms. Right: LES pressure and relaxation are normal in the nutcracker esophagus. Swallow-induced contractions are peristaltic but associated with high-amplitude and occasionally long-duration wave forms.

ability of spontaneous spike activity.[43] These findings may represent impaired non-cholinergic–nonadrenergic inhibitory neural mechanisms. An imbalance between excitatory and inhibitory innervation could conceivably lead to simultaneous, repetitive contractions. Despite these studies, there is little documentation of neuropathologic lesions from smooth muscle segments obtained at the time of myotomy. Disrupted vagal fibers within the esophageal wall have been noted by electron microscopy but ganglion cells have not been observed to be reduced or damaged.[44] To further complicate the matter, simultaneous contractions frequently may be recorded in asymptomatic healthy subjects. Approximately 15% of dry swallows may be followed by simultaneous contractions[32] and emotional stresses may produce simultaneous contractions.[45] Thus, DES may represent a heterogeneous group of pathophysiologic mechanisms. In some patients, it may be nothing more than a transient aberrant motor activity resulting from stressful environmental factors. In others, it may be part of a spectrum of evolving esophageal smooth muscle denervation which terminates in achalasia.

3.2.3. Nutcracker Esophagus

In 1977, Brand et al.[46] reported that 41% of noncardiac chest pain patients with abnormal esophageal manometry showed a pattern of high-amplitude peristaltic contractions. Two years later, Benjamin et al.[47] confirmed these observations and coined the term *nutcracker esophagus*. Subsequently, this manometric diagnosis has been found in 27 to 48% of patients with noncardiac chest pain having abnormal esophageal motility reported from many areas of the country.[31,42,48–50]

The nutcracker esophagus represents the prototype of the new EMDs described as the result of our improved technology and better understanding of the range of normal esophageal pressures. By definition, the nutcracker esophagus is a descriptive term for the manometric finding in patients with chest pain and/or dysphagia characterized by average distal esophageal peristaltic pressures greater than two standard deviations above a well-documented normal range (Fig. 3). In our laboratory, this is defined by average peristaltic pressures (mean of ten wet swallows) exceeding 180 mm Hg as defined by studies in 95 healthy subjects ranging in age from 22 to 79 years.[32]

From a statistical standpoint, there is no doubt that these high-amplitude peristaltic pressures represent a deviation from the normal contraction parameters seen in asymptomatic healthy adults. However, this gives us no assurance that these ''abnormal contractions'' represent an aberrant physiologic state that causes chest pain. Although high-amplitude esophageal contractions may be found more frequently in patients with noncardiac chest pain, these individuals are usually asymptomatic when the diagnosis is made. The barium swallow[51] and radionuclide transit studies[3] are usually normal as the result of orderly peristalsis propelling the bolus along the esophagus. Occasionally a defect in esophageal transit is seen but this likely results from intermittent simultaneous contractions.[52] Furthermore, chest pain improvement does not predictably correlate with amplitude reduction by either calcium channel blockers[15] or surgical myotomy.[16] Therefore, the relationship of chest pain and high-amplitude esophageal peristaltic contractions does not appear to be causal.

Comparable to DES, the nutcracker esophagus may be a heterogeneous disorder. Several patients with the nutcracker esophagus have evolved to diffuse esophageal spasm[53] and even achalasia (Don Gerhardt, personal communication). Furthermore, recent studies suggest that high-amplitude contractions may represent a primary esophageal response to environmental stressors.[54] Although occasional patients have undergone surgical myotomy for this disorder, reports are not available about muscle histology or neurophysiology. Therefore, many questions remain unanswered about the nutcracker esophagus.

3.2.4. Hypertensive LES

This manometric finding in patients with chest pain and dysphagia was first described by Code et al. from the Mayo Clinic.[55] These patients were characterized by increased resting LES pressure associated with normal LES relaxation and normal peristalsis. A subsequent report by Garrett and Godwin[56] also found that these patients had excessively large and prolonged contractions of the sphincter following relaxation, a phenomenon called the "hypercontracting or hyperreacting sphincter." It is quite likely that some of these patients belong to the subsequently described motility disorder, nutcracker esophagus. In our laboratory, hypertensive LES is defined by sphincter pressure exceeding two standard deviations above the normal range (> 45 mm Hg).[32] In our experience, hypertensive LES is an uncommon disorder accounting for 4% of chest pain patients and 2% of dysphagia patients with EMDs.

It is not clear why hypertensive LES should produce symptoms of chest pain and dysphagia. Recently, we have observed that residual LES pressure after relaxation is significantly elevated in these patients [6.3 ± 1.0 mm Hg (± S.E.)] compared to control subjects (1.1 ± 0.3 mm Hg).[57] However, barium esophagrams and upright solid esophageal emptying studies revealed no delay in liquid or solid bolus transport or emptying. Gastroesophageal reflux and psychologic factors have been suggested as possible causes of hypertensive LES. Like many of the other EMDs, histologic and neuropharmacologic studies are not available from resected esophageal specimens.

3.2.5. Nonspecific EMDs

When evaluating a large number of patients for potential esophageal motility abnormalities, a frequent finding is the presence of esophageal contraction patterns that are outside the range of normal findings, yet do not readily fit into the more clearly defined categories of the other EMDs (Table II). We have placed these miscellaneous abnormalities into the general classification of "nonspecific EMDs." These patterns represent a broad spectrum of abnormalities, and the true clinical significance remains to be elucidated. In some cases, these findings are clearly a precursor to the eventual development of a more defined primary motility disorder. We have seen at least one patient who has shown a transition from a nonspecific motility disorder to DES and later classic achalasia.

3.3. Secondary EMDs

In addition to the primary EMDs, a variety of secondary esophageal motility problems may occur as the result of systemic conditions. Many of these patients have severe disturbances of motility but relatively few symptoms. Esophageal manometry is the best test to evaluate the presence of these secondary EMDs.

3.3.1. Collagen Vascular Diseases

The esophagus may be affected by almost any collagen vascular disease, though involvement is most commonly seen with progressive systemic sclerosis (PSS), poly-myositis, and mixed connective tissue disease. PSS (also known as scleroderma) is a disease characterized by fibrosis and degenerative changes in many organs of the body. The esophagus is involved in 75 to 85% of all patients with PSS. Pathologic changes of PSS, which are confined to the lower two-thirds (smooth muscle portion) of the esophagus, give rise to diminished to absent lower esophageal peristalsis and an incompetent LES.[59] Thus, the most common esophageal symptoms attributed to PSS are heartburn and regurgitation. Polymyositis (termed dermatomyositis when accompanied by the classic skin changes) is a diffuse inflammatory disease of striated muscle characterized by sym-metrical muscle weakness and atrophy of the proximal muscle groups. The esophagus is involved in 60 to 70% of cases.[60] Since the upper third of the esophagus is primarily involved in polymyositis, oropharyngeal contractions and proximal esophageal peristalsis may be impaired. Some reports also suggest lower esophageal dysfunction.[60] Cine-radiography studies will commonly show nasopharyngeal reflux, tracheal aspiration, disorganized pharyngeal emptying, and vallecular pooling. Mixed connective tissue dis-ease represents a mixture of clinical features found in PSS, polymyositis, and systemic lupus erythematosus, and diagnosed by the presence of high titers of a circulated antibody for a nuclear ribonucleoprotein antigen. More than 60% of patients have esophageal involvement by either manometry or barium esophagram.[61] The manometric findings are a mixture of the two previous diseases.

3.3.2. Endocrine and Metabolic Disorders

Diabetes mellitus, especially in conjunction with peripheral neuropathy, can produce a myriad of motility abnormalities. Pathophysiologic changes are the result of degener-ative effects of diabetes on the autonomic nervous system rather than smooth muscle dysfunction. The most frequently described manometric abnormalities include decreased amplitude of peristalsis and LES pressure, reduction in primary peristalsis, and increased repetitive or spontaneous contractions.[62,63] More recently,[64] an increased incidence of peristaltic double-peaked waves has been described in diabetics with peripheral neuropa-thy. The significance of this finding remains to be determined, since double-peaked waves frequently occur in normals.[32] The clinical importance of any of these motility abnor-malities is uncertain, since most diabetic patients are asymptomatic. Esophageal motor abnormalities have been reported in both hyperthyroidism and hypothyroidism. An in-crease in velocity of esophageal peristalsis has been described in patients with Graves's disease.[65] On the other hand, patients with myxedema may have a decrease in peristaltic amplitude, velocity, primary peristalsis, or LES pressure.[66] Manometric abnormalities attributed to amyloidosis include a decrease in LES pressure, a decrease in both upper and lower esophageal peristaltic amplitude, simultaneous contractions, and even an achalasia-like picture. In the largest series reported, greater than 60% of patients with systemic amyloidosis had esophageal motility abnormalities.[67] These derangements have been attributed to random deposition of amyloid in the muscles and nerves of the esophagus.

3.3.3. Neuromuscular Disorders

Myotonic dystrophy, myasthenia gravis, multiple sclerosis, Parkinson's disease, cerebral vascular diseases, and amyotrophic lateral sclerosis may affect motility in the esophageal body as well as the oropharynx and UES.[68] As a result of neurologic involvement and muscle wasting, the motility changes are usually seen in the striated muscle portion of the esophagus but smooth muscle involvement has been reported. Manometric abnormalities include decreased contraction amplitude, simultaneous and repetitive waves, impaired LES relaxation, and even patterns consistent with DES.

3.3.4. Chronic Idiopathic Intestinal Pseudoobstruction (CIIP)

This is a syndrome characterized by intermittent symptoms and signs of intestinal obstruction without evidence of actual mechanical blockage. Pathophysiologic changes may be the result of either a neuropathy or myopathy involving the gastrointestinal smooth muscle. One report suggests that at least 85% of all patients with CIIP have abnormal findings by esophageal manometry.[69] Most patients exhibit aperistalsis and variable abnormalities in the LES which mimic achalasia. However, many patients with CIIP do not exhibit dysphagia and those who do apparently do not respond to the usual treatment for achalasia.[69]

3.3.5. Chagas's Disease

This disease is caused by a protozoan, *Trypanosoma cruzi,* commonly found in South America. Chagas's disease affects multiple organs, including the myenteric plexus of the gastrointestinal tract, and produces esophageal manifestations identical to achalasia. Manometry, which may be abnormal even prior to symptoms, reveals a pattern indistinguishable from primary achalasia.[70]

3.3.6. Gastroesophageal Reflux Disease

Although intermittent dysphagia is common, EMDs aside from LES dysfunction are rare in reflux patients. Acid perfusion studies occasionally evoke abnormal esophageal contractions,[8] but acid-induced heartburn or pain usually is not associated with dysmotility.[9] Patients with peptic strictures[71] or Barrett's esophagus[72] frequently have very low LES pressures and decreased amplitude of distal esophageal contractions. However, normal peristalsis usually persists although simultaneous, repetitive contractions and aperistalsis have been reported.[72] Resolution of esophagitis does not improve these EMDs, suggesting they result from smooth muscle fibrosis or irreversible nerve damage.[73] All patients being considered for antireflux surgery should be evaluated by manometry. An alternative diagnosis can rarely be made. More importantly, preoperative manometry allows assessment of the adequacy of peristaltic pressures in the esophageal body. If the patient has severely disordered or weak peristalsis, a traditional fundoplication may result in postoperative dysphagia due to defective esophageal clearing. Therefore, the surgeon may wish to perform a "loose" fundoplication or a gastropexy.

3.3.7. Aging and the Esophagus

Based on radiographic[74] and manometric studies[75] performed in the early 1960s, it was initially felt that the aging process produced certain patterns of esophageal dysfunction, i.e., "presbyesophagus." These studies in a group of nonagenarians demonstrated decreased primary peristalsis, simultaneous contractions, decreased LES relaxation, and increased spontaneous contractions. However, patients with systemic disorders such as diabetis mellitus or other neurologic diseases were not necessarily excluded. Later studies in healthy elderly patients without systemic diseases and peripheral neuropathies have found minimal evidence of esophageal dysfunction—primarily a decrease in the amplitude or force of esophageal contractions and a slight decrease in the frequency of primary peristalsis.[76,77] Therefore, severe motility abnormalities, when encountered in the elderly, are most often due to systemic disease rather than to the aging process.

4. DIAGNOSTIC STUDIES

4.1. Radiology

Patients presenting with dysphagia and esophageal chest pain initially should be evaluated by radiographic studies of the esophagus. The conventional barium esophagram using a double contrast technique is the best method for this examination. In the body of the esophagus, its greatest value is to rule out structural lesions associated with dysphagia. Mucosal changes of esophagitis, if present, are highly specific for reflux disease.[78] Spontaneous reflux and hiatus hernia are supportive of an acid-induced motility disorder but must be interpreted with caution as both may be seen in normals. Depending on the type of EMD, the diagnostic accuracy of the barium esophagram will vary. This point is illustrated by our recent experience with radiographic and manometric examinations of the esophagus in 172 patients with dysphagia.[79] As shown in Table III, overall radiographic sensitivity for identifying an EMD was 56% (37 of 66) but increased to 89% by excluding

Table III. Radiographic Diagnosis of Esophageal Motility
Disorders Detected by Manometry

Manometry diagnosis	No. of patients	
	Total	Diagnosed radiographically
Nonspecific EMDs	26	12 (46%)
Achalasia	19	18 (95%)
Nutcracker esophagus	12	0 (0%)
Diffuse esophageal spasm	7	5 (71%)
Scleroderma	2	2 (100%)
Total	66	37 (56%)

the nutcracker esophagus and nonspecific EMDs. In 106 manometrically normal patients, radiographic specificity was 91% with 10 false-positive diagnoses of nonspecific motor disorders. Fluoroscopic observation and video tape recording greatly aid in evaluating oropharyngeal swallowing disorders and the UES. Permanent motion recording techniques allow the films to be slowly played back and studied in order to identify many of the subtle abnormalities associated with oropharyngeal dysphagia.

4.2. Fiberoptic Endoscopy

Endoscopic evaluation of the esophagus has little value in the routine assessment of EMDs. Its major role is to help evaluate possible structural lesions in patients with dysphagia and to rule out distal esophageal carcinoma simulating achalasia.

4.3. Radionuclide Transit Studies

Radionuclide scintigraphy, in which a gamma camera is used to follow a bolus of technetium sulfur colloid down the esophagus, is a new, safe, and relatively sensitive test of esophageal function. Transit time can be measured and a statement made about the pattern of bolus movement. Abnormal peristalsis and delayed emptying are readily detected. Russell et al.[80] found liquid radionuclide transient studies performed in the supine position to be 100% sensitive in 15 patients with identified motility disorders. In addition, 9 of 15 patients with dysphagia and normal esophageal manometry were found to have transit abnormalities. Achalasia and scleroderma had similar adynamic bolus transit patterns (Fig. 4) and were distinguished by their emptying times. Both were easily discriminated from the chaotic, to-and-fro pattern seen with diffuse esophageal spasm (Fig. 4). False-positives may result from double swallows, unrecognized gastroesophageal reflux, or residual activity in an unsuspected hiatal hernia.[81] False-negatives occur from intermittent esophageal dysmotility or EMDs associated with orderly peristalsis such as the nutcracker esophagus and hypertensive LES.[2] For these reasons, the radionuclide transit study never fulfilled its initial promise as a simple screening test for suspected EMDs. Solid food scintigraphy with the patient in an upright position is the study that most approximates normal food ingestion. This measure of LES relaxation and esophageal emptying is an excellent means of assessing the success of treatment in achalasia.[82] We also have found it to be a useful adjunct to the barium esophagram in the diagnosis of early achalasia where apparent complete LES relaxation may confuse the diagnosis.[35]

4.4. Esophageal Manometry

Manometric evaluation of the esophagus is the definitive test for the diagnosis of EMDs. The development of constant-perfusion, low-compliance systems has made it possible to accurately measure pressures in the esophageal body and sphincters. Accurate measurement of LES pressure can be accomplished using the rapid pull-through or station pull-through techniques. Motility in the body of the esophagus is measured using at least three catheter ports 5 cm apart. An accurate evaluation of amplitude, duration, and velocity of peristaltic contractions can be made with wet swallows of water given every 30 sec. UES basal pressures and coordination can be readily assessed, but perfused systems

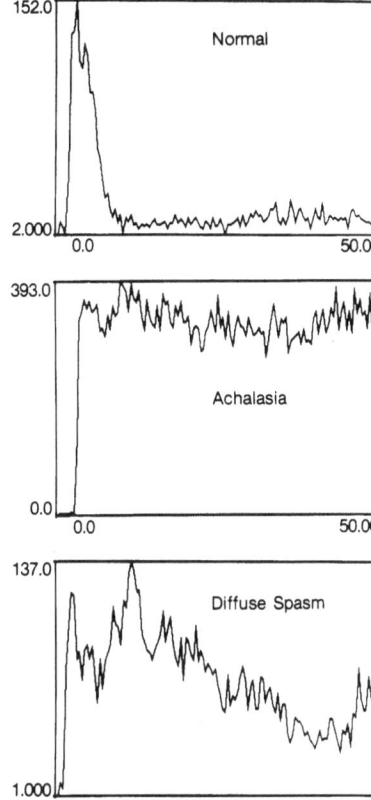

Figure 4. Esophageal radionuclide liquid transit studies in a normal subject (top) and patient with achalasia (middle) and diffuse esophageal spasm (bottom). Radioactivity counts are on vertical axis and time in seconds on horizontal axis. Normal transit time is less than 15 sec. Achalasia has an adynamic bolus transit pattern with delayed emptying time. In contrast, diffuse esophageal spasm demonstrates a chaotic, to-and-fro pattern with delayed transit time.

do not accurately record pharyngeal pressures. Esophageal manometry has its limitations. Although accurately recording esophageal pressures, this technique *does not* reliably evaluate other important aspects of esophageal function, i.e., bolus movement or esophageal emptying.

In our recent 3-year experience with 1161 patients referred for esophageal manometry,[42] EMDs were significantly more prevalent in patients evaluated for dysphagia (132/251, 53%) than in patients evaluated for noncardiac chest pain (255/910, 28%). The nutcracker esophagus was the commonest motility disorder seen in patients with noncardiac chest pain but was infrequent in patients with dysphagia. In contrast, achalasia was common in patients with dysphagia but rare in patients with noncardiac chest pain (Fig. 5).

4.5. Provocative Tests

The majority of patients with suspected esophageal chest pain have normal esophageal motility. Even when an EMD is defined, patients usually are asymptomatic. Therefore, one cannot be certain that the esophagus is the source of pain. Hence, a number of physical or pharmacologic means have been tried to induce dysmotility and chest pain. This is analogous to treadmill testing to elicit EKG changes and chest pain in patients with

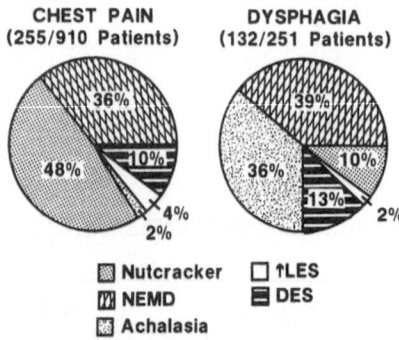

CHEST PAIN
(255/910 Patients)

DYSPHAGIA
(132/251 Patients)

■ Nutcracker □ ↑LES
▨ NEMD   ▤ DES
▨ Achalasia

Figure 5. Incidence of esophageal motility disorders in patients with noncardiac chest pain (left) and dysphagia (right). NEMD, nonspecific esophageal motility disorder; ↑ LES, hypertensive lower esophageal sphincter; DES, diffuse esophageal spasm. Reprinted with permission from Annals of Internal Medicine 106:594, 1987.

suspected angina. Intravenous ergonovine has been shown to produce increased esophageal contractions and reproduce chest pain, but the risk of undesirable cardiac side effects has limited its routine use in the esophageal laboratory.[83,84] Intravenous edrophonium (Tensilon) has emerged as the most popular and potentially most helpful pharmacologic test for esophageal chest pain. Recent experiences with edrophonium have indicated a positivity rate (defined as reproduction of the patient's chest pain) of 24% in one large series[85] using a dose of 80 μg/kg and a positivity rate of 35% in a smaller study with a dose of 10 mg.[86] Edrophonium has not caused chest pain in over 150 healthy subjects.[85] We believe a positive Tensilon test indicates that the esophagus is the source of the patient's chest pain. However, it may not specifically identify the pathophysiology of the pain. The changes in esophageal contractile activity after edrophonium have not predictably distinguished patients with chest pain from healthy subjects.[85–87] Furthermore, a positive Tensilon response can occur in patients with reflux esophagitis.[87] A recent report has indicated that an exceptionally high positive response rate can be obtained using repeated large doses of bethanechol.[88] In a study of 87 patients with noncardiac chest pain, 77% experienced a reproduction of their atypical chest pain following two subcutaneous injections of bethanechol (50 μg/kg) separated by 15 min. However, over half of these patients experienced troubling side effects during the testing procedure.

Other innovative provocative tests have included inflation of an esophageal balloon and measurements of motility during food ingestion. We found that balloon distension produced chest pain in 18/30 (60%) patients, but only 6/30 (20%) healthy volunteers.[19] Balloon pressures and esophageal contractions did not distinguish chest pain patients from control subjects. However, patients were observed to have pain at lower volumes of balloon distension, suggesting the presence of a lowered pain threshold. Mellow et al.[89] found that food ingestion frequently brought out dysphagia and EMDs missed by standard manometry. In a study of 54 patients, dysphagia occurred during food ingestion alone in 21 patients versus 2 patients with water swallows alone. In addition, all but 2 of the patients with food-provoked dysphagia had a motility abnormality seen within 30 sec of reporting their symptoms.

4.6. 24-hr Motility Testing

The critical test in evaluating patients with recurring chest pain should be to identify abnormal esophageal function at the time of spontaneous pain events. To this end, the concept of ambulatory prolonged monitoring of intraesophageal activity has evolved. Intraesophageal pH monitoring has shown that gastroesophageal reflux is a common cause of esophageal chest pain. The technology for ambulatory intraesophageal pressure monitoring has lagged behind pH monitoring but is now emerging as a research tool. Janssens et al.[13] originally reported findings for a group of 60 patients with noncardiac chest pain in which 24-hr esophageal pressures and pH monitoring revealed that 21 patients had an abnormal esophageal episode (30% motility, 19% reflux, 43% both) at the time of a pain event. This report is somewhat confusing since the criteria for an abnormal motility episode were not clearly defined. Using a more defined requirement for abnormal pressures based on an individual standard established for each patient from the 24-hr recording, we[14] found that only 12% of pain events were associated with abnormal motility, 20% with reflux episodes, and an additional 4% with both abnormal motility and reflux. In the remaining 64% of chest pain episodes, no esophageal abnormalities could be identified. Patients frequently were found to experience multiple chest pain episodes over the 24-hr study, *only some* of which were associated with a fall in intraesophageal pH or an abnormal contraction pattern. These preliminary reports suggest that EMDs may not be as common a cause of esophageal chest pain as previously reported. Furthermore, the complex nature of these patients' chest pains may account for their generally poor response to conventional medical therapies.

5. APPROACH TO THE DIAGNOSIS OF EMDs

The diagnostic evaluation of a patient with suspected EMD should be directed by the patient's primary complaint of either dysphagia or chest pain (Fig. 6). All patients with dysphagia should initially be evaluated by a barium esophagram with fluoroscopic observation or video tape recording of the swallowing mechanism. Identification of an anatomic cause of dysphagia generally will be followed by endoscopy. The presence of a normal esophagram or aberrant bolus activity should suggest a functional disorder. Esophageal manometry will be required to precisely define the presence of an EMD. Radionuclide scintigraphic studies may be required to assess the impact of abnormal esophageal pressures on bolus movement or esophageal emptying. If chest pain is the predominant symptom, the diagnostic approach should differ somewhat. Because of the potentially more serious prognosis, coronary artery disease should be ruled out initially. An upper gastrointestinal series with barium esophagram (or perhaps endoscopy) should follow to identify peptic ulcer disease and esophagitis as the possible cause of chest pain. If these studies are unrevealing, esophageal manometry with provocative tests (Bernstein and Tensilon) are performed. Prolonged ambulatory pH and/or pressure studies also may be done to better define the presence of gastroesophageal reflux and the relationship between EMDs and chest pain.

6. PSYCHOLOGIC ABNORMALITIES IN EMDs

The gastrointestinal tract is a sensitive organ of emotional expression. Although the stomach and colon have been the traditional sites for investigation of emotional influences on motility, clinical experience and experimental observations indicate that esophageal

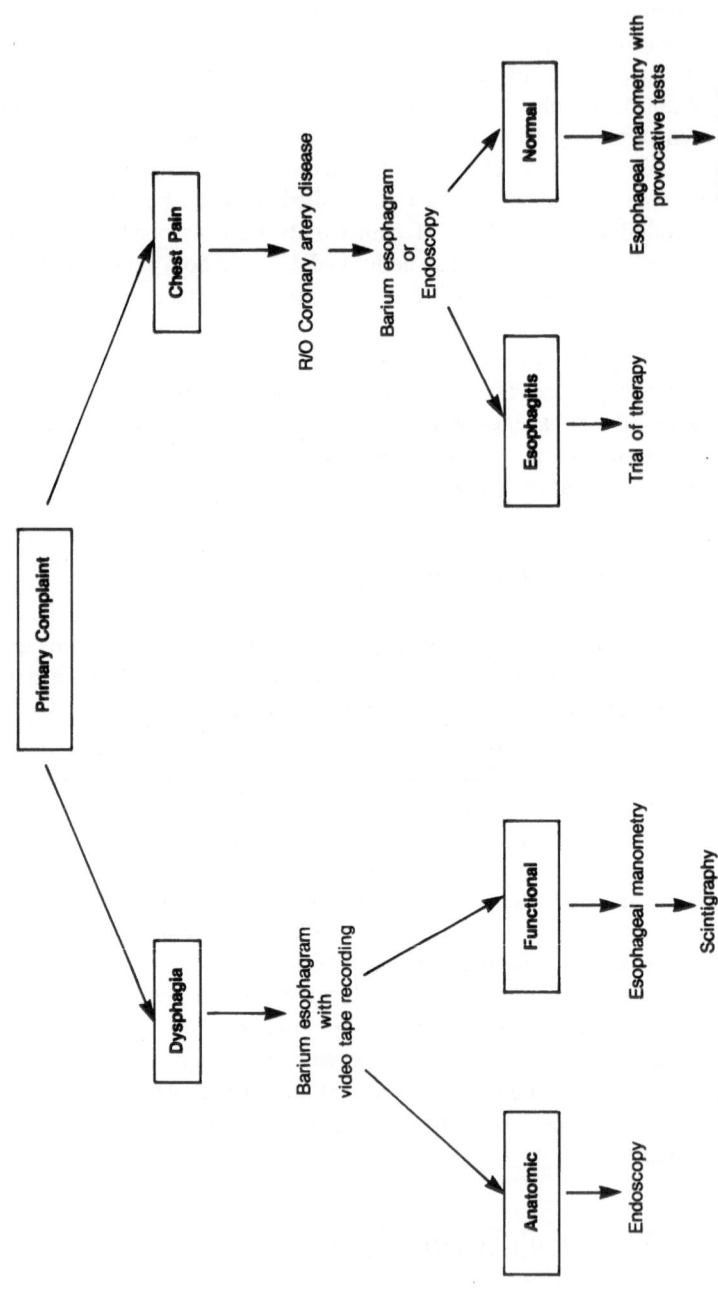

Figure 6. Algorithm for the evaluation of esophageal motility disorders directed by the patient's primary complaint of either dysphagia or chest pain.

function is also affected by emotional stimuli. Kronecker and Meltzer reported in 1883 that psychic upset induced esophageal contractions.[90] In 1892, Sir William Osler[91] wrote: "Esophagismus (esophageal spasm) is met with in hysterical patients and hypochondriacs. . . . The idiopathic form is found in females of a marked neurotic habit. . . ." Uncontrolled observations have found that stressful interviews commonly elicit uncoordinated esophageal contractions.[92]

Two recent studies of patients with EMDs have renewed interest in the association between psychologic stress and esophageal motility abnormalities. Clouse and Lustman [93] found that 21 of 25 patients (84%) with abnormal distal esophageal contractions received a psychiatric diagnosis (primarily depression, anxiety, and somatization) during a structured psychiatric interview. In contrast, only 4 of 13 patients (31%) with normal manometric patterns were given psychiatric diagnoses. In our laboratory, we[94] administered the Millon Behavioral Health Inventory to patient groups with chest pain and the nutcracker esophagus, the irritable bowel syndrome, and those with benign structural esophageal abnormalities as well as to healthy controls. Both the nutcracker esophagus and irritable bowel patient groups had significantly higher scores than all other groups on the Somatic Anxiety and Gastrointestinal Susceptibility Scales. This pattern suggested that these patients tend to show excessive concern regarding somatic functions and react to psychologic stress with increases in the frequency and severity of gastrointestinal symptoms. Similar results have been found in patients with chest pain and a hypertensive LES.[57]

Chest pain patients with EMDs have been found to have lower pain thresholds for esophageal balloon distension,[19] an effect similar to rectal balloon studies in irritable bowel patients.[95] In both groups, this abnormal sensory perception appears to be independent of gut contractile activity or increased wall tension. However, it is unknown to what extent this altered pain perception results from one or more of the following causes: dysfunction of the afferent nervous system, disordered central processing by the brain, or environmental and emotional factors that modify the verbal report of pain. Preliminary studies[96] indicate that esophageal balloon distension can evoke changes in electrical potentials over the cerebral cortex where central processing of internal and external stimuli occurs. Furthermore, conditioning can improve the perception of stimuli from internal organs so that a person senses physiologic changes he or she was not aware of previously, i.e., "selective perception."[97] Anxiety coupled with depression serves as a source of selective perception. The patient becomes progressively more anxious, which leads to more somatic symptoms, which in turn leads to more anxiety, more selective perception, and a vicious cycle (Fig. 7).

These investigations have demonstrated an association between psychologic stress and EMDs. However, they have not produced any evidence of a cause-and-effect nature. One approach to revealing the direction of this relationship is to administer psychologic stressors to individuals in the laboratory while monitoring esophageal pressures. Older studies demonstrated that simultaneous esophageal contractions may be induced in healthy individuals by administering stressful interviews[45] or noxious acoustic stimuli.[98] Using modern manometric instruments, we have recently evaluated the effects of stress on esophageal motility in healthy individuals[99] and esophageal chest pain patients.[54] In both studies, significant increases in esophageal contraction amplitude were the primary response to laboratory stressors including unpredictable bursts of white noise and difficult cognitive problems. After controlling for baseline pressure differences, patients with the

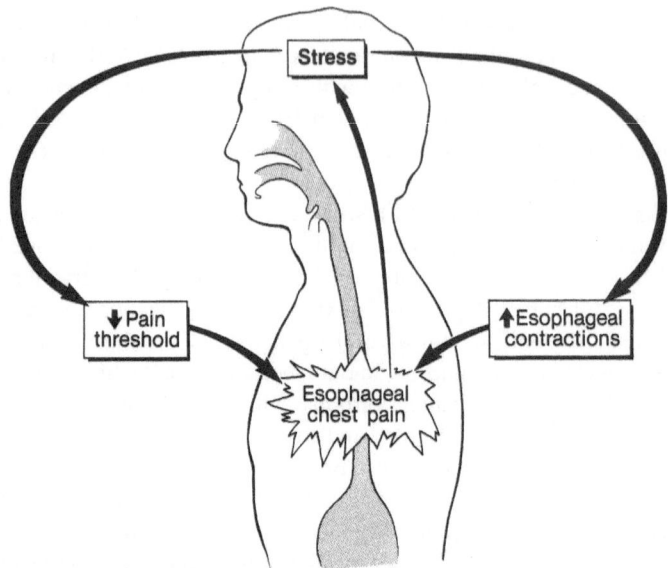

Figure 7. Hypothetical interaction between psychologic stress, lowered visceral pain threshold, and increased esophageal contraction amplitude in the pathogenesis of esophageal chest pain.

nutcracker esophagus demonstrated significantly greater increases in contraction amplitude than did control subjects. Moreover, four of the nine patients with normal baseline esophageal manometric values increased their contraction amplitudes into the nutcracker range during the cognitive problems. Contrary to earlier reports, our studies did not reveal an increase in the frequency of simultaneous contractions during stress.

Other intriguing clinical observations lend support to our laboratory studies. During 24-hr ambulatory pressure monitoring, we have observed that abnormal motility will often occur *after* the onset of chest pain.[14] In 7 of 15 chest pain episodes associated with high-amplitude or prolonged-duration contractions, these abnormal waves began 6 to 20 contractions (up to 10 min) after the patients complained of chest pain. In another report,[100] 9 of 14 patients undergoing the stress of acute alcohol withdrawal were found to have esophageal pressures meeting the manometric criteria for nutcracker esophagus. One month after alcohol abstinence, their esophageal pressures had returned to normal values. Therefore, EMDs such as the nutcracker esophagus and possibly DES and hypertensive LES may in some patients simply be manometric markers of a clinical stress syndrome rather than being directly responsible for symptoms.

7. MEDICAL AND SURGICAL THERAPIES

7.1. Disorders of the UES

It must be remembered that isolated UES dysfunction is an uncommon disorder. Therefore, successful therapy must involve correction of the underlying cause of the deglutition problem. Unfortunately, the majority of neuromuscular causes of oropharyngeal dysphagia are not treatable. Patients with Parkinson's disease, myasthenia gravis, polymyositis, metabolic myopathies, and possibly mononeuritis multiplex may improve with appropriate drug therapy (e.g., L-dopa, anticholinesterases, steroids). Cricopharyngeal myotomy has been advocated in neuromuscular diseases involving the pharynx, but are much less often successful than when used in patients with isolated UES dysfunction. Patients submitted to surgery for Zenker's diverticulum frequently undergo cricopharyngeal myotomy.[28] The basis for inclusion of a myotomy is the theory that Zenker's diverticulum is due to malfunction of the UES. As previously discussed, manometric studies supporting this concept are equivocal. There are no good controlled studies of the relative benefit of diverticulectomy with and without myotomy.

7.2. Achalasia

The goal of therapy in achalasia is to partially destroy the high-pressure LES. If emptying is improved, esophageal stasis and its consequences are reduced. Even though peristalsis rarely returns, the patient feels as if deglutition is normal.

The calcium channel blocker nifedipine, taken sublingually before meals, decreases LES pressure and temporarily improves the symptoms associated with achalasia. However, placebo-controlled clinical studies are not available. In my experience, nifedipine is useful as a temporizing agent in patients with mild symptoms or as definitive therapy in the elderly or patients with contraindications to pneumatic dilatation or surgical myotomy. Otherwise, pneumatic dilatation should be the initial therapy for most patients with achalasia. When properly performed, the success rate of pneumatic dilatation nearly approaches that of surgery and the likelihood of subsequent gastroesophageal reflux is less, the duration of hospitalization is shorter, and overall morbidity is considerably less than that of the Heller myotomy. Indications for primary surgical treatment of achalasia should include: (1) several unsuccessful attempts at pneumatic dilatation; (2) inability to exclude esophageal carcinoma; and (3) children and psychotic patients who are unable to cooperate.

Pneumatic dilatation involves distending a balloon positioned in the LES to the point that the sphincter muscles are torn without rupturing the esophagus. Preferred balloon dilators include the Brown–McHardy, or if a guide wire is necessary due to esophageal tortuosity, the Rider–Moeller or Microvasive achalasia balloon systems. Balloons are available in diameters ranging from 2.9 to 5.0 cm. Initial dilatations are performed with smaller diameter balloons and increased if repeated procedures are required. The largest studies indicate that 60 to 95% of patients have good clinical results (usually defined as no further dysphagia) after pneumatic dilatation.[102] The incidence of esophageal perforation ranges from 1 to 16% with the majority of these cases being small, localized perforations which can be treated with medical therapy. Gastroesophageal reflux is not a significant postdilatation problem, occurring in less than 7% of patients.

Most modern forms of surgical therapy for achalasia are variations on an esophageal myotomy, first performed by Heller in 1913. This operation involves incising the circular muscle fibers down to the mucosa and allowing the mucosa to protrude through. Most of the current variations are related to the length of the myotomy. Classic achalasia does not require a long myotomy. In an attempt to prevent gastroesophageal reflux after a myotomy, some workers now recommend that it be combined with various types of antireflux procedures. However, this should be discouraged as a fundoplication in a patient with achalasia may lead to severe and prolonged dysphagia. In the follow-up studies of esophageal myotomy, approximately 80% of patients have a good clinical result.[102] The most common problem is the high incidence of postoperative reflux. Although this can be demonstrated in as many as 50% of subjects after esophageal myotomy, it causes symptoms in less than 15% of patients.

7.3. Painful EMDs

Treatment for patients with esophageal chest pain has been a major dilemma for clinicians for many years. Although most of the prior literature categorized this under the topic of therapy for DES, the current approaches also apply to the other primary EMDs (nutcracker esophagus, hypertensive LES, nonspecific motility disorders) as well as to patients with decreased esophageal pain thresholds. Many therapies have been proposed (Table IV), but most have not been examined in placebo-controlled trials.

Because chest pain similar to that produced by motility disorders can be caused by gastroesophageal reflux, it is important to carefully exclude this disorder. This may require a trial of good antireflux therapy for a period of 1 to 2 months. This is particularly important since many of the other therapies, aimed at decreasing esophageal contraction pressures, may exacerbate reflux.

Many patients will favorably respond to confident reassurance based on careful diagnostic studies. With the report that their symptoms are not due to cardiac disease and are caused by an esophageal problem, improvement may be noted. We have observed that this supportive approach results in better patient acceptance of their symptoms, less limitation in life-style, and frequently a decrease or resolution of their chest pain.[15,103] Considering that other therapies are often less than satisfactory, simple reassurance during office visits and telephone conversations may be the simplest, safest and most cost-effective approach to these patients.

Smooth muscle relaxants, including nitrates,[104] anticholinergics,[105] and hydrala-

Table IV. Treatment for Painful Esophageal Motility Disorders

- Exclude gastroesophageal reflux
- Reassurance—key treatment
- Smooth muscle relaxants
    Nitrates
    Anticholinergics
    Hydralazine
    Calcium channel blockers
        Diltiazem
        Nifedipine
- Anxiolytics/antidepressants
    Biofeedback/behavioral modification
- Bouginage—pneumatic dilatation
- Surgery—*rarely* required

zine,[106] have been reported to decrease esophageal pressures. Some success in patients with painful EMDs has been reported, but these observations are uncontrolled and the majority of patients do not benefit from these drugs. Recently, the calcium channel blockers, diltiazem and nifedipine, have been studied in patients with EMDs. A dramatic dose–response effect on esophageal contraction pressures in patients with the nutcracker esophagus has been demonstrated with nifedipine.[107] Diltiazem has been shown to decrease amplitude and duration of peristaltic contractions.[12] However, these changes were observed only with the highest tested dose (150 mg by mouth). Unfortunately, two placebo-controlled studies have shown that nifedipine was no better than placebo in relieving chest pain in patients with the nutcracker esophagus[15] or DES.[108] Reports with diltiazem are conflicting, with one preliminary study indicating a possible effect[109] and another showing a lack of therapeutic efficacy.[110] These studies confirm that decreases in esophageal pressures alone may not improve chest pain.

Anecdotal reports have suggested that anxiolytics or antidepressants may be effective in patients with a clear stress relationship to the precipitation of their painful EMDs. A recent placebo-controlled study supports these observations. Clouse et al.[111] found that low-dose trazodone (Desyrel, 100–150 mg/day) decreased symptoms associated with EMDs without changing esophageal pressures. Behavioral modification programs and biofeedback may also be beneficial.[112,113] Contribution of emotional factors should be sought in all patients with esophageal chest pain. A simple discussion about the relationship between emotional factors and the patient's symptoms may be very helpful. More disturbed patients will require psychotropic drugs or referrals to a psychiatrist or psychologist.

Some physicians find that the passage of a 50 French dilator will promote relief from dysphagia and chest pain in patients with EMDs. In our experience, the effects of bouginage dilatation are minimal but can be produced with either a large dilator (54 French) or a much smaller "placebo" dilator (24 French).[114] It has been suggested that DES and hypertensive LES might be treated with pneumatic dilatation.[115] This procedure should be reserved for patients who have severe dysphagia and documented delay in distal esophageal emptying. A long surgical myotomy may help some patients with painful EMDs. However, surgical series are small, the overall good to excellent results only approach 50%, and the follow-up periods have usually been short. Patients with DES seem to do better than those with the nutcracker esophagus or hypertensive LES.[16] In our experience, failure of all medical regimens is quite unusual. Over the last 10 years, we have not needed to refer a single patient for surgical myotomy.[116] In support of this conservative approach, Tom DeMeester has stated: "The creation of a defect to correct a defect can never restore the function of an organ to normal."[117]

7.4. Secondary EMDs

Many of the secondary EMDs are not associated with symptoms and therefore do not need treatment. Patients with scleroderma require vigorous treatment of their gastroesophageal reflux to prevent severe esophagitis and peptic strictures. Esophageal symptoms related to mixed connective tissue disease[61] and polymyositis[60] may respond to steroid therapy. Patients with underlying thyroid disease experience resolution of their esophageal symptoms with correction of their thyroid dysfunction.[65,66] Unfortunately, the majority of neuromuscular disorders are not treatable. If patients have severe oropha-ryngeal dysphagia with frequent pulmonary aspiration and pneumonias, placement of a surgical or percutaneous endoscopic gastrostomy may be required. Symptomatic EMDs attributed to myasthenia gravis or Parkinson's disease may respond to anticholinesterases or L-dopa. Chronic idiopathic intestinal pseudoobstruction may produce an achalasia-like picture. However, patients usually do not complain of dysphagia, and those symptomatic individuals do not apparently respond to the usual treatment for achalasia.[69]

8. FUTURE PERSPECTIVES

Great strides have been made in identifying the potential importance of EMDs as a cause of dysphagia and noncardiac chest pain. However, many questions still are un-answered. Despite the relatively simple appearance of the esophagus, there remain many mysteries about the pathophysiologic causes of EMDs. Improved methods of assessing esophageal smooth muscle function and the relationship to symptoms must be developed. We still have little understanding about the complex interaction between internal esopha-geal stimuli, emotional states, and environmental factors that contribute to patients' complaints of chest pain and dysphagia. Until these questions are resolved, our therapeu-tic armamentarium will be less than perfect. One would hope that application of newer technology and multidisciplinary approach involving collaborative efforts by basic scien-tists, gastroenterologists, psychologists, and pain researchers will reveal new understand-ing and possible solutions to these problems.

ACKNOWLEDGMENTS. Supported in part by Public Health Services Grant AM 34200-01A1 from the National Institutes of Health. The excellent secretarial assistance of Kathy Myers was invaluable in the preparation of the manuscript.

REFERENCES

1. Dodds WJ: 1976 Walter B. Cannon lecture: Current concepts of esophageal motor function: Clinical implications for radiology. Am J Roentgenol 128:549–561, 1977
2. Richter JE, Blackwell JN, Wu WC, et al: Relationship of radionuclide liquid bolus transport and esophageal manometry. J Lab Clin Med 109:217–224, 1987
3. Kahrilas PJ, Dodds WJ, Hogan WJ: Effect of peristaltic dysfunction on esophageal volume clearance. Gastroenterology 94:73–80, 1988
4. Watson WC, Sullivan SN: Hypertonicity of the cricopharyngeal sphincter: A cause of globus sensation. Lancet 2:1417–1419, 1974
5. Malcolmson KG: Radiological findings in globus hystericus. Br J Radiol 39:583–586, 1966
6. Lehtinen V, Puhakka H: A psychosomatic approach to globus bystericus syndrome. Acta Psychiatr Scand 53:21–25, 1976
7. Alban-Davies H, Jones DB, Rhodes J, et al: Angina-like esophageal pain: Differentiation from cardiac pain by history. J Clin Gastroenterol 7:477–481, 1985
8. Siegel CI, Hendrix TR: Esophageal motor abnormalities induced by acid perfusion in patients with heartburn. J Clin Invest 42:686–695, 1963
9. Richter JE, Johns DN, Wu WC, et al: Are esophageal motility abnormalities produced during the intra-esophageal acid perfusion test? J Am Med Assoc 253:1914–1917, 1985
10. Mellow MH, Simpson AG, Watt L, et al: Esophageal acid perfusion in coronary artery disease: Induction of myocardial ischemia. Gastroenterology 83:306–312, 1983

11. Mellow M: Symptomatic diffuse esophageal spasm: Manometric follow-up and response to cholinergic stimulation and cholinesterace inhibition. Gastroenterology 73:237–240, 1977
12. Richter JE, Spurling TJ, Cordova CM, et al: Effects of oral calcium blocker, diltiazem, on esophageal contractions. Dig Dis Sci 29:649–656, 1984
13. Janssens J, Vantrappen G, Ghillebert F: 24 hour recording of esophageal pressure and pH in patients with non-cardiac chest pain. Gastroenterology 90:1978–1984, 1986
14. Peters LF, Maas LC, Petty D, et al: Spontaneous non-cardiac chest pain: Evaluation by 24 hour ambulatory esophageal motility and pH monitoring. Gastroenterology 94:878–886, 1988
15. Richter JE, Dalton CB, Bradley LA, et al: Oral nifedipine in the treatment of non-cardiac chest pain in patients with the nutcracker esophagus. Gastroenterology 93:21–28, 1987
16. Ellis FH, Crozier RE, Shea JA: Long esophagomyotomy for diffuse esophageal spasm and related disorders. Surgery (in press)
17. Meyer GW, Castell DO: Human esophageal response during chest pain induced by swallowing cold liquids. Am Med Assoc, 246:2057–2059, 1981
18. Kaye MD: Anomalies of peristalsis in idiopathic diffuse oesophageal spasm. Gut 22:217–222, 1981
19. Richter JE, Barish CF, Castell DO: Abnormal sensory perception in patients with esophageal chest pain. Gastroenterology 91:845–852, 1986
20. Hunt PS, Connell AM, Smiley TB: The cricopharyngeal sphincter in gastric reflux. Gut 11:303–306, 1970
21. Gerhardt DC, Shock TJ, Bordeaux RA, et al: Human upper esophageal sphincter; response to volume, osmotic and acid stimuli. Gastroenterology 75:268–274, 1978
22. Gerhardt DC, Castell DO, Winship DH, et al: Esophageal dysfunction in esophagopharyngeal regurgitation. Gastroenterology 78:893–897, 1980
23. Vantrappen G, Hellmans J: Diseases of the esophagus. Berlin, Springer-Verlag, 1974, pp 399–421
24. Kilman WJ, Goyal RK: Disorders of pharyngeal and upper esophageal sphincter motor function. Arch Intern Med 136:592–601, 1976
25. Reichert TJ, Bluestone CD, Stool SE, et al: Congenital cricopharyngeal achalasia. Ann Otol Rhinol Laryngol 86:603–610, 1977
26. Hellmans J, Agg HO, Pelemans A, et al: Pharyngoesophageal swallowing disorders and the pharyngoesophageal sphincter. Med Clin North Am 90:107–112, 1981
27. Marguilies SI, Bruut PW, Donner MW, et al: Familial dysautonomia, a cineradiographic study of the swallowing mechanism. Radiology 90:107–112, 1968
28. Ellis FH, Schlegel JF, Lynch VP, et al: Cricopharyngeal myotomy for pharyngo-esophageal diverticulum. Ann Surg 170:340–349, 1969
29. Duranceau A, Rheault MJ, Jamieson GG: Physiologic response to cricopharyngeal myotomy and diverticulum suspension. Surgery 94:655–662, 1983
30. Knuff TE, Benjamin SB, Castell DO: Pharyngoesophageal (Zenker's) diverticulum: A reappraisal. Gastroenterology 82:734–736, 1982
31. Clouse RE, Staiano A: Contraction abnormalities of the esophageal body in patients referred for manometry. Dig Dis Sci 28:784–791, 1983
32. Richter JE, Wu WC, Johns DN, et al: Esophageal manometry in 95 healthy adult volunteers. Dig Dis Sci 32:583–592, 1987
33. Cohen S: Esophageal motility disorders and their response to calcium channel antagonists. The sphinx revisited. Gastroenterology 93:201–203, 1987
34. Bondi JL, Godwin DH, Garrett JM: "Vigorous" achalasia: Its clinical interpretation and significance. Am J Gastroenterol 58:145–154, 1972
35. Katz PO, Richter JE, Cowan R, et al: Apparent complete lower esophageal sphincter relaxation in achalasia. Gastroenterology 90:978–983, 1986
36. Tucker JH, Snape WJ, Cohen S: Achalasia secondary to carcinoma. Manometric and clinical features. Ann Intern Med 89:315–318, 1978
37. Cassella RR, Brown AL, Sayre GP, et al: Achalasia of the esophagus: Pathologic and etiologic considerations. Ann Surg 160:474–479, 1964
38. Vantrappen G, Helleman J: Oesophageal spasm and other muscular dysfunction. Clin Gastroenterol 11:453–477, 1982
39. Holloway RH, Dodds WJ, Helm JF, et al: Integrity of cholinergic innervation of the lower esophageal sphincter in achalasia. Gastroenterology 90:924–929, 1986
40. Richter JE, Castell DO: Diffuse esophageal spasm: A reappraisal. Ann Intern Med 100:242–245, 1984

41. DiMarino AJ, Cohen S: Characteristics of lower esophageal sphincter in symptomatic diffuse esophageal spasm. Gastroenterology 66:1–6, 1974
42. Katz PO, Dalton CB, Richter JE, et al: Esophageal testing in patients with non-cardiac chest pain and/or dysphagia. Ann Intern Med 106:593–597, 1987
43. Ouyang A, Reynolds JC, Cohen S: Spike-associated and spike independent esophageal contractions in patients with symptomatic diffuse esophageal spasm. Gastroenterology 84:907–913, 1983
44. Gillies M, Nicks R, Skyring A: Clinical, manometric and pathological studies in diffuse oesophageal spasm. Br Med J 2:527–530, 1967
45. Rubin J, Nagler R, Spiro HM, et al: Measuring the effect of emotions on esophageal motility. Psychosom Med 24:170–176, 1962
46. Brand DL, Martin D, Pope CE: Esophageal manometrics in patients with angina-like chest pain. Am J Dig Dis 22:300–305, 1977
47. Benjamin SB, Gerhardt DC, Castell DO: High amplitude, peristaltic esophageal contractions associated with chest pain and/or dysphagia. Gastroenterology 77:478–483, 1979
48. Herrington JP, Burns TW, Balart LA: Chest pain and dysphagia in patients with prolonged peristaltic contractile duration of the esophagus. Dig Dis Sci 29:134–140, 1984
49. Traube M, Abibi R, McCallum RW: High amplitude peristaltic esophageal contractions associated with chest pain. J Am Med Assoc 250:2655–2659, 1983
50. Orr WC, Robinson MG: Hypertensive peristalsis in the pathogenesis of chest pain. Am J Gastroenterol 77:604–607, 1982
51. Ott DJ, Richter JE, Wu WC, et al: Radiologic and manometric correlation in "nutcracker esophagus." Am J Roentgenol 147:692–695
52. Benjamin SB, O'Donnell JK, Hancock J, et al: Prolonged radionuclide transit in "nutcracker esophagus." Dig Dis Sci 28:775–779, 1983
53. Narducci F, Bassotti G, Graburri M, et al: Transition from nutcracker esophagus to diffuse esophageal spasm. Am J Gastroenterol 80:242–244, 1985
54. Anderson KO, Dalton CB, Bradley LA, et al: Stress: A modulator of esophageal pressures in healthy volunteers and non-cardiac chest pain patients. Dig Dis Sci 34:83–91, 1989
55. Code CF, Schlegel JF, Kelley ML, et al: Hypertensive gastroesophageal sphincter. Mayo Clin Proc 35:391–399, 1960
56. Garrett JM, Godwin DH: Gastroesophageal hypercontracting sphincter. J Am Med Assoc 208:992–998, 1969
57. Waterman DC, Dalton CB, Ott D, et al: The hypertensive lower esophageal sphincter: What does it mean? Clin Res 36:14A, 1988
58. Turner R, Lipshutz W, Miller W, et al: Esophageal dysfunction in collagen vascular disease. Am J Med Sci 261:191–199, 1973
59. Cohen S, Laufer I, Snape WJ, et al: The gastrointestinal manifestations of scleroderma; pathogenesis and management. Gastroenterology 79:155–166, 1980
60. Jacob H, Berkotitz D, McDonald E, et al: The esophageal motility disorder of polymyositis. A prospective study, Arch Intern Med 143:2262–2264, 1983
61. Winn D, Gerhardt D, Winship D, et al: Esophageal function in steroid treated patients with mixed connective tissue disease. Clin Res 24:545A, 1976
62. Mandelstam P, Siegel CI, Lieber A, et al: The swallowing disorders in patients with diabetic neuropathy-gastroenteropathy. Gastroenterology 56:1–2, 1969
63. Hollis JB, Castell DO, Braddon RL: Esophageal function in diabetes mellitus and its relation to peripheral neuropathy. Gastroenterology 73:1098–1102, 1977
64. Loo FD, Dodds WJ, Soergel KH, et al: Multipeaked esophageal peristaltic pressure waves in patients with diabetic neuropathy. Gastroenterology 88:485–491, 1985
65. Meshkinpour H, Afrasiabi MA, Valenta LJ: Esophageal motor function in Grave's disease. Dig Dis Sci 24:159–161, 1979
66. Christensen J: Esophageal manometry in myxedema. Gastroenterology 52:1130A, 1967
67. Rubinow A, Buradoff R, Cohen AS, et al: Esophageal manometry in systemic amyloidosis. A study of 30 patients. Am J Med 75:951–956, 1983
68. Scobey MW: Secondary motility disorders, in Castell DO, Richter JE, Dalton CB (eds): Esophageal Motility Testing. Amsterdam, Elsevier, 1987, pp 172–176

69. Schuffler MD, Pope CE II: Esophageal motor dysfunction in idiopathic intestinal pseudoobstruction. Gastroenterology 70:677–682, 1976
70. Bettarello A, Pinotti HW: Oesophageal involvement in Chaga's disease. Clin Gastroenterol 5:103–117, 1976
71. Ahtaridis G, Snape WJ, Cohen S: Clinical and manometric findings in benign peptic strictures of the esophagus. Dig Dis Sci. 24:858–861, 1979
72. Burgess JN, Payne WS, Anderson HA, et al: Barrett's esophagus. The columnar-epithelial-lined lower esophagus. Mayo Clin Proc 46:728–734, 1971
73. Echardt VF: Does healing of esophagitis improve esophageal motor function? Dig Dis Sci 33:161–165, 1988
74. Zboralske FF, Amberg JR, Soergel KH: Presbyesophagus: Cineradiographic manifestations. Radiology 82:463–467, 1964
75. Soergel KH, Zboralske FF, Amberg JR: Presbyesophagus: Esophageal motility in nonagenarians. J Clin Invest 43:1472–1479, 1964
76. Hollis JB, Castell DO: Esophageal function in elderly men. A new look at "presbyesophagus." Ann Intern Med 80:371–374, 1974
77. Khan TA, Shragge BW, Crispin JS, et al: Esophageal motility in the elderly. Am J Dig Dis 22:1049–1054, 1977
78. Ott DJ, Gelfand DW, Wu WC: Reflux esophagitis: Radiographic and endoscopic correlation. Radiology 130:583–588, 1979
79. Ott DJ, Richter JE, Chen YM, et al: Esophageal radiography and manometry: Correlation in 172 patients with dysphagia. Am J Roentgenol 149:307–311, 1987
80. Russell COH, Hill LD, Holmes ER, et al: Radionuclide transit: A sensitive screening test for esophageal dysfunction. Gastroenterology 80:887–892, 1981
81. Blackwell JN, Richter JE, Wu WC, et al: Esophageal radionuclide transit test: Potential false positive results. Clin Nucl Med 9:679–683, 1984
82. Holloway RH, Krosin G, Lange RC, et al: Radionuclide esophageal emptying of a solid meal to quantitative results of therapy for achalasia. Gastroenterology 84:771–776, 1983
83. Alban-Davies H, Kaye MD, Rhodes J: Diagnosis of oesophageal spasm by ergometrine provocation. Gut 23:89–97, 1982
84. Eastwood GL, Weiner BH, Dickerson J: Use of ergonovine to identify esophageal spasm in patients with chest pain. Ann Intern Med 94:768–771, 1981
85. Richter JE, Hackshaw BT, Wu WC, et al: Edrophonium: A useful provocative test for esophageal chest pain. Ann Intern Med 103:14–21, 1985
86. Lee CA, Reynolds JC, Ouyang A, et al: Esophageal chest pain: Value of high-dose provocative testing with edrophonium chloride in patients with normal esophageal manometries. Dig Dis Sci 32:682–688, 1987
87. Nasrallah SM, Hendrix EA: Comparison of hypertonic glucose to other provocative tests in patients with non-cardiac chest pain. Am J Gastroenterol 82:406–409, 1987
88. Nostrant TT, Saves J, Haber T: Bethanechol increases the diagnostic yield in patients with esophageal chest pain. Gastroenterology 91:1141–1146, 1986
89. Mellow M, Orr W, Allen M, et al: Food ingestion as a provocative stimulus in patients with chest pain or dysphagia. Am J Gastroenterol 80:835A, 1985
90. Kronecker H, Meltzer S: Der schluckmechanismus, seine erregung und seine hemmung. Arch Anat Physiol (Suppl) 7:328–362, 1883
91. Osler W: The Principles and Practice of Medicine, ed 1. New York, Appleton, 1892
92. Wolf S, Almy TP: Experimental observations on cardiospasm in man. Gastroenterology 13:401–421, 1949
93. Clouse RE, Lustman PJ: Psychiatric illness and contraction abnormalities of the esophagus. N Engl J Med 309:1337–1392, 1983
94. Richter JE, Obrecht WF, Bradley LA, et al: Psychological comparison of patients with nutcracker esophagus and irritable bowel syndrome. Dig Dis Sci 31:131–138, 1986
95. Ritchie J: Pain from distention of the pelvic colon by inflating a balloon in the irritable colon syndrome. Gut 14:125–132, 1973
96. Castell DO, Wood JD, Freiling F, et al: Cerebral electrical potentials evoked by balloon distention of the human esophagus. Abstract submitted to American Gastroenterological Association, 1988

97. Kellner R: Hypochondriasis and somatization. J Am Med Assoc 258:2718–2722, 1987
98. Stacher G, Schmeierer C, Landgraf M: Tertiary esophageal contractions evoked by acoustic stimuli. Gastroenterology 44:49–54, 1979
99. Young LD, Richter JE, Anderson KO, et al: The effects of psychological and environmental stressors on peristaltic esophageal contractions in healthy volunteers. Psychophysiology 24:132–141, 1987
100. Keshavarzian A, Iber FL, Ferguson Y: Esophageal manometry and radionuclide emptying in chronic alcoholics. Gastroenterology 92:751–757, 1987
101. Bortolotti M, Labo G: Clinical and manometric effects of nifedipine in patients with esophageal achalasia. Gastroenterology 80:39–44, 1981
102. Wong RKH, Johnson LF: Achalasia, in Castell DO, Johnson LF (eds): Esophageal Function in Health and Disease. Amsterdam, Elsevier, 1983, pp 99–117
103. Ward BW, Wu WC, Richter JE, et al: Long-term follow-up of symptomatic status of patients with non-cardiac chest pain: Is diagnosis of esophageal etiology helpful? Am J Gastroenterol 82:215–218, 1987
104. Orlando RC, Bozymski EM: Clinical and manometric effects of nitroglycerin in diffuse esophageal spasm. N Engl J Med 289:23–24, 1973
105. Blackwell JN, Dalton CB, Castell DO: Oral pirenzepine does not affect esophageal pressures in man. Dig Dis Sci 31:230–235, 1986
106. Mellow MH: Effect of isosorbide and hydralazine in painful primary esophageal motility disorders. Gastroenterology 83:364–370, 1982
107. Richter JE, Dalton CB, Buice RG, et al: Nifedipine: A potent inhibitor of contractions in the body of the human esophagus. Gastroenterology 89:549–554, 1985
108. Alban-Davies H, Lewis MJ, Rhodes J, et al: Trial of nifedipine for prevention of oesophageal spasm. Digestion 36:81–83, 1987
109. Spurling TJ, Cattau EL, Hirszel R, et al: A double blind crossover study of the efficacy of diltiazem on patients with esophageal motility dysfunction. Gastroenterology 88:1596A, 1985
110. Frachtman RL, Botoman VA, Pope CE: A double-blind crossover trial of diltiazem shows no benefit in patients with dysphagia and/or chest pain of esophageal origin. Gastroenterology 90:1420A, 1986
111. Clouse RE, Lustman PJ, Eckert TC, et al: Low-dose trazodone for symptomatic patients with esophageal contraction abnormalities: A double-blind, placebo controlled trial. Gastroenterology 92:1027–1036, 1987
112. Latimer PR: Biofeedback and self-regulation in the treatment of diffuse esophageal spasm: A single-case study. Biofeedback Self-Regul 6:181–189, 1981
113. Shabsin HS, Katz PO, Schuster M: Behavioral treatment of intractable chest pain in a patient with vigorous achalasia. American Journal of Gastroenterology 83: 970–973, 1988
114. Winters C, Artnak EJ, Benjamin SB, et al: Esophageal bougienage in symptomatic patients with the nutcracker esophagus. J Am Med Assoc 252:3630–366, 1984
115. Ebert EC, Ouyang A, Wright SH, et al: Pneumatic dilatation in patients with symptomatic diffuse esophageal spasm and lower esophageal sphincter dysfunction. Dig Dis Sci 28:481–485, 1983
116. Richter JE, Castell DO: Surgical myotomy for nutcracker esophagus. To be or not to be. Dig Dis Sci 32:95–96, 1987
117. DeMeester TR: Surgery for esophageal motor disorders. Ann Thorac Surg 34:225–228, 1982

8

Functional Causes of Disturbed Gastric Function

Andre Dubois

1. NORMAL PHYSIOLOGY

The stomach is a reservoir placed between the esophagus and the small intestine. It allows short-term storage of food, initiates peptic digestion, and ensures a timely delivery of liquefied and partly digested nutrients to the small intestine. To better understand functional disorders of the stomach, it is necessary to have a good knowledge of gastric anatomy and physiology.

1.1. Functional Anatomy (Fig. 1)

The distal or lower esophageal sphincter, also called cardia, represents the transition between the esophagus and the stomach. It relaxes to allow passage of food, and contracts to prevent gastroesophageal reflux.

The proximal stomach may be divided in a fundus and a corpus, but no clear anatomical differences exist between these two portions in humans. The proximal stomach relaxes during feeding, allowing accommodation of the cavity to food and secretions with only a very small increase in intraluminal pressure (receptive relaxation). In addition, peristaltic waves that travel across the corpus and the distal stomach are initiated in a pacemaker located in the proximal stomach. Because its mucosa contains acid-secreting parietal cells, it has also been named oxyntic gland area (from the Greek *oxynein:* to make acid).

The antrum, or distal stomach, has stronger muscles than the proximal stomach with which it cooperates to propel gastric contents in an aboral direction. In addition, coordination of the motility of the antrum and of the pylorus promote grinding of the particulate matter, sieves nutrients, and prevents excessive duodenogastric reflux.

Andre Dubois • Laboratory of Gastrointestinal and Liver Studies, Digestive Diseases Division, Department of Medicine, Uniformed Services University of the Health Sciences, Bethesda, Maryland 20814.

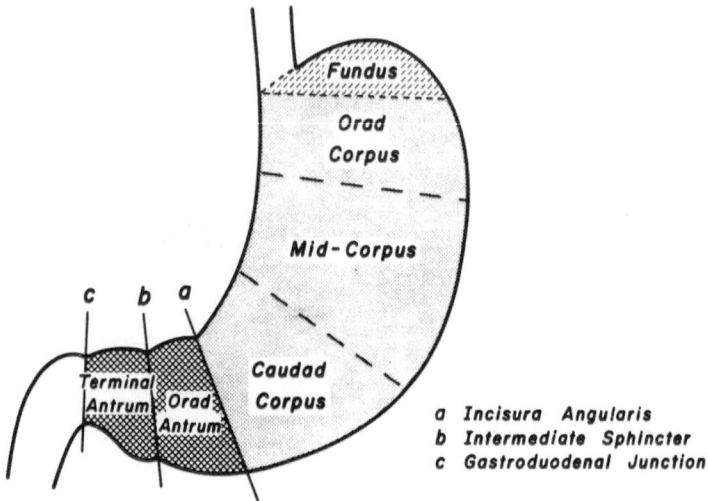

Like the rest of the digestive tube, the gastric smooth muscles are composed of two main layers. The outer, longitudinal muscle is in continuity with the pylorus while the inner, circular muscle exists only up to the distal antrum. In addition, the stomach contains a third, inner layer of muscle which is found immediately beneath the mucosa of the proximal stomach. This oblique muscle appears to be in continuity with the muscles of the lower esophageal sphincter.[1]

1.2. Gastric Electrical and Motor Activity

Classical knowledge of normal gastric motility has been reviewed by Szurzewski[2] and Sarna.[3]

In brief, gastric electrical activity is characterized by the presence of slow waves, also called electrical control activity (ECA), or basic electric rhythm (BER) or pacesetter potential (PSP). These membrane potentials may be recorded every 12 sec (5 cpmdogs) to 20 sec (3CPM;primates), both intra- and extracellularly, and in the presence as well as in the absence of contractions (Figs. 2 and 3). In the absence of mechanical contraction, extracellular electrical activity appears as a succession of triphasic waves, with a large negative potential preceded and followed by a smaller positive deflection (Fig. 3, left waves). When the stomach contracts, this triphasic event is followed by a "second potential" (or plateau potential) which is typically a 4- to 8-sec positive or negative deflection in most of the stomach (Fig. 2, G and H; Fig. 3, middle waves). In the terminal antrum, fast action potentials [spikes or electrical response activities (ERA)] are superimposed on the second potential (Fig. 3, right waves). These spikes are thought to reflect the Ca^{2+} ion fluxes associated with mechanical contractions. Acetylcholine and adrenergic agonists respectively stimulate and inhibit the spikes (ERA) but not the ECA. Both ECA and ERA propagate along the greater curvature at a speed that progressively increases from 0.1 cm/sec in the corpus to 4 cm/sec in the distal antrum (Fig. 4).

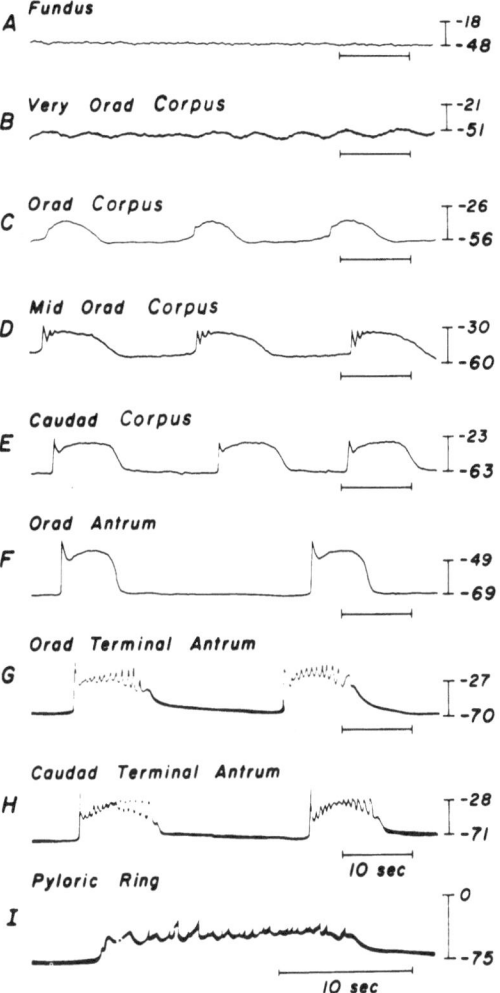

Figure 2. Examples of intracellular recordings of resting membrane potentials and spontaneous action potentials in different regions of the stomach. Note that spikes are present only in the terminal antrum, and that they appear as slower events than in the duodenum. From Szurzewski[116] with permission.

Contractile activity of the stomach is principally manifested by tonic contractions in the proximal stomach and by phasic contractions in the antrum. The tone of the fundus and corpus may be recorded using large balloons inflated in the proximal stomach, demonstrating that swallowing is immediately followed by receptive relaxation and accommodation of food in the stomach without accompanying increase of intragastric pressure. No electrical activity is recorded from the proximal stomach during gastric relaxation, but this could be due to technical defects. In the corpus, the phasic contractions may be superimposed on tonic contractions, but the amplitude of these waves and their characteristics may be related to the pressure applied by the balloon onto the gastric mucosa. In the distal stomach, peristaltic waves progressing toward the pylorus may be

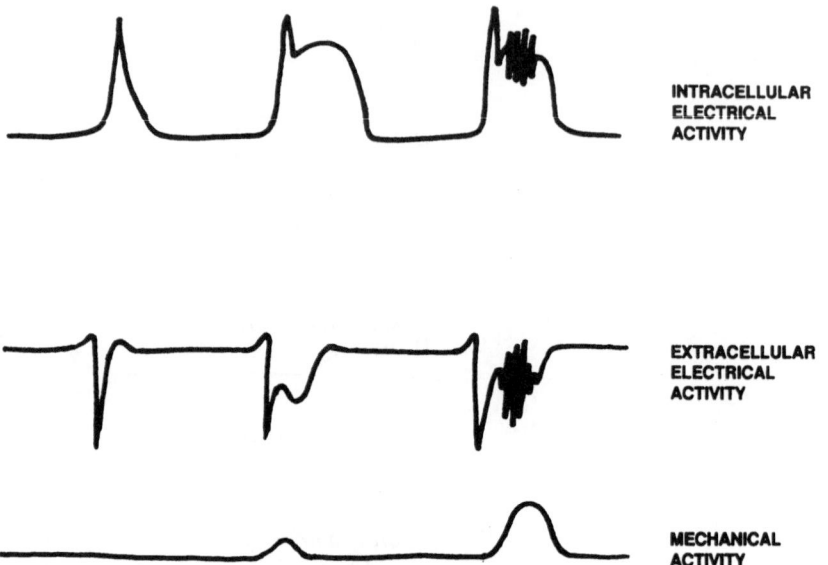

Figure 3. Schematic representation of electrical and mechanical activity of the stomach. Note that the action potentials illustrated in the middle and on the right are accompanied by mechanical activity, whereas the membrane potentials on the left are not. The action potentials on the right are typical of the prepyloric antrum, whereas the other membrane potentials may be found in the rest of the stomach.

observed using either cineradiography, intraluminal balloons, perfused catheters, or intra- and extraluminal strain gauges (force transducers). Although the mechanical contractions propagate at a speed that increases distally, their amplitude does not differ in the proximal and distal antrum, at least when measured with extraluminal force transducers. In contrast, intraluminal transducers or continuously perfused catheters demonstrate distal increase in the amplitude of the pressure wave, which is probably caused by the fact that intraluminal pressure is inversely proportional to the diameter of the cavity.

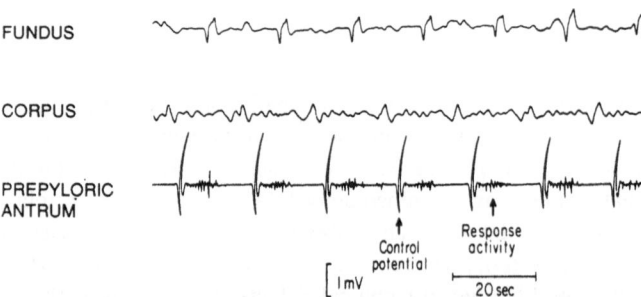

Figure 4. Electrical activity recorded in a patient after recovery from postoperative ileus. Note the propagation of the electrical control activity (ECA, slow waves) in an aboral direction, and that the electrical response activities (ERA, spikes) are present only in the prepyloric antrum. After Sarna et al.[117] with permission.

1.3. Gastric Emptying in Relation to Gastric Motility

1.3.1. The Fasting Stomach

Although gastric emptying is usually studied only after meals, it is a continuous process which goes on even during fasting. Fasting gastric emptying has two functions. First, it permits the continuous transfer of gastric secretions and swallowed saliva to the duodenum. Second, it allows the emptying of undigestible solids greater than approximately 25 mm or 1 inch in diameter, which occurs at the end of the postprandial period concurrently with bursts of spikes and powerful phase III contractions. These bursts precede the intestinal migrating myoelectric (or motor) complexes (MMC) and are thought to be initiated by cyclic variations of plasma motilin concentration. However, it has also been contended that changes in gastrointestinal motility are responsible for the changes of the plasma motilin concentration.

1.3.2. Gastric Filling

During swallowing of food or liquids, the stomach relaxes and can accommodate large volumes with very little increase in intragastric pressure. This relaxation occurs mostly in the proximal stomach, and recording of electrical potentials during gastric relaxation failed to demonstrate a typical event reflecting this activity. Section of the vagus nerve abolishes gastric relaxation, but the neurotransmitter responsible for this response has not been identified. It is neither noradrenergic nor cholinergic, and is therefore called nonadrenergic noncholinergic (see below).

1.3.3. Mixing and Grinding of Food (Fig. 5)

During the early stages of the digestion of a meal, antral contractions are usually weak; as filling of the stomach progresses, powerful antral peristaltic waves are initiated in the area of the incisura. These nonocclusive waves progress toward the pylorus, pushing the gastric contents that are lining the stomach mucosa into the duodenum. Larger particles tend to accumulate away from the gastric walls, in a zone where the flow is reversed. As a result, the larger particles are pressed between the ring of contraction to flow back and to be dispersed into the proximal stomach. There, the slow tonic contractions of the corpus again propel the particles toward the antrum where they are caught by the next peristaltic wave. This to-and-fro motion produces trituration of food and explains both the sieving and the grinding of particles which are known to occur after consumption

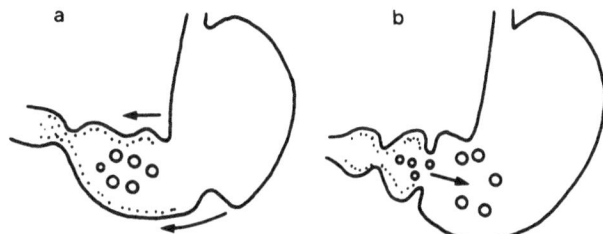

Figure 5. Schematic illustration of the effect of antral peristaltic activity on the movements of particles in the stomach. (a) Antral peristaltic wave pushes small particles into the duodenum. (b) Large particles which cannot pass through the pylorus flow back into the gastric corpus. From Dubois[118] with permission.

of solid food. It is worth noting that grinding may occur through the effect of rapid flow of particles through a small opening, even in the absence of a totally occlusive contraction wave.

1.3.4. Emptying

Gastric emptying occurs concurrently with mixing and grinding during the postprandial period. Liquids are emptied exponentially, i.e., at a rate that is proportional to the intragastric volume. To express emptying of liquids independently of the stimulatory effect of gastric distension, one should use the fractional rate of emptying, which is equal to the rate of emptying divided by the intragastric volume.[4] Since 99% of the solids are emptied only after having been ground to particles of less than 2 mm, solids are emptied more slowly than liquids and at a rate inversely proportional to the diameter of the particles present in the stomach (Fig. 6). Thus, the delay between emptying of liquids and that of solids probably results from the fact that solids need to be processed by the stomach before being emptied. In addition, the chemical composition of food affects emptying as discussed below. Large (> 5-mm diameter), indigestible solids are retained by the stomach during the entire digestive period (Fig. 6), and are emptied by MMCs after all digestible food has left the stomach. In addition, the maximum diameter of the particles that can be emptied from the stomach is 25 mm or less because the pylorus has limited distensibility.

The electrical and mechanical activity of the stomach during the grinding and emptying phases of gastric digestion are complex and appear less organized than fasting MMCs. Because a better knowledge of gastric activity during the immediate postprandial period would be required to enhance our understanding of gastric functional diseases, more studies should concentrate on this question.

1.3.5. Duodenogastric Reflux

The rate and direction of flow through the pylorus must depend on the difference between intragastric and intraduodenal pressures, although this has not been proven experimentally. Whatever the cause of movements of gastroduodenal contents, some of the duodenal fluids may enter the stomach under physiologic conditions, both postpran-

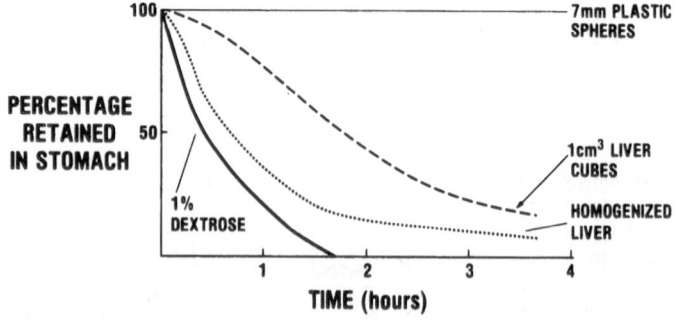

Figure 6. Schematic representation of the emptying of particles of various sizes and of liquids from the stomach. From Dubois[118] with permission.

dially and during fasting. Postprandial reflux is probably not damaging, since food and gastric secretion dilute and neutralize duodenal fluids. During fasting, however, reflux of duodenal, pancreatic, and biliary enzymes may cause significant damage to the gastric mucosa.

1.4. Regulation of Gastric Motility

The functioning of the stomach is controlled by impulses that can be triggered by external (visual, olfactory, auditory, motion) or internal (e.g., pneumonia, peritoneal irritation) stimuli perceived by the central nervous system and conveyed to the stomach through nervous or humoral mechanisms. In addition, gastric emptying is delayed when the acidity and caloric concentration of the gastroduodenal contents increase, an effect mediated by neurohumoral vectors released following stimulation of chemoreceptors located in the wall of the stomach and duodenum. Similarly, gastroduodenal mechanoreceptors mediate the stimulation of gastric motility induced by distension of the stomach, as well as the inhibition produced by overdistension. It is worth noting that hormones and neurotransmitters which affect gastric motility may stimulate the gastric antrum while inhibiting the corpus. In addition, their effect on the movements of the gastric contents within and out of the stomach results from the complex integration of each of these actions. Therefore, only *in vivo* studies of gastric emptying allow the precise definition of the pathophysiologic effect of various transmitters. In addition, in vivo and in vitro studies of mechanical and electrical activity of the stomach permit the analysis and the interpretation of these effects.

1.4.1. Nervous Factors

The nervous control of the stomach relies on extrinsic nerves, which connect the central nervous system to the stomach, and on intramural myenteric plexus.

1.4.1a. Extrinsic Nerves

i. Vagus Nerves. The right and left vagi originate from numerous rootlets from the lateral sides of the medulla oblongata. Below the diaphragm, they lie anteriorly and posteriorly to the esophagus and stomach. At the level of the lower esophageal sphincter, both trunks give rise to branches innervating the anterior and posterior walls of the stomach. The anterior trunk gives off pyloric branches traveling within the lesser omentum (nerve of Latarjet), while the posterior aspect of the distal antrum and the pylorus are innervated by the celiac branch. Vagus nerves contain approximately 80% afferent fibers and 20% motoneurons. Afferent fibers conduct potentials from gastric mechano- and chemoreceptors to the central nervous system, while the motor fibers are either preganglionic cholinergic, postganglionic noradrenergic, or nonadrenergic noncholinergic. Preganglionic parasympathetic nerves synapse with the myenteric (Auerbach) and submucosal (Meissner) plexus (see below). Their stimulation increases gastric contractility and peristalsis, relaxes the pylorus, and enhances gastric emptying of both solids and liquids. Postganglionic noradrenergic nerves also innervate the myenteric and submucosal plexus; in addition, a number of noradrenergic nerve endings are present in the circular muscles and near the mucosal cells. Stimulation of mucosal receptors produces relaxation of the stomach, inhibition of gastric motility, and contraction of the pyloric sphincter, thus resulting in an inhibition of gastric emptying of both solids and liquids. Nonadrenergic, noncholinergic nerves contain several neurotransmitters that vary according to the species, but the neurotransmitter that is responsible for gastric relaxation is not yet defined. Vasoactive intestinal polypeptide (VIP), ATP (purinergic), or serotonin may be involved, but so far, none of these substances has satisfied all the required criteria. The stimulation of these nerves produces relaxation of the stomach and allows accommodation of food.

ii. Splanchnic Nerves. These contain mostly postganglionic noradrenergic nerves originating in the thoracic chains and the celiac and mesenteric ganglia, and their branches follow the blood vessels to the gastric wall. Cholinergic nerves are probably also present since electrical stimulation of the peripheral end of the cut splanchnic nerves produces atropine-sensitive contraction of the stomach. Sensory nerves are also traveling along these tracts to convey impulses from the stomach to the central nervous system.

1.4.1b. Myenteric Plexus. The organization of the myenteric plexus resembles in many respects that of the central nervous system and is extremely complex. In the stomach, like in other parts of the gut, the nerve terminals contain and release various neurotransmitters (e.g., acetylcholine, one or several peptides). The cholinergic preganglionic axons appear to synapse with a number of intramural nerves that contain one or more neurotransmitters. Postganglionic noradrenergic nerves present in these myenteric plexuses innervate the smooth muscle both indirectly by synapsing with myenteric ganglia, and directly by entering the inner circular muscle (but not the longitudinal outer layer). The functionally defined nonadrenergic noncholinergic nerves have been difficult to characterize morphologically.

1.4.2. Hormonal Factors

Many hormones have been found to modify gastric motor activity, but their physiological role or their involvement in gastric pathology is often difficult to establish.

1.4.2a. Secretin. This hormone, which was the first to be described, is known to delay gastric emptying of liquids.[5,6] Since secretin is released by infusion of physiological amounts of acid into the duodenum, it could play a role in the normal regulation of gastric emptying. Generally, secretin relaxes fundic and antral smooth muscle and contracts the pylorus, which may occur because secretin decreases the responsiveness of gastric smooth muscle to other neural and homonal stimuli.

1.4.2b. Cholecystokinin (CCK). Like secretin, CCK delays gastric emptying at very low doses and may also play a physiological role in the regulation of gastric emptying and secretion.[5,7] Both homones also suppress gastric secretion which could further decrease intragastric digestion, thereby delaying grinding and emptying of solid food. CCK may suppress emptying by inhibiting the spontaneous contraction of gastric muscle, or by increasing the contractility of antral circular muscles.

1.4.2c. Gastrin. The gastrins and their analogue pentagastrin delay gastric emptying through relaxation of the fundus and contraction of the antrum.[8,9] However, these actions occur only after administration of pharmcologic doses, suggesting that gastrin may not play a physiological role in the regulation of gastric motility.

1.4.2d. Motilin. Motilin is the only gastrointestinal peptide that has been found to stimulate gastric emptying.[10] This effect appears to result from a direct effect on the smooth muscles of both the proximal and the distal stomach. Plasma motilin concentrations are higher at the time of initiation of the gastric MMCs, but it is still unclear whether motilin initiates these MMCs or if the MMCs release motilin.

1.4.2e. Other Hormones. VIP, gastric inhibitory polypeptide, pancreatic polypeptide, and glucagon have been found to alter gastric smooth muscle activity but their physiological role in the regulation of gastric emptying is unknown. More studies will be needed before such a role can be established.

1.4.3. Paracrine Mechanisms

Little is known about the effect of the release of local agents on gastric emptying. Prostaglandins E, F, and I have been found in significant amounts in the stomach wall and in the gastric juice. Since prostaglandins have a major effect on gastric emptying, they could play a role in the physiological and pathological regulation of gastric motility.[11]

2. FUNCTIONAL DISORDERS OF GASTRIC MOTILITY AND EMPTYING

Functional symptoms may be attributed to disorders of the stomach on the basis of the location of the complaints described by patients, i.e., if they seem to originate in the upper abdomen. In fact, many upper abdominal symptoms are probably caused by alterations of gastric motility resulting in either decreased or accelerated gastric emptying, as suggested as early as 1943 by Wolf.[12] However, it is only recently that a number of studies have addressed this question, and it is often difficult to predict the abnormality of gastric function which causes a specific symptom. For example, postprandial bloating is usually believed to be caused by gastric retention and depressed gastric motility. However, rapid gastric emptying may cause bloating symptoms because it produces distension of the small intestine. Furthermore, slow gastric emptying may be due to enhanced, noncoordinated gastric motility, much like constipation is usually associated with colonic hypermotility. In addition, only extreme cases of gastric retention are obvious clinically and can be recognized with the qualitative tests usually available. It is likely that milder cases of gastric retention also produce symptoms, but at present these can be detected only by special laboratory techniques. Finally, physicians should remember that normal gastric emptying can produce symptoms of gastric retention if associated with gastric hypersecretion: normal subjects receiving pentagastrin have increased intragastric volume, but patients with Zollinger–Ellison syndrome usually have normal intragastric volumes, only because they have markedly enhanced gastric emptying.[4] In contrast, some patients with Zollinger–Ellison syndrome have gastric distension because of normal emptying associated with marked gastric hypersecretion.[13] In the latter case, symptoms of gastric distension completely disappear after treatment with cimetidine, which does not modify emptying but markedly decreases gastric fluid output. Similarly, gastric retention in patients with duodenal ulcer may be more or less severe depending on the degree of gastric hypersecretion.[14] Thus, it may not be enough to make the diagnosis of delayed gastric emptying solely on the basis of exaggerated intragastric volume either in the basal state or after a saline load test. Strong evidence in favor of symptoms being caused by gastric retention can be provided by intragastric[4] or intraduodenal[15] dye dilution techniques as well as by radionuclide imaging using technetium-tagged solid meals mixed with indium-labeled liquids.[16] After water or saline meals, fractional emptying rates of less than 10%/min (i.e., half-life > 6 min) strongly suggest slow gastric emptying. Regarding solid meals, however, the variability of their composition makes standardization of emptying relatively difficult, but fractional emptying rates of less than 0.5%/min (i.e. half-life > 140 min) after chicken liver meal[16] suggest the diagnosis of decreased gastric emptying. If these sophisticated tests are not available, the steak and barium test meal[17,18] can be used, and gastric retention should be suspected if barium is still present in the stomach 5 hr after ingestion of the meal in man. Unfortunately, results obtained with this technique have not been compared with those provided by other techniques or with symptoms.

In this review, I will discuss the most frequently encountered nonorganic causes of disturbed gastric function: diabetes, primary anorexia nervosa, collagen diseases, dyspepsia, gastric dysrhythmias (tachygastria and tachyarrhythmia), and idiopathic intestinal pseudoobstruction.

2.1. Diabetic Gastroparesis

2.1.1. Epidemiology

Most patients with diabetes mellitus report intermittent nausea, vomiting, and postprandial abdominal discomfort, but a minority of them may be totally asymptomatic.[19] Even in the absence of any abdominal complaint, however, gastric emptying is delayed in 20–30% of diabetics,[20] although the frequency of subclinical gastric stasis may be greater in patients with peripheral neuropathy.

2.1.2. Etiology and Pathophysiology

Diabetic gastroparesis is believed to be caused by defective vagal innervation related to autonomic neuropathy.[19] Axonal degeneration and segmental demyelination similar to those observed in peripheral nerves appear to involve vagal preganglionic fibers. At a later stage of the disease, postganglionic sympathetic nerves are also involved, but the myenteric plexus appears to remain normal. However, the extent of the neuropathy does not always correlate with gastric symptoms, and other factors such as hyperglycemia, diabetic ketoacidosis, or electrolyte imbalance probably play an important role.[21,22] Furthermore, the variability of the symptoms and of decreased gastric emptying may be related to fluctuations of hyperglycemia.[23–25] Finally, gastric dysfunction is relevant to the management of diabetes mellitus, because the difficulty in controlling the blood sugar levels of some patients receiving insulin could be related to the slow rate at which food enters the intestine, and because vomiting may lead to diabetic ketoacidosis.

2.1.3. Clinical Presentation

The vague abdominal discomfort, nausea, and vomiting experienced by many diabetics after meals are probably related to diabetic gastroparesis[19] although gastric stasis may be present in the absence of clinical symptoms. In addition, some patients with diabetic "thoracic radiculopathy" report intense upper abdominal pain associated with weight loss, nausea, and vomiting, which often disappear after 6 to 18 months.[26] Occasional formation of gastric bezoar may result from a combination of gastric stasis and hypo- or anacidity.[27] Finally, other digestive symptoms not related to stomach dysfunction (e.g., esophageal dysmotility, diarrhea, bacterial overgrowth) may cause clinically important complications.

2.1.4. Diagnosis

Upper GI series demonstrate a stomach containing retained food and devoid of peristalsis, although there is no pyloric obstruction,[28,29] and gastric emptying of barium[28,29] and solid radioopaque markers[23] is often markedly decreased. Studies with radionuclide imaging and technetium- and indium-labeled meals demonstrated decreased gastric emptying in only 3 of 29 well-controlled diabetic patients[30] and in 3 of 6 diabetics with autonomic neuropathy.[23] In another study, radionuclide imaging demonstrated that gastric emptying of solids, but not of liquids, was delayed in 16 insulin-dependent diabetics with neuropathy compared to 18 healthy controls, although only 10 patients complained of chronic nausea and vomiting.[31]

Delayed gastric emptying is often associated with low acid output[22,30] and with a lower than expected incidence of duodenal ulcer but not of gastric ulcer, which suggests that abnormalities of emptying or secretion of acid could play a role in the pathophysiology of duodenal ulcer. In this respect, the normal emptying observed in some diabetic patients could be related to their decreased acid secretion, since low intragastric acid may increase an otherwise inhibited gastric emptying, but no information is available regarding this possibility.

In addition to the measurements of gastric emptying as described above, intragastric manometry may provide useful information to differentiate *gastroparesis diabeticorum* from other gastric functional diseases. Intragastric pressure measured during graded distension of the stomach has demonstrated insufficient receptive relaxation.[32] Furthermore, amplitude of gastric contractions was suppressed or reduced,[32] and fasting phase III MMCs were reduced in amplitude, nonpropagated, or even absent[33,34] (Fig. 7). Finally, episodes of prolonged and intense pyloric contractions were observed in 14 of 24 diabetics but only in 1 of 12 healthy individuals.[35] These anomalies probably play an important role in the slowing of gastric emptying, but the exact mechanism remains to be fully determined.

2.1.5. Differential Diagnosis

The presence of gastric symptoms in patients with diabetes should always be investigated aggressively. Mechanical outlet obstruction due to gastric cancer should be ex-

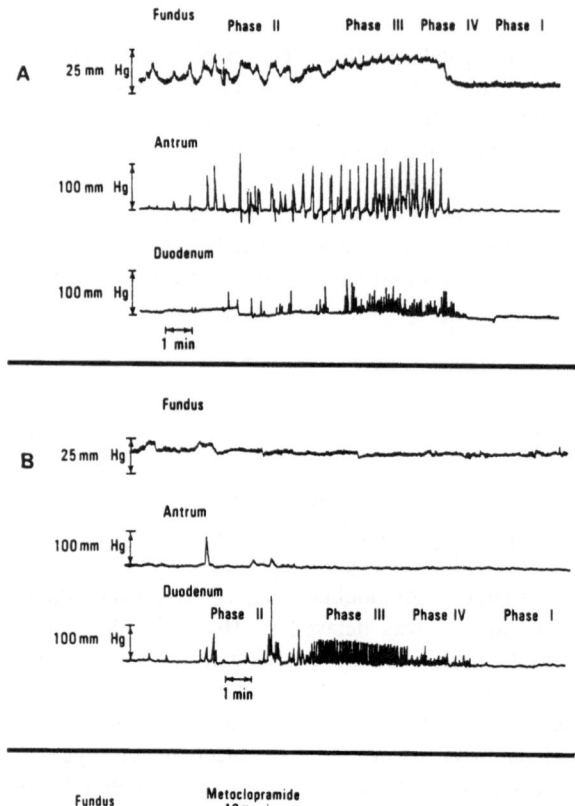

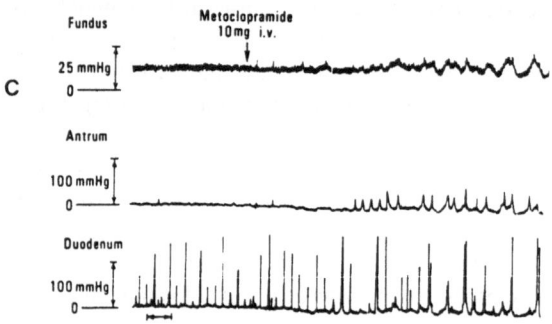

Figure 7. Fundic, antral, and duodenal motor activities in a healthy control (A), in an untreated patient with diabetic gastroparesis (B), and in a similar patient after treatment with metoclopramide (C). Note the absence of strong contractions in the stomach of the diabetic subject, and the increase of activity after metoclopramide. After Malagelada et al.[33] with permission.

cluded by upper GI series or gastroscopy, and the presence of an extragastric tumor should be investigated, especially when abdominal pain, weight loss, nausea, and vomiting are reported by the patient.

2.1.6. Treatment

Treatment of diabetic gastroparesis should first aim at restoring normal plasma glucose levels. In addition, a high-fiber diet may regularize gastric emptying, allow a timed delivery of nutrients into the duodenum, and facilitate balancing insulin requirements.[36] Treatment with prokinetic agents should be reserved for those patients who do not experience sufficient improvement of their subjective symptoms of gastric retention once their diabetes is well equilibrated. In those cases, bethanechol and/or metoclopramide may be administered because they have been shown to increase gastric motility and gastric emptying.[33,34,37,38] However, it should be noted that bethanechol, but not metoclopramide, increased antral motility in diabetics with gastroparesis; furthermore, the increased antral motility induced by metoclopramide in nongastroparetic patients was suppressed by atropine, suggesting that metoclopramide is effective only if cholinergic neurons are intact. An interesting trial has been made with metoclopramide suppositories, which appear to be effective even if marked gastric stasis precludes oral administration of the medication.[39] However, treatment with metoclopramide should be closely monitored because this medication may cause extrapyramidal dystonia and diarrhea.[40] The peripheral dopamine antagonist domperidone has been shown to improve gastric emptying, cutaneous electrogastrogram, and subjective symptoms of gastric stasis after a 2- to 6-month delay.[41] In another study, intravenous domperidone increased gastric emptying of solids acutely, but chronic oral administration increased only the emptying of liquids and not of solids.[42] Recent studies have demonstrated that cisapride, a new non-antidopaminergic prokinetic agent,[43] is also effective in increasing both gastric motility and gastric emptying in diabetics, while not producing clinically significant side effects.[23,44–46] In one of those studies, cisapride improved subjective symptoms and the control of glycemia, and also decreased mean half-time gastric emptying by 50% after 4 months of treatment.[44] Both domperidone and cisapride are currently used in many clinical trials and are available for compassionate use in individual cases.

2.2. Collagen Diseases

2.2.1. Epidemiology

Progressive systemic sclerosis (PSS or scleroderma), polymyositis, and systemic lupus erythematosus (SLE) may affect the stomach by producing atrophy of gastric smooth muscle cells and replacement by connective tissue. Up to 50% of patients with SLE may experience gastric symptoms.[47] The exact frequency of gastric infiltration in PSS and polymyositis is not established, although it appears less frequent than esophageal involvement, which has been found in up to 96% of patients.[48]

2.2.2. Etiology and Pathogenesis

The degenerated and atrophic smooth muscle cells lose their ability to contract[49] which results in slow gastric emptying in many patients with scleroderma.

2.2.3. Clinical Presentation

Patients with PSS, dermatomyositis and SLE often present with anorexia, nausea, vomiting, and abdominal pain, the cause of which is unclear.[47,50–52] Pyloric stenosis may also occur, resulting in gastric retention.

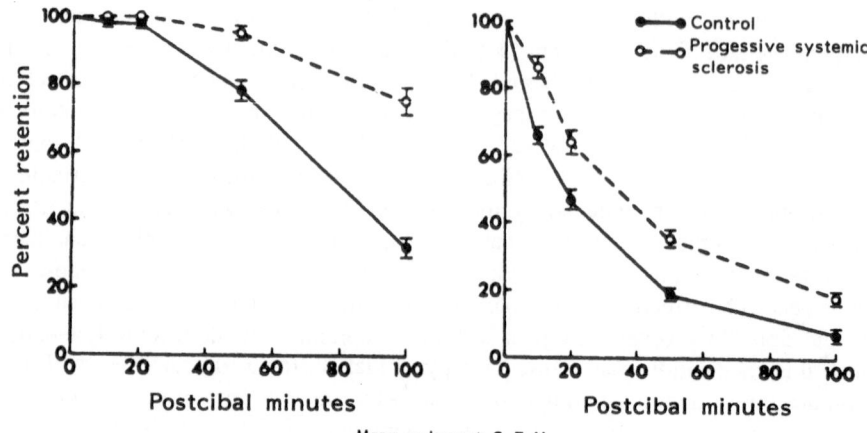

Figure 8. Gastric emptying of solids (left) and liquids (right) in patients with progressive systemic sclerosis and in healthy controls. Note that the slowing of gastric emptying is similar for solids and liquids. From Maddern et al.[55] with permission.

2.2.4. Diagnosis

Radiological methods have shown that the early phase of gastric emptying appears normal or rapid, but that small amounts of barium are often retained for many hours in the stomach.[53] Patients with PSS have decreased antral and intestinal motility index, and 3 of 15 patients did not demonstrate cycling MMCs.[54] In addition, gastric emptying of solids and liquids is significantly decreased in patients with PSS[55] (Fig. 8) and with polymyosite/dermatomyosite.[56] Finally, plasma motilin was found to be significantly higher in PSS during each phase of the interdigestive cycle,[54] suggesting that hypersecretion of the peptide represents a feedback attempt to stimulate sluggish GI motility.

2.2.5. Differential Diagnosis

Patients with collagen diseases may present with symptoms that suggest a malignancy; therefore, a careful evaluation is warranted and no treatment should be undertaken until this possibility is excluded. In addition to routine laboratory tests, upper GI series, esophageal and GI manometry, and radionuclide imaging may be helpful.

2.2.6. Treatment

Metoclopramide and bethanechol significantly increase GI motility in PSS patients, but the response to metoclopramide is greater in the absence of GI involvement.[54] Similarly, cisapride was recently shown to enhance gastric emptying in patients with PSS.[57]

2.3. Primary Anorexia Nervosa

2.3.1. Epidemiology

The incidence of primary anorexia nervosa (PAN) appears to have increased in recent years and is currently estimated at about 0.5/100,000.[58,59] PAN has a reported mortality rate of 7–21%, some of which may be related to gastric dysfunction.[60]

2.3.2. Etiology and Pathophysiology

The exact cause of this disease remains to be defined, and most studies have concentrated on the neuropsychiatric and endocrine symptomatology, although altered GI function appears to play an important role in the pathophysiology of PAN. Acute gastric dilatation was observed in patients with PAN during refeeding,[61–64] and early radiological studies have demonstrated dilatation of the duodenum without noticeable slowing of gastric emptying.[63] Because of its complexity, a multidisciplinary approach is required to improve our understanding of the pathophysiology of this disease.[65]

A dye dilution technique demonstrated that a majority of patients with PAN had a decrease of both gastric secretion and gastric emptying, which resulted in nearly normal fasting and postpentagastrin gastric volumes[66] (Fig. 9). After a water load, the decrease of fluid output by the stomach was insufficient to compensate for the decreased emptying of liquids, and post-water load gastric volumes were therefore greater than normal in most subjects,[66] which explains acute gastric dilatation if refeeding is performed without controlling gastric emptying. Subsequent studies using radionuclide imaging confirmed these findings and demonstrated that gastric emptying of solids was also delayed.[67–71] In addition, measurements of gastric electrical and mechanical activity in patients with PAN demonstrated impaired antral contractility and the presence of increased episodes of gastric dysrhythmia,[71] although the latter abnormality was not observed by others.[70] These findings suggest that postprandial epigastric fullness frequent in anorexia nervosa could be related to a treatable gastric dysfunction (see below) and not simply be the result

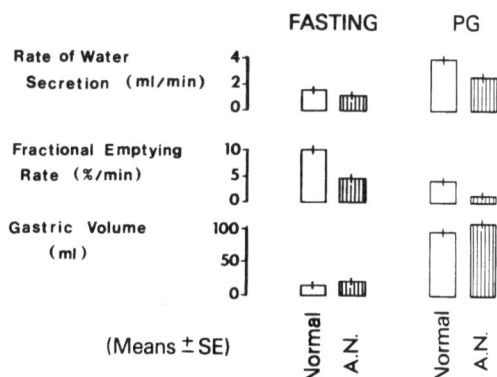

Figure 9. Fasting and postpentagastrin (PG) gastric secretion of water, gastric fractional emptying rate, and volume of intragastric contents in healthy controls compared to patients with primary anorexia nervosa. Note that, although gastric emptying is inhibited in anorexia nervosa, the concurrent decrease of gastric secretion prevents a significant increase of intragastric volume. Based on data published in Dubois et al.[66]

of abnormal sensations related to their psychiatric disorder. Finally, postprandial blood levels of norepinephrine and neurotensin were decreased whereas those of other peptides were normal, and autonomic cardiovascular function was impaired,[71] suggesting that complex neurohumoral abnormalities are present.

2.3.3. Clinical Presentation

As indicated by its name, PAN is characterized by a loss of appetite, although a number of subjects present with bulimia, gorging of foods, and subsequent vomiting. Acute gastric dilatation may be observed in patients with PAN during refeeding,[61-64] which suggests that realimentation should be progressive and prudent. Neuropsychiatric and endocrine symptoms of PAN are highly complex and have been reviewed recently.[65]

2.3.4. Diagnosis

The diagnosis of PAN rests essentially on psychiatric evaluation and on the exclusion of other causes of anorexia and cachexia. In addition, the presentation usually occurs in young females in whom other disorders are not frequent. Finally, the gastroenterologist with an interest in psychotherapy may provide invaluable help in defining the existence of a decrease of gastric emptying which can be objectively diagnosed and treated (see below).

2.3.5. Differential Diagnosis

As with other functional disorders of the stomach, the presence of anorexia, epigastric fullness, nausea, vomiting, and weight loss should prompt extensive investigations to exclude the presence of a malignancy. In addition, manometry and radionuclide imaging will permit the characterization of another nonorganic gastric disease, as described in the present chapter. Finally, the presence of endogenous or reactive depression as well as acute infections may cause symptoms that are very similar to those of PAN, and careful psychiatric and laboratory evaluation should be performed to ascertain the correct diagnosis.

2.3.6. Treatment

Cholinergic agonists such as bethanechol have been shown to be effective in acutely stimulating gastric emptying.[72] In addition, metoclopramide and domperidone have been found to improve gastric emptying.[73] Finally, intravenous cisapride was shown to increase slow gastric emptying and to enhance antral contraction amplitude in PAN.[70] In the coming years, it can be expected that an effective treatment of the gastric symptoms of PAN will help in the long-term management of this primarily psychiatric disease.

2.4. Dyspepsia

2.4.1. Epidemiology

Dyspepsia is one of the most common symptoms encountered in the practice of gastroenterology. It is the final diagnosis in over 50% of patients referred for functional

GI diseases, which in turn represents 40 to 70% of patients who consult their primary care physician for a GI complaint. Because functional GI disorder is estimated to be present in 10 to 40% of the general population, dyspepsia appears to represent a major cause of disability.[74]

2.4.2. Etiology and Pathophysiology

Increased or decreased gastroduodenal motility, as well as increased or decreased gastric secretion have been reported as possible pathogenic factors of this syndrome.[75-77] The most probable pathophysiological theory, however, is that the chronic idiopathic gastric stasis of functional dyspepsia is attributable to two different alterations of gastroduodenal motility: gastric hypomotility or duodenal dysmotility. For example, in a group of 18 patients with unexplained dyspepsia, 10 had gastric hypomotility, while the remaining 8 had duodenal hypermotility.[78] The cause of the hypomotility remains unclear and could be related to insufficient acetylcholine release by nerve endings or excessive inhibition by sympathetic or peptidergic neurons. In contrast, the duodenal dysmotility type of nonulcer dyspepsia may be due to hypersecretion of endogenous opioids, or hypersensitivity of duodenal opiate receptors, because naloxone was recently found to improve gastric emptying only in patients with gastric dysmotility[78] (Fig. 10). This observation suggests that a causal therapy of some of the patient suffering from this syndrome could be achieved with an opiate antagonist. This concept bears similarities with the observation that gastric motility and gastric emptying may be altered by numerous noxious stimuli as well as in various disease states, and that endogenous opiates could play a role in the mediation of these events. Vestibular stimulation[79] and cold pressor test[80] increase plasma β-endorphin, decrease gastric emptying, and cause alterations of gastric motility similar to those induced by intraarterial injections of Met-enkephalin.[81] The suppression of antral motility induced by cold or labyrinthine stimulation is prevented by naloxone, but it is not known whether the involvement of opioid mechanisms is at the central or peripheral level since naltrexone was not used in this study.[80]

2.4.3. Clinical Presentation

Symptoms of nonulcer dyspepsia are similar to those reported by patients with peptic ulcer disease, but differ in that epigastric pain is usually aggravated by food and milk, and in that anorexia, nausea, vomiting, and weight loss are more pronounced.[74] Gastric stasis is usually found in subjects with idiopathic dyspepsia.[82] However, the extent of the slowing of gastric emptying does not appear to correlate with the intensity of subjective symptoms.[83] In addition, although endoscopic appearance of the gastroduodenal mucosa may be normal, differential mucosal neutrophil cell count is significantly increased in dyspeptic patients compared to healthy controls.[84] Finally, a possible role of *Campylobacter pylori*-like organisms (CPLO) in nonulcer dyspepsia should be investigated because CPLO were found in 71% of dyspeptic patients.[85] These observations suggest that inflammation of the gastroduodenal mucosa and/or intragastric microorganisms may account for some of the symptoms of patients with nonulcer dyspepsia.

2.4.4. Diagnosis

After routine but comprehensive history and physical examination, the physician should obtain complete blood count, chemistries, electrolytes, serum amylase and lipases, upper GI and lower endoscopy, and barium radiographic studies. If these analyses exclude an organic cause (e.g., cancer, reflux esophagitis, or peptic ulcer disease), the diagnosis of nonulcer dyspepsia may be made. In addition, specialized gastroduodenal manometry and gastric emptying measurements may be helpful, because interdigestive gastric activity fronts are absent in almost all patients with nonulcer dyspepsia and delayed gastric emptying, and duodenal activity fronts are present in only half of them.[86]

2.4.5. Differential Diagnosis

Ulcerlike symptoms may be reported in gastric ulcer, duodenal ulcer, irritable bowel syndrome, gastroesophageal reflux, and gallstones. Symptoms of nonulcer dyspepsia are considered by some authors to be similar to those described by patients with peptic ulcer diseases.[87,88] However, others found significant differences when computer-aided studies were performed.[89] Patients with nonulcer (or essential) dyspepsia were slightly younger, and a majority of them were female.[74] In addition, this diagnosis was more likely (1) if food or milk aggravated the patient's upper abdominal pain, (2) if the pain was not severe, (3) if there was no history of night pain waking the patient from sleep, (4) if there was no vomiting, and (5) if there was no history of marked weight loss.[74] The symptoms of nausea, vomiting, bloating, and pain are also present in about 70% of patients with chronic idiopathic intestinal obstruction.[90] However, gastric emptying is normal in those subjects,[91] and abnormalities of motility are largely confined to the small intestine.[90]

2.4.6. Treatment

In earlier years, the treatment of nonulcer dyspepsia was disappointing.[92] Antacids and cimetidine appeared to be ineffective,[93] but preliminary trials have shown that the

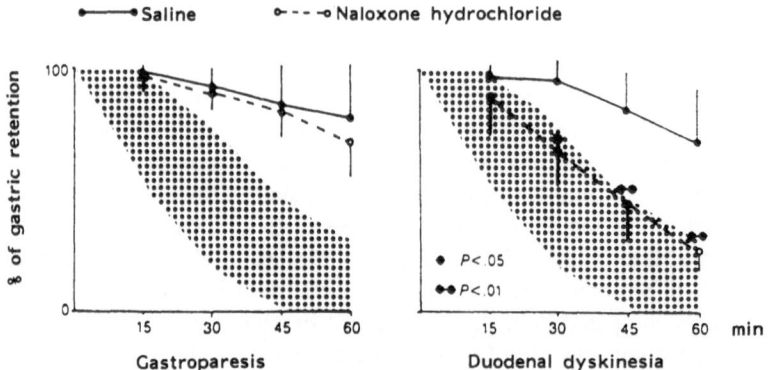

Figure 10. Percentage of marker retained in the stomach in two groups of patients with dyspepsia (solid lines) compared to healthy controls (stippled areas). Treatment with naloxone (broken lines) does not improve gastric emptying in patients with gastroparesis (left), whereas naloxone restores normal emptying in patients with duodenal dyskinesia (right). From Narducci et al.[78] with permission.

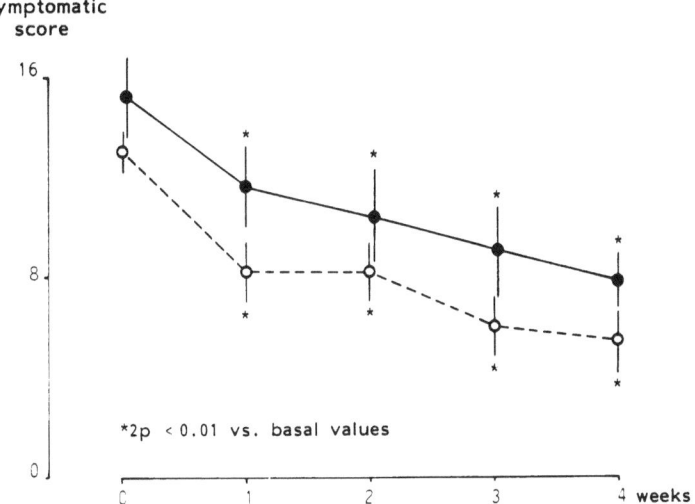

Figure 11. Effect of clebopride (●) and metoclopramide (○) given during a 4-week period on dyspeptic symptoms. Values are means ± SE. From Corinaldesi et al.[94] with permission.

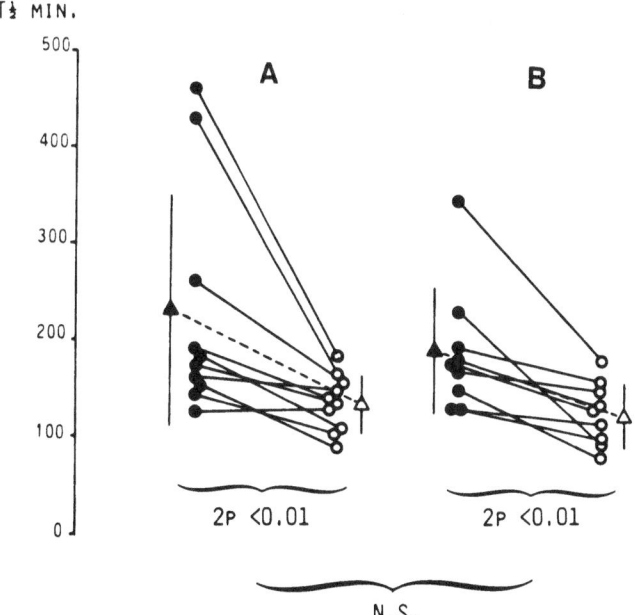

Figure 12. Gastric half-emptying-time for solids before (●) or after (○) 4-week treatment with clebopride (A) and metoclopramide (B) in patients with functional dyspepsia. Values are means ± SE. N.S. = nonsignificant · From Corinaldesi et al.[94] with permission.

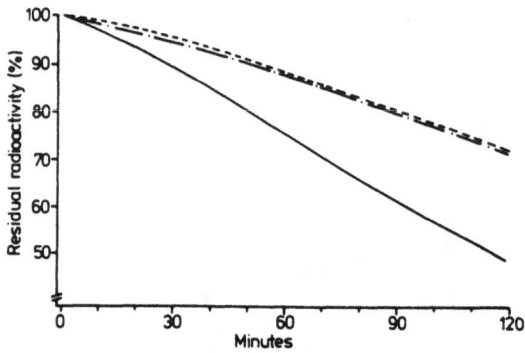

Figure 13. Percentage of solids remaining in the stomach over time before (-----) or after a 2-week treatment with placebo (· — ·) and cisapride (———) in patients with functional dyspepsia. From Corinaldesi et al.[97] with permission.

selective muscarinic receptor antagonist pirenzepine produced a greater reduction of symptoms than did placebo.[92] Naloxone prevented gastric stasis in patients with duodenal dysmotility, but had no effect on gastric emptying in patients with gastric hypomotility[78] (Fig. 10). However, the cause of gastric hypomotility observed in some patients with nonulcer dyspepsia is not yet established, and empiric therapies must be investigated in order to clarify and treat this disabling condition. Gastrokinetic agents such as metoclopramide have improved subjective symptoms and have increased slow gastric emptying in patients with dyspepsia[94] (Figs. 11 and 12), but the side effects of this medication have to be considered before proposing this type of therapy.[40] Novel gastrokinetic agents such as domperidone, clebopride, and cisapride have been shown to increase gastric emptying which correlated with a concurrent decrease of the symptoms of nonulcer dyspepsia[94–97] (Figs. 13 and 14). Furthermore, domperidone and cisapride may become standard care of dyspepsia because clinical studies have shown that they significantly improved the symptoms of these patients.[98–101]

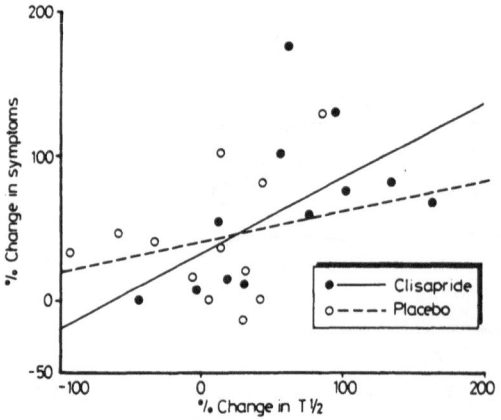

Figure 14. Correlation between % changes from control values of dyspeptic symptom scores, and of gastric emptying half-time. Note that the % changes in symptom scores are significantly correlated with % changes in gastric emptying after cisapride ($r = 0.69$; $p < 0.025$), but not after placebo ($r = 0.12$; NS). From Corinaldesi et al.[97] with permission.

2.5. Gastric Dysrhythmia

2.5.1. Epidemiology

During the past decade, a new motility disorder of the stomach characterized by nausea, vomiting, and gastric and intestinal dysrhythmia has been described.[102,103] Although the frequency is unknown, the syndrome may be the cause of the gastric symptoms of patients with PAN,[71] and a number of patients with nonulcer dyspepsia may, in fact, suffer of gastric dysrhythmia. However, because the relation between these syndromes is not established, gastric dysrhythmia is presented as a separate section in this review.

2.5.2. Etiology and Physiopathology

The first reported patient with irregular antral myoelectrical activity was a case of carcinomatous invasion of the gastric myenteric plexus.[104] Gastric tachygastria associated with unexplained gastric stasis was later described as a clinical entity in a 5-month-old boy[102] and in a 26-year-old female.[105] In the last two cases, it is possible that there was a myopathy characterized by a failure of Ca^{2+} channels to open (J. H. Szurzewski, personal communication), or a shift in Ca^{2+} or voltage dependence of Ca^{2+}-activated K^{+} channels (K. Sanders, personal communication). In one of these patients, in vitro electrophysiological studies of the surgical specimen demonstrated 9–12/min slow waves with a normal upstroke but no subsequent plateau potential and weak contractions; after a 60-min in vitro incubation of the preparation with 10^{-5} M indomethacin, the force of contraction was increased by more than 1000%, the frequency was reduced to 3–4/min, and a normal plateau potential was observed. Finally, all abnormalities could be reproduced by exposing the muscle to 10^{-6} M PGE_2,[105,106] suggesting that tachygastria was related to hyperproduction of prostaglandins in this patient (Fig. 15). Subsequent reports demonstrated that gastric dysrhythmia may be produced in dogs by intraarterial injections of Met-enkephalin, epinephrine, or PGE_2.[102,107,108] Studies using indomethacin suggest that the dysrhythmic action of opioids and epinephrine, but not of glucagon, may be prostaglandin-dependent.[108] Similar alterations of the frequency of gastric waves have been recorded in humans by using cutaneous electrogastrography after intravenous injection of glucagon,[109] during motion sickness,[110,111] and in pregnant women with nausea.[112] The exact cause of this syndrome is unknown, but ectopic pacemakers have been observed in patients with autonomic dysfunction or with gastric cancer.[104]

2.5.3. Clinical Presentation

In this syndrome, ectopic antral pacemakers are firing at rapid rates of 4–10 cycles/min (tachygastria), or at an irregular and rapid frequency[113,114] (tachyarrhythmia) (Fig. 16). These abnormal electrical potentials may conflict with the natural gastric pacemaker, capture the antral smooth muscle, uncouple the gastric corpus and antrum, and destroy the usual orderly patterns of aborally directed gastric peristalis. The pacesetter potentials generated by the ectopic pacemaker are propagated in a reverse direction, i.e., orally from the antral site of origin toward the body of the stomach. Action potentials and

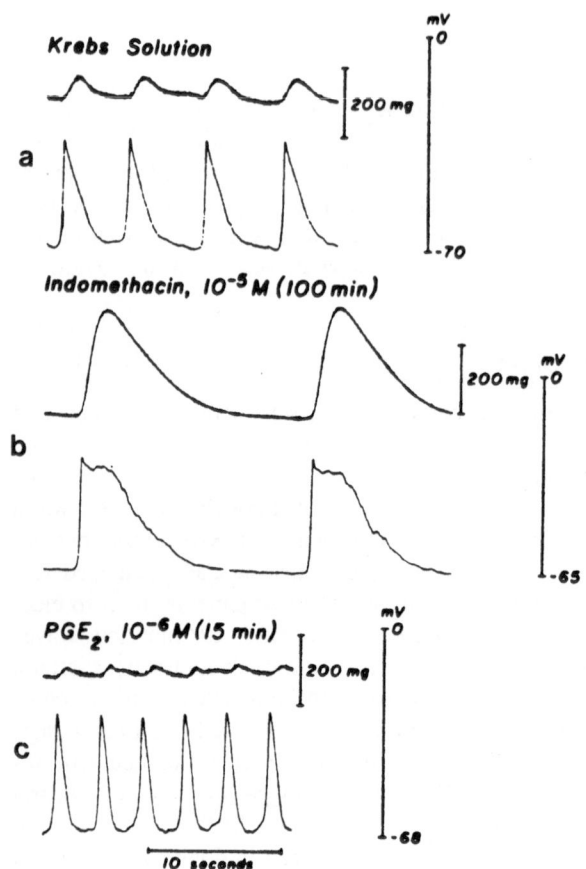

Figure 15. Mechanical (top tracing, each panel) and electrical (bottom tracing, each panel) activities of a strip of gastric muscle isolated from a patient with gastric pseudoobstruction. (a) Spontaneous activity; (b) after 1-hr incubation with indomethacin; (c) after addition of PGE_2. From Sanders et al.[106] with permission.

contractions phased by such orally moving cycles also propagate in an aboral direction. Furthermore, dysrhythmia per se appears to inhibit the strength of antral contractions, much like cardiac arrhythmia reduces cardiac output.[107] Therefore, normal gastric propulsion is impaired, and gastric stasis, distension, nausea, and vomiting result.

2.5.4. Diagnosis

This condition cannot be diagnosed by conventional methods and is easily confused with a psychosomatic illness. Thus, gastric dysrhythmia should be suspected in the presence of unexplained gastric stasis which should be documented by measurements of gastric emptying. In addition, recording of mucosal and/or cutaneous electrogastrogram may help to define a gastric dysrhythmia and to treat this condition (see below).

2.5.5. Differential Diagnosis

All other functional disorders of the stomach may cause symptoms similar to those of gastric dysrhythmia and these other diagnoses should be carefully evaluated. As stated

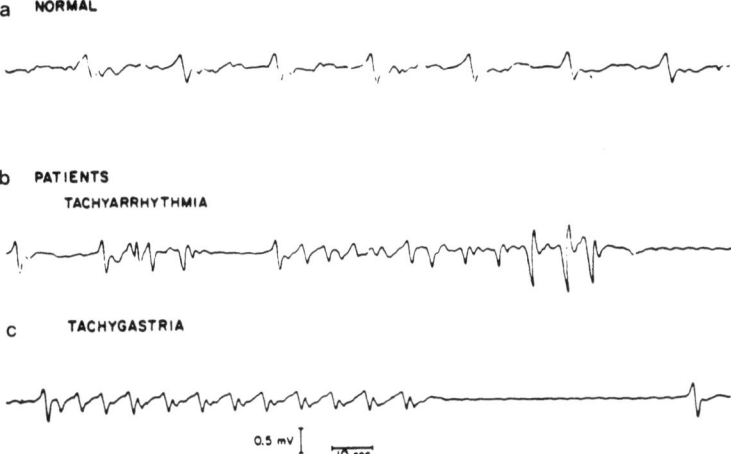

Figure 16. Gastric myoelectrical activity as recorded using peroral suction mucosal electrodes. (a) Tracing obtained in a healthy control; (b) example of tachyarrhythmia; (c) example of tachygastria. Both b and c show period of electrical silence after dysrhythmia. From You et al.[112] with permission.

above, an electrogastrogram may be the only reliable method to exclude or to demonstrate gastric dysrhythmia.

2.5.6. Treatment

The treatment of gastric dysrhythmia is not established. Based on the first cases reported,[103,106] an inhibitor of prostaglandin synthesis such as indomethacin should be tried, although many cases have been treated surgically. In addition, the potential of the new gastrokinetic agents such as domperidone and cisapride has not been fully evaluated and may prove beneficial.

2.6. Idiopathic Intestinal Pseudoobstruction

Little is known about abnormalities of gastric emptying in this syndrome, although radiological studies suggested that emptying was slower than normal in a third of the cases.[114] A recent scintigraphic study demonstrated that, even in the absence of abnormalities in the upper GI series, 50% of the patients had delayed emptying of solids and accelerated emptying of liquids.[115] In addition, MMCs originating in the stomach were either absent or occurred less frequently than normal, phase I was absent or shorter, and the distinction between fasted and fed pattern was lost.

3. GENERAL CONCLUSIONS

A majority of the patients referred to gastroenterologists complain of a functional GI disease. This means that, even after extensive investigations, no organic explanation for the patient's symptoms will be found. With the progress of our understanding of the regulation of GI functions and of its alterations, it can be expected that the cause of these "functional" disorders will be elucidated. At this time, however, we have to treat these conditions based on incompletely verified hypotheses, while continuing our search for a possible "organic" cause for these "functional" symptoms.

REFERENCES

1. Rayl JE, Balison JR, Thomas HF, et al: Combined radiographic, manometric and histologic localization of the lower esophageal sphincter. J Surg Res 13:307–314, 1972
2. Szurzewski JH: Electrical basis for gastrointestinal motility, in Johnson LR (ed): Physiology of the Gastrointestinal Tract. New York, Raven Press, 1987, vol 2, pp 383–422
3. Sarna SK: In vivo myoelectric activity: Methods, analysis and interpretation, in Wood JD (ed): Handbook of Physiology: Gastrointestinal Motility and Circulation. Bethesda, American Physiological Society, 1988
4. Dubois A, Van Eerdewegh P, Gardner JD: Gastric emptying and secretion in Zollinger–Ellison syndrome. J Clin Invest 59:255–263, 1977
5. Chey MJ, Hitanant S, Hendricks J, et al: Effect of secretin and cholecystokinin on gastric emptying and gastric secretion in man. Gastroenterology 58:820–827, 1970
6. Kleibeuker JH, Beekhuis H, Piers DA, et al: Retardation of gastric emptying of solid food by secretin. Gastroenterology 94:122–126, 1988
7. Debas HT, Farooq O, Grossman MI: Inhibition of gastric emptying is a physiological action of cholecystokinin. Gastroenterology 68:1211–1217, 1975
8. Hunt JN, Ramsbottom N: Effect of gastrin II on gastric emptying and secretion during a test meal. Br Med J 4:386–390, 1967
9. Cooke AR, Chvasta TE, Weisbrodt NW: Effect of pentagastrin on emptying and electrical motor activity of the dog stomach. Am J Physiol 223:934–938, 1972
10. Debas HT, Yamagishi Y, Dryburgh FR: Motilin enhances gastric emptying of liquids in dogs. Gastroenterology 73:777–780, 1977
11. Dubois A: E prostaglandins and the stomach. Pathophysiological mediators or therapeutic agents? Adv Prostaglandin Thromboxane Ser 8:1581–1585, 1979
12. Wolf S: The relations of gastric function to nausea in man. J Clin Invest 22:877–882, 1943
13. Mignon M, Bonnefond AN, Gratton J, et al: Repeated vomiting of gastric juice in a patient with Zollinger–Ellison syndrome: Modifying influence upon clinical features. Dig Dis Sci 26:752–754, 1981
14. Dubois A, Price SF, Castell DO: Gastric retention in duodenal ulcer disease, a reappraisal. Am J Dig Dis 23:993–997, 1978
15. Malagelada JR, Longstreth GF, Summerskill WHJ, et al: Measurement of gastric functions during digestion of ordinary solid meals in man. Gastroenterology 70:203–210, 1976
16. Meyer JH, MacGregor IL, Gueller R, et al: ^{99m}Tc-tagged chicken liver as a marker of solid food in the human stomach. Am J Dig Dis 21:293–304, 1976
17. Stordy SN, Greig JH, Bogogh A: The steak and barium meal. Am J Dig Dis 14:463–469, 1969
18. Raskin H: Barium-burger roentgen study for unrecognized, clinically significant, gastric retention. South Med J 64:1227–1235, 1971
19. Goyal RK, Spiro HM: Gastrointestinal manifestations of diabetes mellitus. Med Clin North Am 55:1031–1044, 1971
20. Kassander P: Asymptomatic gastric retention in diabetes. Ann Intern Med 48:797–812, 1958
21. Campbell IW, Heading RC, Tothill P, et al: Gastric emptying in diabetic autonomic neuropathy. Gut 18:462–467, 1977
22. Feldman M, Corbett DB, Ramsey EJ, et al: Abnormal gastric function in long-standing, insulin-dependent diabetic patients. Gastroenterology 77:12–17, 1979
23. Feldman M, Smith HJ, Simon TR: Gastric emptying of solid radioopaque markers: Studies in healthy subjects and diabetic patients. Gastroenterology 87:895–902, 1984
24. Isal JP, Dehan R, Bergmann JF, et al: Parallel evolution of gastric emptying and severity of the disease in diabetics. Gastroenterology 88:147A, 1985
25. Aylett P: Gastric emptying and change in the blood sugar level as affected by glucagon and insulin. Clin Sci 22:171–178, 1962

26. Longstreth GF, Newcomer AD: Abdominal pain caused by diabetic radiculopathy. Ann Intern Med 86:166–168, 1977
27. Brady PG, Richardson K: Gastric bezoar formation secondary to gastroparesis diabeticorum. Arch Intern Med 137:1729, 1977
28. Hodges FJ, Rundles RW, Hanelin J: Roentgenologic study of the small intestine. Dysfunction associated with neurological diseases. Radiology 49:659–674, 1947
29. Gramm HP, Reuter K, Castello P: The radiologic manifestations of diabetic gastric neuropathy and its differential diagnosis. Gastroenterol Radiol 3:151–155, 1978
30. Scarpello JHB, Barber DC, Hague RV, et al: Gastric emptying of solid meals in diabetics. Br Med J 2:671–673, 1976
31. Loo FD, Palmer DW, Soergel KH, et al: Gastric emptying in patients with diabetes mellitus. Gastroenterology 86:485–494, 1984
32. Liavag I, Tonjum S: Gastric retention in diabetes mellitus. Acta Chir Scand 137:593–597, 1971
33. Malagelada JR, Rees WDW, Mazzota LJ, et al: Gastric motor abnormalities in diabetic and postvagotomy gastroparesis: Effect of metoclopramide and bethanechol. Gastroenterology 78:286–293, 1980
34. Fox S, Behar J: Pathogenesis of diabetic gastroparesis: A pharmacologic study. Gastroenterology 78:757–763, 1980
35. Mearin F, Camilleri M, Malagelada JR: Pyloric dysfunction in diabetes with recurrent nausea and vomiting. Gastroenterology 90:1919–1925, 1986
36. Jenkins DJA, Leeds AR, Gassul MA: Decrease in postprandial insulin and glucose concentrations by guar and pectin. Ann Intern Med 86:20–23, 1977
37. Brownlee M, Kroopf SS: Metoclopramide for gastroparesis diabeticorum. N Engl J Med 291:1257–1258, 1974
38. Snape WJ, Battle WM, Schwartz SS, et al: Metoclopramide to treat gastroparesis due to diabetes mellitus. Ann Intern Med 96:444–446, 1982
39. Trapnell BC, Mavko LE, Birskovich LM, et al: Metoclopramide suppositories in the treatment of diabetic gastroparesis. Arch Intern Med 146:2278–2279, 1986
40. Schulze-Delrieu K: Metoclopramide. Gastroenterology 77:768–779, 1979
41. Koch KL, Stern WR, Stewart WR, et al: Effect of long term domperidone therapy on gastric electromechanical activity in symptomatic patients with diabetic gastroparesis. Gastroenterology 90:1497A, 1986
42. Horowitz M, Harding P, Chatterton BE, et al: Acute and chronic effects of domperidone on gastric emptying in diabetic autonomic neuropathy. Dig Dis Sci 30:1–9, 1985
43. Reboa G, Arnulfo G, Di Somma C, et al: Prokinetic effects of cisapride on normal and reduced antroduodenal motility and reflexes. Curr Ther Res 36:18–23, 1984
44. Champion MC, Gulanchyn K, O'Leary T, et al: Cisapride is effective in long term therapy of diabetic gastroparesis. Am J Gastroenterol 81:855A, 1986
45. Horowitz M, Maddox A, Harding P, et al: Effect of cisapride on gastric and esophageal emptying in insulin-dependent diabetes mellitus. Gastroenterology 92:1899–1907, 1987
46. Feldman M, Smith HJ: Effect of cisapride on gastric emptying of indigestible solids in patients with gastroparesis diabeticorum: A comparison with metoclopramide and placebo. Gastroenterology 92:171–174, 1987
47. Hoffman BI, Katz WW: The gastrointestinal manifestations of systemic lupus erythematosus: A review of the literature. Semin Arthritis Rheum 9:237–247, 1980
48. Orringer MB, Dabich L, Zarafonetis CJD, et al: Gastroesophageal reflux in esophageal scleroderma: Diagnosis and implications. Ann Thorac Surg 22:120–130, 1976
49. Cohen S, Laufer I, Snape WJ Jr, et al: The gastrointestinal manifestations of scleroderma: Pathogenesis and management. Gastroenterology 79:155–166, 1980
50. Brown CH, Shirey EK, Haserick JR: Gastrointestinal manifestations of systemic lupus erythematosus. Gastroenterology 31:649–655, 1956
51. Feldman F, Marshak RH: Dermatomyositis with significant involvement of the gastrointestinal tract. Am J Roentgenol 90:746–752, 1963
52. Case Records of the Massachusetts General Hospital: Case 47-1976. N Engl J Med 295:1187–1193, 1976
53. Peachy RDG, Creamer B, Pierce JW: Sclerodermatous involvement of the stomach and the small and large bowel. Gut 10:285–292, 1969

54. Rees WDW, Leigh RJ, Christofides ND, et al: Interdigestive motor activity in patients with systemic sclerosis. Gastroenterology 83:575–580, 1982

55. Maddern GJ, Horowitz M, Jamieson GG, et al: Abnormalities of esophageal and gastric emptying in progressive systemic sclerosis. Gastroenterology 87:922–926, 1984

56. Horowitz M, McNeil JD, Maddern GJ, et al: Abnormalities of gastric and esophageal emptying in polymyosite/dermatomyosite. Gastroenterology 90:434–439, 1986

57. Horowitz M, Maddern GJ, Maddox A, et al: Effect of cisapride on gastric and esophageal emptying in progressive systemic sclerosis. Gastroenterology 93:311–315, 1987

58. Halmi KA: Anorexia nervosa: Demographic and clinical features in 94 cases. Psychosom Med 36:18–26, 1974

59. Kendell RE, Hall DJ, Hailey A, et al: The epidemiology of anorexia nervosa. Psychol Med 3:200–203, 1973

60. Soures JA: Anorexia nervosa: Nosology, diagnosis, developmental patterns and power-control dynamics, in Kaplan G, Labovici S (eds): Adolescence Psychosocial Prospectives. New York, Basic Books, 1969

61. Russell GFM: Acute dilatation of the stomach in anorexia nervosa. Br J Psychiatry 112:203–207, 1966

62. Evans DS: Acute dilatation and spontaneous rupture of the stomach. Br J Surg 55:940–942, 1968

63. Scobie BA: Acute gastric dilatation and duodenal ileus in anorexia nervosa. Med J Aust 2:932–934, 1973

64. Jennings KP, Klidjian AM: Acute gastric dilatation in anorexia nervosa. Br Med J 2:477–478, 1974

65. Pirke KM, Ploog D (eds): The Psychobiology of Anorexia Nervosa. Berlin, Springer-Verlag, 1984

66. Dubois, A, Gross HA, Ebert MH, et al: Altered gastric emptying and secretion in primary anorexia nervosa. Gastroenterology 77:319–323, 1979

67. Holt S, Ford MJ, Grant S, et al: Abnormal gastric emptying in primary anorexia nervosa. Br J Psychiatry 139:550–552, 1981

68. McCallum RW, Grill BB, Lange R, et al: Definition of a gastric emptying abnormality in patients with anorexia nervosa. Dig Dis Sci 30:713–722, 1985

69. Stacher G, Kiss A, Wiesnagrotzki S, et al: Oesophageal and gastric motility disorders in patients categorised as having primary anorexia nervosa. Gut 27:1120–1126, 1986

70. Stacher G, Bergmann H, Wiesnagrotzki S, et al: Intravenous cisapride accelerates delayed gastric emptying and increases antral contraction amplitude in patients with primary anorexia nervosa. Gastroenterology 92:1000–1006, 1987

71. Abell TL, Malagelada JR, Lucas AR, et al: Gastric electromechanical and neurohormonal function in anorexia nervosa. Gastroenterology 93:958–965, 1987

72. Dubois, A, Gross HA, Richter JE, et al: Effect of bethanechol on gastric functions in primary anorexia nervosa. Gastroenterology 26:598–600, 1981

73. Russel DM, Friedma ML, Feiglin DHI, et al: Delayed gastric emptying and improvement with domperidone in a patient with anorexia nervosa. Am J Psychiatry 140:1235–1236, 1983

74. Talley NJ, McNeil D, Peper DW: Discriminant value of dyspepsia symptoms: A study of the clinical presentation of 221 patients with dyspepsia of unknown cause, peptic ulceration, and cholelithiasis. Gut 28:40–46, 1987

75. Spiro HM: Moynihan's disease? The diagnosis of DU. N Engl J Med 291:567–569, 1974

76. Thompson WG: Functional dyspepsia, in The Irritable Gut. Baltimore, University Park Press, 1979

77. Malagelada J, Stanghellini V: Manometric evaluation of functional upper gut symptoms. Gastroenterology 88:1223–1231, 1985

78. Narducci F, Bassotti G, Granata MT, et al: Functional dyspepsia and chronic idiopathic gastric stasis. Role of endogenous opiates. Arch Intern Med 146:716–720, 1986

79. Thompson DG, Richelson E, Malagelada JR: Perturbation of gastric emptying and duodenal motility through the central nervous system. Gastroenterology 83:1200–1206, 1982

80. Stanghellini V, Malagelada JR, Zinsmeister AR, et al: Stress-induced gastroduodenal motor disturbances in humans: Possible humoral mechanisms. Gastroenterology 85:83–91, 1983

81. Kim CH, Azpiroz F, Malagelada JR: Characteristics of spontaneous and drug induced gastric dysrhythmias in a chronic canine model. Gastroenterology 90:421–427, 1986

82. Jian R, Ducrot F, Piedeloup C, et al: Measurement of gastric emptying in dyspepsia patients: Effect of a new gastrokinetic agent (cisapride). Gut 26:352–358, 1985

83. Da Rocha AFG, Zuccaro AM, Marquiotti M: Relationship between severity of clinical symptoms and

delay in gastric emptying in chronic gastritis; studied with ^{99m}Tc-DTPA scintigraphy. Eur J Nucl Med 12:91–95, 1986

84. Toukan AU, Kamal MF, Amr SS, et al: Gastroduodenal inflammation in patients with non-ulcer dyspepsia: A controlled endoscopy and morphometric study. Dig Dis Sci 30:313–320, 1985

85. Rauws EAJ, Langenberg W, Houthoff HJ, et al: Campylobacter pyloridis-associated chronic antral gastritis. A prospective study of its prevalence and the effect of antibacterial and antiulcer treatment. Gastroenterology 94:33–40, 1988

86. Labo G, Bortolotti M, Vezzadini P, et al: Interdigestive gastroduodenal motility and serum motilin levels in patients with idiopathic delay in gastric emptying. Gastroenterology 90:20–26, 1986

87. Greenlaw R, Sheahan DG, De Luca V, et al: Gastroduodenitis. A broader concept of peptic ulcer disease. Dig Dis Sci 25:660–672, 1980

88. De Luca VA, Winnan GG, Sheahan DG, et al: Is gstroduodenitis part of the spectrum of peptic ulcer disease? J Clin Gastroenterol 3(suppl 2):17–22, 1981

89. Horrocks JD, de Dombal FT: Clinical presentation of patients with 'dyspepsia': Detailed symptomatic study of 360 patients. Gut 19:19–26, 1978

90. Stanghellini V, Camilleri M, Malagelada JR: Chronic idiopathic intestinal pseudo-obstruction: Clinical and intestinal manometric findings. Gut 28:5–12, 1987

91. Camilleri M, Brown ML, Malagelada JR: Impaired transit of chyme in chronic intestinal pseudo-obstruction. Gastroenterology 91:619–626, 1986

92. Soll AH, Isenberg JI: Duodenal ulcer diseases, in MH Sleisinger, JS Fortran (eds): Gastrointestinal Disease. Philadelphia, Saunders, 1983, pp 625–672

93. Nyren O, Adami HO, Bates S, et al: Absence of therapeutic benefit from antacids or cimetidine in non-ulcer dyspepsia. N Engl J Med 314:339–343, 1986

94. Corinaldesi R, Stanghellini V, Raiti C, et al: Effect of chronic oral administration of clebopride and metoclopramide on gastric emptying of solids in patients with functional dyspepsia. Curr Ther Res 38:790–797, 1985

95. Corinaldesi R, Stanghellini V, Zarabini GE, et al: The effect of domperidone on the gastric emptying of solid liquid phases of a mixed meal in patients with dyspepsia. Curr Ther Res 34:982–986, 1983

96. Jian R, Ducrot F, Piedeloup C, et al: Measurements of gastric emptying in dyspeptic patients: Effect of a new gastrokinetic agent (cisapride). Gut 26:352–358, 1985

97. Corinaldesi R, Stanghellini V, Raiti C, et al: Effect of chronic oral administration of cisapride on gastric emptying of a solid meal and on dyspeptic symptoms in patients with idiopathic gastroparesis. Gut 28:300–305, 1987

98. Rosch, W: Cisapride in non-ulcer dyspepsia. Results of a placebo-controlled trial. Scand J Gastroenterol 22:161–164, 1987

99. Davis RH, Clench JR, Mathias JR: Effects of domperidone in patients with gastric stasis: A double-blind placebo-controlled study. Gastroenterology 92:1364A, 1987

100. McCallum RW, Plankey MW, Fisher KL: Chronic oral cisapride therapy increases solid meal gastric emptying and improves symptoms in patients with gastric stasis. Gastroenterology 92:1525A, 1987

101. Camilleri M, Abell TL, Brown ML, et al: Motor transit and symptomatic effects of cisapride in patients with upper gut dysmotility. Gastroenterology 92:1337A, 1987

102. Telander RL, Morgan KG, Kreulen DL, et al: Human gastric atony with tachygastria and gastric retention. Gastroenterology 75:497–501, 1978

103. You CH, Lee KY, Chey WY, et al: Electrogastrographic study of patients with unexplained nausea, bloating, and vomiting. Gastroenterology 79:311–314, 1980

104. Nelsen TS, Kohatsu S: Clinical electrogastrography and its relationship to gastric surgery. Am J Surg 116:215–222, 1968

105. Sanders KM, Menguy R, Chey W, et al: An explanation for human tachygastria. Gastroenterology 76:1274A, 1979

106. Sanders KM, Bauer AJ, Publicover NG: Regulation of antral gastric slow wave frequency by prostaglandins, in Roman C (ed): Gastrointestinal Motility. Lancaster, MTP Press, pp 77–85

107. Kim CH, Zinsmeister AR, Malagelada JR: Effect of gastric dysrhythmia on postcibal motor activity of the stomach. Dig Dis Sci 33:193–199, 1988

108. Abell TL, Malagelada JR: Glucagon-evoked gastric dysrhythmias in humans shown by an improved electrogastrographic technique. Gastroenterology 88:1932–1940, 1985

109. Stern RM, Koch KL, Leibowitz HW, et al: Tachygastria and motion sickness. Aviat Space Environ Med 56:1074–1077, 1985
110. Stern RM, Koch KL, Stewart WR, et al: Spectral analysis of tachygastria recorded during motion sickness. Gastroenterology 92:92–97, 1987
111. Koch KL, Creasy GW, Dwyer A, et al: Gastric dysrhythmia and neausea of pregnancy. Dig Dis Sci 32:917A, 1987
112. You CH, Lee KY, Chey WY: Gastric electromyography in normal and abnormal states in humans, in Chey WY (ed): Functional Disorders of the Digestive Tract. New York, Raven Press, 1983, pp 167–173
113. You CH, Chey WY: Study of electromechanical activity of the stomach in humans and dogs with particular attention to tachygastria. Gastroenterology 86:1410–1418, 1984
114. Schuffler MD, Rohrmann CA, Templeton FE: The radiological manifestations of idiopathic intestinal pseudoobstruction. Am J Roentgenol 127:729–736, 1976
115. Mayer EA, Elashoff J, Hawkins R, et al: Gastric emptying of a mixed solid–liquid meal in patients with intestinal pseudoobstruction. Dig Dis Sci 33:10–18, 1988
116. Szurzewski JH: Electrical basis for gastrointestinal motility, in Johnson LR (ed): Physiology of the Gastrointestinal Tract. New York, Raven Press, 1981, pp 1435–1466
117. Sarna SK, Bowes KL, Daniel EE: Postoperative gastric electrical control activity in man, in Proceedings of the IVth International Symposium on Gastrointestinal Motility. Vancouver, Mitchell Press, pp 73–83, 1973
118. Dubois A: The stomach, in Christensen J, Wingate D (eds): A Guide to Gastrointestinal Motility. Boston, Wright, 1983

9

Functional Disorders of the Small Intestine

John E. Kellow and Sidney F. Phillips

1. INTRODUCTION

The small intestine handles a large volume of oral and secretory fluids, perhaps 10 liters or more daily.[1] Mechanisms for its transit and absorption are finely regulated, and disorders of function that may give rise to symptoms in the functional bowel diseases could involve abnormal motor activity or disturbed absorption and/or secretion.

Incoordinated or exaggerated contractions of smooth muscle may lead to pain or, by retarding the propulsion of gas or fluid contents, could provoke distension. Under these circumstances, diarrhea should also be anticipated. Motor dysfunction will alter rates of transit through the small intestine; rapid transit, for example, will diminish contact between intestinal contents and mucosa, and could increase the volume and rate of ileocecal flow, thus overwhelming the "salvage capacity" of the large intestine. Malabsorption of individual dietary or endogenous components (e.g., fat, carbohydrate, bile acids) can also provoke secretion or impair the absorption of water and electrolytes.[1-4]

Although the abdominal pain and alterations of bowel habit which occur in the irritable bowel syndrome (IBS) have traditionally been attributed to disorders of the colon, there are ample mechanisms whereby such symptoms may also emanate from the small intestine.[5] Supportive evidence for such a concept includes balloon distension of the small intestine, which provokes characteristic pain in some patients with IBS, although there can be a wide referral of such discomfort.[6] In the case of altered patterns of defecation, it is well established that diarrhea can arise from organic diseases which affect the small intestine alone. There is no reason to believe that the same may not apply to functional bowel disease.

This chapter will review evidence that implicates small intestinal dysfunction in the

John E. Kellow • Department of Medicine, Royal North Shore Hospital, St. Leonards, New South Wales 2065, Australia.   *Sidney F. Phillips* • Gastroenterology Unit and Digestive Diseases Care Center, Mayo Clinic, Rochester, Minnesota 55905.

pathogenesis of functional bowel disorders. We believe that these reasons are at least as compelling as those which incriminate the colon. We must first review some aspects of the normal functions of the small bowel. Recent studies of human small bowel motility are of particular relevance to functional disorders; these, perhaps more than disorders of water and electrolyte transport, appeal as being relevant to most functional bowel disorders.

2. MOTOR ACTIVITY OF THE SMALL INTESTINE IN HEALTH

After a meal, the motor activity of the small intestine accomplishes several vital functions: mixing food with digestive secretions, circulation of chyme so that mucosal contact is maximal, and propulsion of contents in a net aboral direction.[7] These postprandial events can now be expanded upon to the interdigestive state. The phenomenon of cyclical motor activity in the fasting small bowel[8] is now well known, and is clearly relevant to the transit and clearance of food and secretions during the interdigestive period. Disorders of both fasting and postcibal motility, therefore, need to be considered separately as possible contributors to the symptoms of IBS.

2.1. Interdigestive Motility

The interdigestive myoelectrical complex and its most dramatic component, the migrating motor complex (phase III or the ''MMC''), were described most clearly in the dog by Szurszewski.[8] The mechanical equivalent of the electrical phenomenon (here referred to as the MMC) has been shown to occur cyclically in the small intestine of many species, including humans.[9-14] The motor (or mechanical) equivalents of the interdigestive myoelectrical cycle (Fig. 1) are: phase I (motor quiescence), phase II (a period of irregular and intermittent contractions), and phase III (a brief sequence of uninterrupted, rhythmic contractions, the MMC). In addition to the periodic appearance of this sequence at any single locus, the entire cycle migrates caudad along the fasting bowel. Thus, the cycle passes from antroduodenum to ileum each 60–120 min in the fasting state.

2.1.1. Regional Variations

Following Szurszewski's description of the interdigestive cycle in the dog, interest in human small bowel motility was reawakened. Recordings were initially limited to the duodenum and proximal jejunum, but have now been extended to the entire small intestine. Indeed, quantitative mapping of MMC cycles along the length of the human small intestine has established several important differences from other species. In humans, about half of the interdigestive cycles begin in the esophagus or stomach, and most of the remainder commence in the proximal small bowel[12]; however, the MMC reaches the terminal ileum only infrequently (Fig. 2). Phase III usually becomes unrecognizable within the active and apparently random motor activity of the proximal ileum.[12] These findings are in contrast to those in species such as the dog, where MMCs traverse the entire small bowel[8]; but they are similar to patterns in both the pig and the rat.[13,14] In these species, up to 50% of MMCs do not reach the terminal ileum. Furthermore, whereas in the dog, ileal motility is highly organized,[15,16] the predominant motor pattern in the

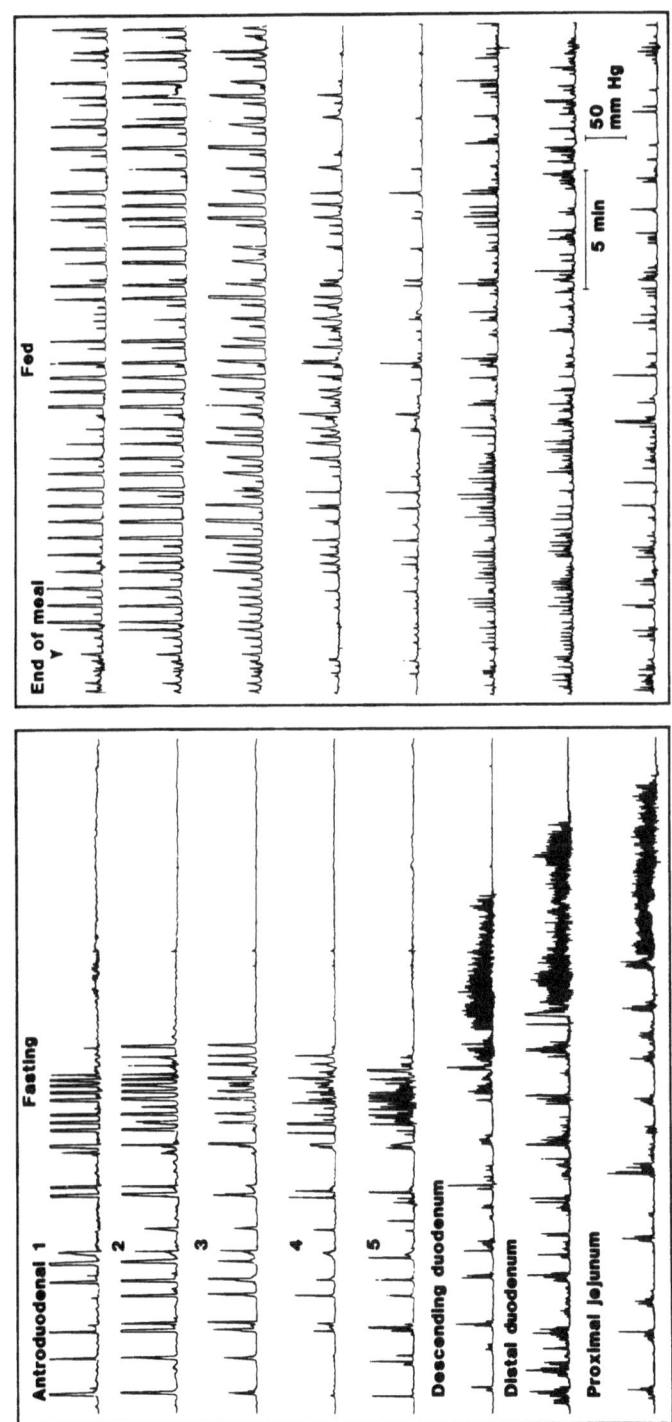

Figure 1. Motility tracing from human stomach and proximal small bowel showing (on left) the fasting sequence of phase II, phase III, and phase I. On the right, the interdigestive cycle is replaced by the "fed pattern." From Malagelada et al.[21] with permission.

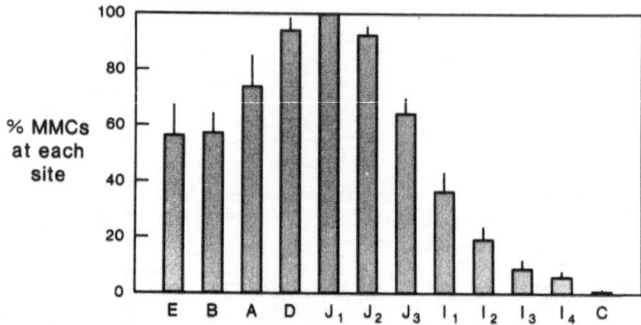

Figure 2. Distribution of interdigestive cycles (identified by the MMC) along the human bowel. Note that about half are seen in the esophagus and gastric body; few are seen in the distal ileum. From Kellow et al.[12] with permission.

human ileum during fasting is that of irregular, apparently random contractions. The velocity of the MMC also slows in the ileum, phase III lasts longer, and the frequency of the maximum contractile rate slows from duodenum to ileum.[9,12]

Prolonged recordings from the human small bowel are now possible owing to the development of fine-bore catheter manometry,[17] radiotelemetry,[18] and techniques employing intraluminal strain gauges.[19] Observations have confirmed the wide variability in the length of the MMC cycle (its periodicity) between and within normal subjects.[9,12,20,21] Certainly, this variability must be kept in mind if failure to record MMCs is to be proposed as an index of disease.[12,20,21]

2.1.2. Other Specific Motor Patterns (Figs. 3 and 4)

Specific motor patterns other than the MMC have also been recognized by prolonged perfused catheter manometry. Continuous, regular bursts of contractions (''clusters''), at times propagated rapidly in an aboral direction, have been noted in the proximal small intestine of apparently healthy subjects.[12,22] Like the MMC, the overall incidence of these ''discrete clustered contractions,'' their duration, and their propagation are in fact quite variable when recordings are made for long periods.[12] This particular pattern appears to represent the mechanical equivalent of the myoelectrical ''minute rhythm.''[23-25] However, the functional significance remains to be established, even though a propulsive potential has generally been assumed. It is relevant to the understanding of disease that ambulatory, outpatient strain-gauge recordings from healthy subjects, maintaining their usual daily activities, also demonstrate that this pattern is relatively infrequent.[26]

In the ileum, another specific motor pattern has been described. It was designated as a ''prolonged propagated contraction'' by Quigley et al.[11]; these striking but infrequent motor events are of relatively long duration (> 12 sec), large amplitude, and they propagate through the ileocecal region rapidly. ''Peristaltic'' waves similar to these have been recorded from the ileum of fasting ileostomates, where they were accompanied by active expulsion of contents.[27] They are also present in the functionally obstructed distal ileum of patients who have undergone endorectal ileoanal operations[28]; such pressure

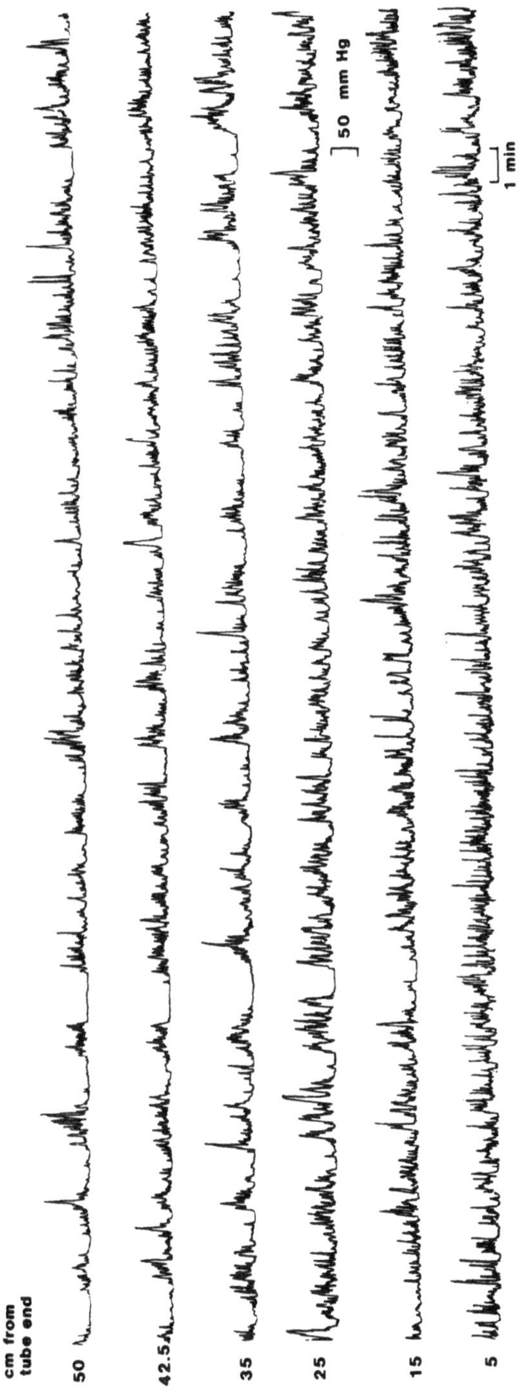

Figure 3. Vigorous phase II activity in human jejunum with "clustering" of pressure waves particularly in the upper three tracings. From Kellow et al.[12] with permission.

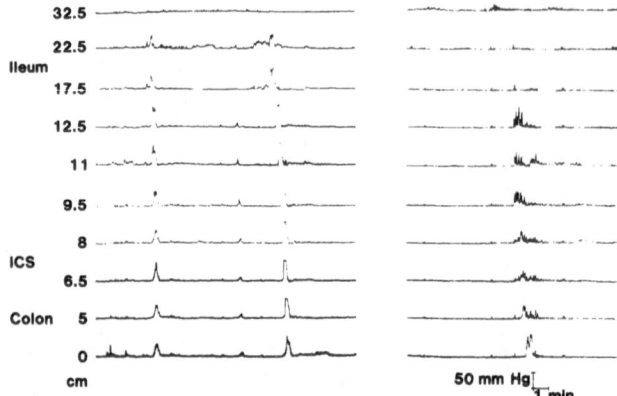

Figure 4. Pressure recordings from human ileum and proximal colon. Rapidly propagated pressure activity is present. On the left, two broad, prolonged pressure waves are seen; on the right, a discrete burst of phasic waves. Both pressure phenomena pass across the ileocolonic sphincter (ICS) into the proximal colon.

waves have been related to the leakage of stool in these patients. Comparable contractions have been recorded in the canine ileum using serosal strain gauges; in the dog, they are clearly propulsive, emptying the ileum of its contents.[29] Clusters and PPCs are provoked by chemical and mechanical physical stimulation of the canine ileum,[30] and similar circumstances can be expected to occur at times in the human ileum.

2.1.3. Circadian Variations

Prominent circadian variations in small bowel motor motility have been demonstrated during prolonged daytime and nighttime recordings. An overall depression of jejunal motor activity during sleep was first noted 40 years ago[31]; this has now been shown to affect a specific phase of the cycle. By radiotelemetry[32,33] or perfused catheter manometry,[5] phase II motility lessens or even disappears in the jejunum and ileum of most healthy subjects during sleep; the colon shows similar changes.[34]

The periodicity of the MMC cycle is significantly shorter at night than during the day, whether recordings are made during a prolonged experimental period of diurnal fasting[12] or in the course of regular meals at home.[21] Thus, despite the variability alluded to earlier, the most frequent cycle length at night is 30–90 min, whereas during the day the distribution is biphasic; the most common cycle lengths are 60–120 and 120–150 min.[12] During prolonged ambulatory recordings, the mean cycle length at night is about 65 min, compared with about 100 min during the day.[21] Variations in the duration and propagation velocity of the MMC, according to the state of wakefulness, have also been demonstrated.[12,20,21] Phase III is longer and its propagation velocity is markedly reduced during sleep. Although a relationship between the phases of cortical sleep and the ultradian rhythm of the MMC has been suggested,[33] such a correlation has not been well characterized. However, the interim conclusion can be reached that higher centers play at least a modulating role in control of the interdigestive cycle.

2.2. Postprandial Motility

Feeding not only blocks temporally the appearance of interdigestive cycles but also interrupts activity fronts, replacing them with a qualitatively different pattern. As in the dog,[35] cyclical patterns of fasting motor activity are replaced by continuous, irregular contractions which are characteristic of the fed state. Vantrappen et al.[10] documented that a 450-kcal breakfast instituted the fed pattern in the jejunum and delayed the MMC for several hours. Observations on postprandial motor activity were extended in other studies, in which recordings from the ileum were also obtained.[9,17]

2.2.1. Influence of Food Components and Regional Variations

In animals, the physicochemical composition of food is more important in determining how long the fed pattern lasts than is the volume or caloric load; fat has a more potent disruptive effect than does carbohydrate, which is in turn more potent than is protein.[36] Oral intake of nutrients does not appear to be essential for disruption of the cycle, since jejunal or ileal infusions of glucose or fat, in dogs, also inhibit MMC.[36] Species differences are present, however, as two different mixed meals—one with and one without fat—disrupted the fasting cycle for equivalent periods of time in humans.[12] As in dogs, the route of administration did not affect the duration of the fed pattern, since oral and intraduodenal meals were equally effective. After a meal, phase III in humans almost always reappears first in the proximal jejunum, the site at which cycles occur most frequently during prolonged periods of fasting.[12]

Few studies have attempted to define in humans the motor response of the terminal ileum to feeding—the "gastroileal reflex."[37] This response, an increase in the incidence of irregular phasic contractions, does not require the stomach for it is seen in animals after the administration of food through a duodenal fistula.[38] The ileal response occurs before food arrives in the distal ileum, is preserved following extrinsic and intrinsic denervation, but is abolished by atropine.[37,38]

2.2.2. Influence of Eating Patterns

Ambulatory recording techniques, which enable meals to be eaten at normal times and in the home environment, have characterized the patterns of motor activity during day and night. Relatively few MMCs occur during a day in which three meals are ingested, although a single activity front usually occurs shortly before the next meal.[39] Furthermore, when subjects pursue their usual activities and select their own meals, free from the environment of a hospital or laboratory, the overall motor pattern depends on the frequency of eating.[21] Thus, more MMCs are seen in subjects who do not eat snacks between meals; those who do may have no diurnal interdigestive cycles.

2.2.3. Relationship between Motility and Transit

Several attempts have been made to correlate motor patterns with flow rates through the human small intestine.[9,10,17] Flow varies during fasting, according to the specific phase of the interdigestive cycle; flow is most pronounced at the time of phase III, the MMC.[9,17] However, flow is not insignificant even during the quiescence of phase I. Flow rates, however, increase postprandially. More detailed analysis of the relationships among motor patterns and flow has required animal models and the use of computer analysis of the contractile events constituting the fed pattern.[39,40] The results suggest that transit is fastest when localized propulsive events are closely coordinated so that they propagate distally. Read et al.[41] investigated the broader relationships among the frequency of contractions in the small bowel and transit time. There was some correlation between the times for 50 and 80% of a solid meal to enter the cecum and the contraction frequency in the proximal jejunum. There was no correlation between transit and the contraction frequency in the ileum.

2.3. Control Mechanisms

The control of small bowel motor activity is still poorly understood, although the central nervous system (CNS), extrinsic (autonomic) nerves, enteric nervous system (ENS), and the humoral factors are all involved. The periodicity and cyclical nature of the MMC is probably generated within the ENS itself, with two main programs reflecting the absence or presence of nutrient in the lumen. However, the effects of sleep and extrinsic denervation (e.g., vagotomy) indicate also that the cycle is modulated by higher centers. The concept of the "brain–gut axis" has arisen for two main reasons: first, because the majority of vagal fibers are sensory and, as such, are afferent projections to the CNS; second, that of the numerous peptides synthesized and released in the gastrointestinal tract, many are also found in the CNS.

Function of the ENS as a "minibrain" that coordinates intestinal motility is more obvious when peristalsis, segmentation, adynamic ileus, and spasm—the local or regional systems of transit—are examined neurophysiologically.[42] Thus, Wood concludes that each of these distinct motility states can be accounted for by intrinsic neural mechanisms and it requires little extrapolation to conceive a pathophysiology of IBS based on neurological "lesions" of the ENS.

2.3.1. Control of Interdigestive Patterns

Variations of human interdigestive motor activity concomitant with the state of wakefulness strongly suggest its modulation by the CNS. There is evidence in animals that variations such as these depend on the extrinsic innervation; vagal blockade significantly shortens or abolishes phase II activity in the duodenum and jejunum,[43] extrinsic denervation affects MMC activity,[44] and the MMC propagates slowly after vagotomy.[45]

On the proposed basis of an intimate relationship between the CNS and the ENS, psychological stress might be expected to modulate the cyclic motor activity generated by the ENS. Effects of mental stress on gastric and colonic motility have been reported on numerous occasions, but there are relatively few studies in the small bowel.[46] Two have examined the effects of mental stress on fasting small bowel motor activity, using the MMC as an index of enteric neural function. McCrae et al.,[47] using radiotelemetry, stressed 11 healthy subjects for 4 hr by "dichotomous listening." Stress interrupted fasting motor complexes and this effect was most marked in subjects who also showed a pronounced cardiovascular response to the stress.

Valori et al.[48] used two different stresses. Enteric motor activity during a day of prolonged, intermittent, low-grade stress was compared with that during a day of normal activities; following this, a night disturbed by short episodes of severe stress was compared with an undisturbed night. The stress induced appropriate cardiovascular and subjective responses. Diurnal stress significantly reduced the incidence of MMCs; however, during intervening periods when no stress was applied, there was no decrease in the number of MMCs. Nocturnal stress was less disruptive of MMCs than was daytime stress. In this study, there was no correlation between the responses of the gut and the cardiovascular system to stress; moreover, the subjective perception of stress did not appear to correlate with its effect on the gut.

2.3.2. Control of Postprandial Motility

The inhibitory effects of food on cycling of the MMC appear to be mediated through humoral and neural pathways. When infused exogenously, the foregut peptides, gastrin, secretin, and cholecystokinin (CCK) disrupt MMCs[49-51]; however, the irregular patterns induced by these peptides are possibly different from those found after feeding.[51] Conversion to the fed state in the distal small intestine could also involve peptides located primarily in the lower gastrointestinal tract, such as neurotensin or enteroglucagon, which are released when chyme reaches the ileum.[52] Despite uncertainties over the role of gastrointestinal peptides in establishing or maintaining the fed pattern, CCK remains a possible candidate.[53] Moreover, it has been implicated in the pathogenesis of functional bowel disorders.[54,55]

In contrast to its established roles in gallbladder motility and pancreatic secretion, the effects of CCK on human gastrointestinal muscle are not well defined. In the stomach, CCK clearly inhibits gastric emptying,[56] but results from in vitro and in vivo approaches to small intestinal muscle have been conflicting. Stimulatory and inhibitory responses have been reported; moreover, interpretations have been greatly hampered by the absence of well-established specific assays for CCK in plasma.[57] Of course, differences may merely indicate regional variations, receptor heterogeneity, or species differences. When the response of the gallbladder was used as a simultaneous "bioassay," intravenous CCK-OP evoked different responses in proximal and distal human small intestine.[58] At "physiological" doses of CCK-OP, amounts which contracted the gallbladder to the same degree as did food, motor activity in the jejunum was increased but that in the ileum was reduced. CCK has been shown to have inhibitory effects in the duodenum of some species,[59,60] while regional differences were also present in the canine small intestine.[61]

The simultaneous onset of the fed pattern along the small bowel may be indicative of neural as well as humoral influences. After vagotomy, initiation of the fed pattern requires larger caloric loads,[49] its onset is delayed,[62] and it is also of shorter duration. The amplitude and frequency of the irregular contractions after vagotomy are decreased. Hall et al.[43] demonstrated that the initiation and maintenance of postprandial motor patterns, with a concurrent inhibition of the fasting cycle, requires an intact vagus. Moreover, during vagal blockade in the fed state, the entire small bowel exhibited migrating electrical spike bursts which were termed "postprandial vagally-independent complexes." These bursts occurred with the same periodicity one would expect of spontaneous MMCs, just as if nutrients had not been administered. The ileum appears to be less sensitive to vagal blockage than is the jejunum.[63]

Despite the temporal relationship of food intake to symptoms in many patients with functional bowel disorders, no studies have reported the effects of psychological stress on postprandial motor activity in the small intestine. Two studies have, however, examined the effects of psychological stress on transit of the meal through the small bowel. Breath hydrogen and scintigraphic techniques were used to determine transit times of a solid[65] or liquid[66] meal under the influence of a dichotomous listening test. In the first, stress accelerated small bowel transit of solids, but in the second, there was no consistent effect on orocecal transit time of the liquid meal.

3. ABSORPTION AND SECRETION IN THE SMALL INTESTINE

3.1. Water and Electrolyte Transport and Nutrient Absorption

The general processes whereby water and electrolytes undergo transepithelial transport in the small intestine are fairly well understood. The epithelium absorbs and secretes water and electrolytes simultaneously; in the jejunum osmotic pressure gradients, imposed upon the gut by the nature of the meal, are rapidly equilibrated.[1] The upper small bowel is freely permeable to water and small solutes and most absorption takes place there, whereas the aqueous "pores" of the ileum are smaller and less permeable; therefore, absorption is slower. At both sites, sodium and chloride ions are absorbed by specific active processes; water follows along osmotic gradients. However, bicarbonate is secreted by the ileal mucosa, whereas it is absorbed in the jejunum.[67,68] There is also evidence of functional differentiation at all loci; the epithelium of the villus tips is responsible for sodium, chloride, and water absorption, while the crypts secrete chloride and water.[69]

The final steps in the assimilation of carbohydrates occur at the digestive–absorptive surface of the small intestine. Hydrolysis of disaccharides at the brush border is a prerequisite for efficient absorption, and some hydrolytic products (e.g., glucose, galactose) are absorbed by active, sodium-dependent transport systems. Fructose is not transported actively but, when ingested as a monosaccharide, is taken up by facilitated diffusion. When taken as one of the components of sucrose, fructose appears to be better absorbed than is fructose alone. It is now recognized that appreciable amounts of carbohydrate escape absorption in the human small intestine. Indeed, all persons fail to assimilate completely the starch in common foods such as corn, potato, oats, and wheat.[2,70] Rice starch seems to be an exception, being relatively well absorbed.[70,71] Some simple carbohydrates, such as fructose, sorbitol, stachyose, and raffinose, also escape complete absorption in the small intestine,[72–74] as does the artificial disaccharide lactulose, which functions this way as a laxative.

The volume of fluid in the lumen of the small bowel is increased by the osmotic activity of unabsorbed carbohydrate, and small bowel transit time is also accelerated. Once unabsorbed, carbohydrate enters the colon where the fecal flora avidly ferment the carbohydrate substrate to produce gases (H_2, methane, and CO_2) as well as the organic acids (acetate, butyrate, propionate). It is an attractive speculation that the consequences of incomplete absorption of carbohydrate could explain many of the features of the IBS (gas, osmotically active moieties in the colon), including rapid transit.

On the other hand, the fat content of a meal does not appear to reduce the time taken for its head to reach the cecum. Indeed, when fat (or protein hydrolysates) is infused into the ileum, small bowel transit times are retarded,[75,76] and the volume of chyme leaving the stomach and traversing the jejunum is thereby reduced. However, this finding raises the concept of excess fat in the ileum predisposing to jejunal stasis, bloating, and distention. The mechanism of this "ileal brake" is unclear; the ileal peptides neurotensin and enteroglucagon and endogenous opiates have been implicated.[75-77] Dietary fatty acids or endogenous bile acids, if absorbed incompletely by the jejunoileum, can be potent colonic secretagogues, and potential mediators of diarrhea.[4]

3.2. Control Mechanisms

As with motor activity, intestinal fluid and electrolyte transport is influenced importantly by neurohumoral controls. Thus, in healthy humans, small intestinal secretion is stimulated by cholinergic agonists[78] and absorption enhanced by adrenergic agonists[79]; receptors for such agents have been demonstrated on intestinal epithelial cells.[80,81] The physiological role of autonomic control of human intestinal mucosal function has been addressed in two reports. In one, vagal stimulation by sham feeding reduced jejunal absorption[82]; in another, however, absorption was unaffected by the same stimulus.[83]

It is likely that nonadrenergic-noncholinergic transmitters also influence intestinal secretion. Regulatory peptides and neuromodulators have been classified as absorptive or secretory agents on the basis of their exogenous effects when applied in vitro. Indeed, for some peptides, specific receptors have been demonstrated on the enterocyte. Such classifications rely on the action of peptides not being blocked by classic adrenergic or cholinergic antagonists; and yet, the neurotoxin tetrodotoxin can be used to demonstrate a mechanism dependent on nerves.[84] The peptides shown to exhibit absorption or to promote secretion include gastrin, secretin, CCK, vasoactive intestinal peptide, gastric inhibitory peptide, and glucagon; many studies, however, have used supraphysiological doses. Exogenous prostaglandins (PG) of the E_1 type stimulate secretion but PGI_2, on the other hand, promotes the absorption of fluid and electrolytes.[85]

Little attention has been paid to the role of psychological factors in epithelial transport. Stress from a dichotomous listening test reduced intestinal absorption of fluid and electrolytes[86] and similar findings were reported by Barclay and Turnberg.[82] The effects were interpreted to indicate mediation by a cholinergic, parasympathetic mechanism, because they were not observed after intravenous atropine. Further, an effect secondary to the influence of stress on intestinal transit was deemed unlikely, since transit times during stress did not differ from those during the control period.

4. FUNCTION OF THE SMALL INTESTINE IN IBS

4.1. Definition and Clinical Picture

Functional disorders are the most common chronic gastrointestinal complaints in developed countries, where they rank equally with the common cold as the leading causes of industrial absenteeism. Several different syndromes, some of which appear to have different pathophysiologies, are now recognized.[87–89] "Spastic colon"[89–91] refers to abdominal pain, usually related to defecation, with periods of constipation, diarrhea, or both. This is now often designated as IBS. Other "functional" syndromes include diarrhea without pain, or constipation occurring as the major (or even sole) symptom and the grouping of complaints commonly attributed to disordered function of the upper gastrointestinal tract, "nonulcer dyspepsia."[92] As has been emphasized,[93] these entities should probably be considered as different from each other and from those in which a major complaint is chronic abdominal pain without any alteration of bowel habit. For our purposes, abdominal pain without bowel disturbance, or bowel disturbance without abdominal pain, will *not be* regarded as representing IBS.

With this background, IBS may be defined as a symptom complex which includes abdominal pain and an altered bowel habit, in the absence of diagnosable organic disease. Such symptoms have long been held to be due to a disturbed colonic motility. Manning et al.[87] identified several symptoms which were more common in IBS than in organic gastrointestinal disease; these were an altered frequency or consistency of stools with the onset of pain, abdominal distension, rectal mucus, and a sensation of incomplete defecation. The more of the above symptoms present, the more likely was a patient to have IBS. Thus, rather than relying only on the exclusion of organic illness, questionnaires have been designed for the positive diagnosis of IBS.[87,94] *Using these criteria, deviations from normal patterns of motility in the small bowel and gallbladder can be detected in IBS.*[5,95] *Indeed, we believe that the case for disordered motility of the small bowel in IBS is as plausible as that for colonic dysfunction.*

In fact, many symptoms that accompany IBS do not immediately suggest disorders of the hindgut. Upper gastrointestinal complaints such as dyspepsia, early satiety, nausea, vomiting, heartburn, and dysphagia are all quite common.[96] Whorwell et al. found such symptoms to be more common in IBS than in healthy controls,[97] and also reported a high prevalence of urinary symptoms such as nocturia, frequency, and incomplete voiding.[98] All of this raises the question of a more diffuse disorder of smooth muscle (or its control) in IBS. Indeed, a motor abnormality of the urinary bladder (detrusor instability[98]), gallbladder,[95,99] and bronchial smooth muscle[100] has been described in patients with IBS. The gallbladder in IBS responds differently from that of controls when stimulated with CCK-OP; moreover, patients with constipation responded more than did normals, while those with diarrhea contracted the gallbladder less.[95] Fasting and residual gallbladder volumes after a meal were twice as great in IBS patients as in controls.[99]

4.2. Motility of the Small Bowel

Though the evidence favors a disorder of small intestinal motility in IBS, this abnormality could represent a dysfunction of the smooth muscle itself, its immediate neural connections within the ENS, or pathophysiology of central control mechanisms. Another major hypothesis is that IBS is an expression of a "sensitive gut," in other words, an abnormality on the sensory side.[100] Thus, important to better understanding of the underlying mechanisms is the recognition of motor patterns which differ from those of the healthy small bowel. Studies directed toward this goal have been facilitated by a greater awareness of possibly different symptom complexes in IBS.

4.2.1. Early Observations

Horowitz and Farrar[101] studied ten patients with functional bowel disorders, using radiotelemetry; at least eight appear to have had symptoms compatable with IBS. They described increased rhythmic bursts of activity in the jejunum; moreover, in at least two patients, symptoms of abdominal discomfort occurred during this motor pattern. Holdstock et al.[102] recorded motor activity from the proximal small intestine of patients with pain and constipation. During an episode of pain, the contractile activity was found to be markedly increased, subsiding again when the pain abated. In postprandial studies, Connell et al.[103] demonstrated ileal hypermotility in one patient who experienced abdominal pain postprandially. Ritchie and Salem,[104] using manometry, recorded reduced motility in the proximal small intestine of six patients with diarrhea ascribed to IBS.

At the time of these descriptions, the periodic nature of fasting motility in the small bowel was not appreciated and most observations were of short duration; thus, any differences observed must now be seen in the light of possible sampling errors. Description of the interdigestive cycle in animals and humans[8,10,12] dictated that more difficult, prolonged recordings (of at least many hours) would be needed; but this new appreciation also provided a firmer basis for their interpretation.

4.2.2. Interdigestive Motility

Following description of the MMC, the first report of small intestinal motor activity in IBS was in a single patient with abdominal pain and diarrhea.[105] Jejunal motility was recorded for 47 hr using a telemetering "radio-pill." During the first 12 hr of fasting, two MMCs were identified, the remainder of the record consisting largely of active but irregular contractions. The patient experienced abdominal pain during the study; these episodes were associated with periods of irregular contractile activity, and pain ceased when normal interdigestive cyclical activity reappeared. Foster et al.[106] also recorded by radiotelemetry abnormal bursts of high-frequency pressure activity in the jejunum of one patient. Kingham et al.[107] undertook more prolonged radiotelemetric recordings of the jejunum in controls and six patients with abdominal pain and other features of IBS. They concentrated on MMCs, which were present, and thought to be normal, in all patients. However, the variable periodicity of the MMC within patient and control groups[9] may have precluded demonstration of any differences between them. All the patients experienced pain at some time during the recordings, but there was no obvious relationship to particular motor patterns.

The first prolonged, perfused catheter manometry in IBS[5] used an assembly which spanned the entire small bowel. In 16 patients with pain and constipation or diarrhea, sensors were positioned in the duodenum, jejunum, ileum, and cecum. Fasting recordings encompassed both day and night, when the patients slept. Despite the variability of motor patterns known to exist in health,[9,12] small intestinal motility in IBS patients deviated in several ways from that of the controls. The cycle length of the MMC in patients with diarrhea was shorter than it was in patients with constipation or in the controls (Table I). This overall difference was due to a more rapid cycling in the diarrhea group during the day; nocturnal cycle lengths were not different among all groups. Within the MMC cycle, phase II activity was longer in IBS than in controls; again, this was only present during the

Table I. Periodicity of Migrating Motor Complexes in Patients
with Irritable Bowel Syndrome[a]

	Periodicity of MMC (min)[b]		
	Overall	Daytime (4:00 AM–8:00 PM)	Nighttime (8:00 PM–4:00 AM)
All patients	86 ± 6[c] (50–130)	97 ± 10 (43–208)	74 ± 5 (48–108)
Predominantly diarrhea	71 ± 6[d] (50–100)	77 ± 10[e] (43–117)	70 ± 7 (48–108)
Predominantly constipation	100 ± 7 (75–130)	118 ± 15 (81–208)	78 ± 6[f] (57–106)
Control subjects	108 ± 7 (66–174)	113 ± 10 (67–218)	91 ± 7 (51–143)

[a]From Kellow and Phillips[5] with permission.
[b]All values are mean ± S.E.M.
[c]p < 0.05 versus control.
[d]p < 0.01 and p < 0.05 versus control and constipation-predominant, respectively.
[e]p < 0.05 versus control and constipation-predominant.
[f]p < 0.05 versus daytime periodicity.

daytime. Other general characteristics of the MMC including its velocity of propagation, regional distribution, extent of propagation, and contractile frequency gradient were not altered in IBS.

Potentially significant was the finding that two specific phase II motor patterns, both of which could be quantified by the recording technique, were more common in IBS than in controls.[5] "Discrete clustered contractions" (DCCs) occupied approximately 30% of the duration of phase II in both groups with IBS (Fig. 5); in controls this pattern was present only infrequently, occupying only 10% of phase II. The maximal amplitude of the pressure waves was also greater in IBS patients than in controls. In about one-fourth of the

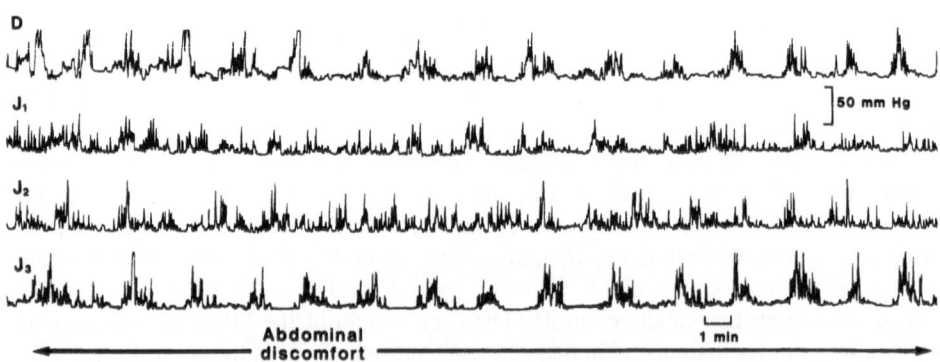

Figure 5. Prominent clusters of pressure waves in the proximal small bowel of a patient with irritable bowel syndrome. This pattern was often accompanied by abdominal symptoms. From Kellow and Phillips[5] with permission.

patients, DCCs were accompanied by abdominal discomfort; in control subjects, DCCs were never symptomatic. The patient studied by Horowitz and Farrar[101] experienced pain during motor event with characteristics similar to DCCs. This motor phenomenon, which appears to be the mechanical equivalent of the "minute rhythms,"[23-25] is assumed to be propulsive, but DCCs could not be related specifically to patients with symptoms of diarrhea or constipation.[5]

The other motor events observed more frequently in IBS were "prolonged propagated contractions" (PPCs). These are high-pressure, monophasic waves which propagate rapidly through the distal small bowel[11,12]; they are peristaltic in nature and clearly are propulsive in the dog.[29] The median number of PPCs in IBS patients was 5 versus 2 in controls, but the most impressive feature was the striking relationship of PPCs with the occurrence of abdominal pain in patients with IBS (Fig. 6). Overall, 61% of PPCs in IBS were symptomatic, compared to 17% in controls; the periumbilical cramping discomfort reported was similar to that experienced regularly by the patients. These findings firmly implicate the small intestine, in particular the ileocecal region, as a site of origin of symptoms in at least some IBS patients. Distinctive and propulsive patterns of ileal motility, which may represent the myoelectrical equivalent of the PPC, have been recorded under conditions of experimental diarrhea in the rabbit.[108,109] Ileal PPCs were no more prominent, however, in the IBS patients with predominant diarrhea.

Kumar and Wingate,[110] using prolonged radiotelemetric recordings, also described bursts of intermittent, irregular or "paroxysmal," jejunal motor activity in IBS. This

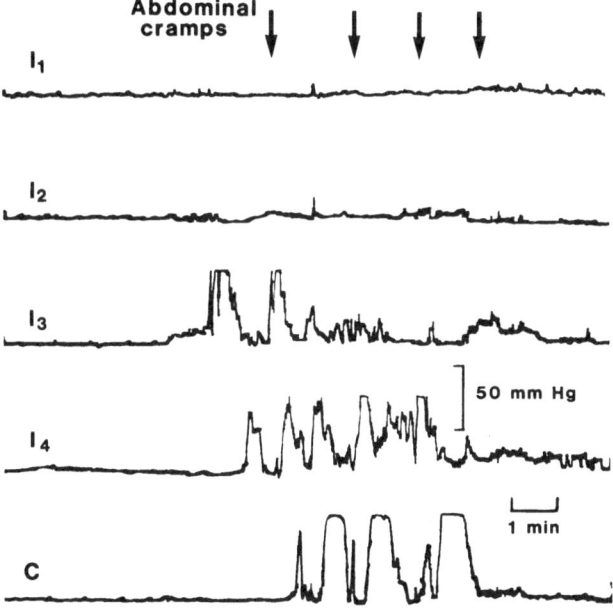

Figure 6. Prominent, high-pressure, "prolonged propagated contractions" in a patient with irritable bowel syndrome. Abdominal cramping pain accompanied this motor pattern. From Kellow and Phillips[5] with permission.

pattern, which appears likely to represent bursts of DCCs, coincided with abdominal pain in some patients and was not observed in controls. In their study of 22 patients, the spontaneous occurrence of this pattern was noted more often in men than women. Eight patients who exhibited this pattern spontaneously were more likely to have presented initially with two or more of the Manning criteria[87] than those in whom the motor abnormalities were observed only after stress.

In a second study from the same unit,[26] the small bowel was monitored continuously for 72 hr using a novel recording system.[21] The technique enabled subjects to pursue their usual daily activities, to select their own meals, and to sleep at home. Intraluminal pressure was recorded using two strain gauge sensors positioned in the duodenum and proximal jejunum; motility was compared in 12 IBS patients and 8 healthy, asymptomatic controls. Patients were subdivided prospectively on the basis of predominant diarrhea or constipation. Their classification was supported by the bowel habits reported during the study period; stool frequency in those with diarrhea was significantly greater than that in the constipation group. Significant motor abnormalities were again observed in the IBS patients, and earlier findings using perfused catheters[5] were generally confirmed. During the day, MMCs occurred more frequently in those with diarrhea (mean cycle length 62 min) than in controls (101 min) or patients with constipation (122 min). Periods of DCCs were also observed in 11 out of 12 IBS patients but in no controls. This "minute-rhythm" activity in IBS accounted for 12% of overall phase II motor activity, and was only present during the day. At night, MMCs occurred regularly in IBS and the patterns of motor activity were not different from those of controls.

These differences in the periodicity of the MMC during the day in IBS patients help explain earlier conflicting reports of (1) more frequent[111] and (2) less frequent[105] inter-digestive cycles in IBS. The inconsistencies presumably relate to patient selection, and to whether diarrhea or constipation predominated. It thus appears that patients with predominant diarrhea have no demonstrable circadian change in the periodicity of the MMC—the diurnal periodicity is similar to the normal, shorter nocturnal cycle length. Interpretations of such a phenomenon are still unclear, but patients with painful diarrhea presumably lack the programming which normally prolongs diurnal cycles, or utilize an inhibitory or counteracting mechanism. Whatever the cause, an exaggerated response to the stress of intubation seems unlikely; if this were the case, a decreased incidence in diurnal MMCs would be expected.[48] Differences in age and gender are not relevant, as in all studies patients with IBS were age and sex matched with controls.[5,26,110]

4.2.3. Postprandial Motility

Though food has been used to provoke colonic dysmotility in IBS,[103] postprandial motility in the small intestine has received little attention. Following a liquid fatty meal, administered directly into the duodenum, typical "fed patterns" were established at each level of the small intestine in all IBS patients.[5] There was a trend for a briefer response in IBS; patients with diarrhea (mean duration of fed pattern, 100 min) and constipation (113 min) had shorter fed patterns than did controls (132 min). During a 3-hr postprandial period, a greater number of PPCs also occurred in IBS patients, and as in the fasting recordings, PPCs were often accompanied by cramping abdominal pain.[5] In two IBS patients, prolonged abdominal discomfort coincided with exaggerated, postprandial motility in the ileum.

Recordings of proximal small bowel motor activity for 72 hr during which free-choice meals were eaten have recently been obtained in IBS[26]; persons were encouraged to continue their usual daily activities. Postprandial patterns in IBS were qualitatively similar to those in the control group. After main meals (one to three per day), however, the fed pattern was briefer in IBS (mean 76 min) than in controls; there were no significant differences between patients with diarrhea and those with constipation. In diarrhea, phase III activity fronts recurred more frequently between meals than in those with constipation or in controls. These findings may be relevant to reports[112,113] of shorter postprandial transit times in IBS patients with diarrhea.

Several groups have examined the transit of liquids and solids through the small bowel in patients with IBS. Corbett et al.[114] administered a liquid meal containing lactulose to 16 patients with IBS and predominant diarrhea. The orocecal transit time was significantly shorter in these patients (mean 54 min) than in 20 controls (93 min). From the same laboratory,[112] the time taken for a solid meal to pass through the stomach, small intestine, and colon was measured in 61 patients with IBS, subdivided according to their presenting symptoms; findings were compared to those from 53 healthy volunteers. Small bowel transit times, determined using the breath-hydrogen technique, were significantly shorter in patients with diarrhea and significantly longer in those with constipation, when compared with controls. Rates of gastric emptying were not different among any of the groups. Despite the overall differences in transit in IBS, virtually all of the patients exhibited transit values that were within the control range. The authors therefore postulated that the colon in IBS was less able to compensate for the effects of widely fluctuant small bowel transit, especially if this was accompanied by large variations in the volume of ileal effluent. Indeed, about half of the IBS patients in the above study reported the onset of pain, particularly localized to the right iliac fossa, coincident with the arrival of meal residues in the cecum. An insight into delayed small bowel transit in patients with constipation is perhaps given by the finding that small intestinal transit is inhibited by colorectal distension.[115,116]

Jian et al.[113] studied the small intestinal transit of a mixed solid and liquid meal, using scintigraphy, in patients with "functional diarrhea." It is unclear whether or not these patients also had abdominal pain, consistent with their classification as IBS. Transit was twice as rapid in the patients as in the controls. A propulsive "gastrocolic reflex" was evident in five of the seven patients, but in none of the controls; unabsorbed residues of the meal appeared to be propelled rapidly through the ileocecal region.

Abnormalities in transit through the ileocecal region in IBS have also been demonstrated by another scintigraphic technique. In this instance,[117] scintiscanning was done 3 hr after the ingestion of bran labeled with technetium; dynamic scanning was then continued after ingestion of a 400-kcal liquid meal. Studies were performed on ten women with IBS; particular importance was placed on the presence of abdominal bloating, but further details of the predominant alteration of bowel habit were not provided. When compared with eight controls, ileal emptying in IBS was significantly slower, peak isotope counts in the cecum were lower, and ileocecal clearance of isotope was less. Delayed transit through the proximal small bowel was judged unlikely to account for the differences, as in both groups the labeled bran had accumulated in the distal small bowel before the meal was given.

The Nottingham group[118,119] compared the transit of two radiolabeled preparations—a nondisintegrating capsule and a multiparticulate formulation—in patients with

IBS, subdivided into those with predominant diarrhea or constipation. The transit of small solids through the small intestine was the same for both patient groups. In the patients complaining of diarrhea, however, the capsule passed through the small intestine at a faster rate than did the particles; such a difference was not found in those with constipation. However, postprandial propulsion of ileocecal contents did not differ in patients with IBS when compared to normal subjects.[118,119]

4.2.4. Role of Neuropeptidergic Control

It has been suggested that patients with IBS may have enteric smooth muscle which is hypersensitive to physiological levels of gastrointestinal peptides, or that the secretion of one or more of these peptides is abnormal.[54] Given the frequent relationship of IBS symptoms to eating, and the known release of many peptides after food, the hypothesis is attractive. However, the overlapping distributions of peptides along the gut, the interacting mechanisms of their release, and the multiple actions of each make their contributions to disease states very difficult to evaluate.

Besterman et al.[120] measured fasting and postprandial levels of peptides in 42 patients with IBS. No abnormalities were found in the fasting levels or postprandial release of gastrin, insulin, VIP, motilin, and enteroglucagon when the patients were considered as a homogeneous group. However, although basal concentrations of GIP were normal in all groups, patients with predominant constipation had an increased response to the meal when compared to controls. Similarly, basal levels of neurotensin in IBS did not differ from those in controls, but patients with predominant diarrhea had an elevated postprandial response. In an earlier study in 27 patients,[121] gastrin release was measured; no significant differences in fasting and stimulated levels of gastrin were found. Levels of gastrin, motilin, and pancreatic polypeptide after an oral water load were compared in 40 patients with functional bowel disorders and controls.[122] Nine patients with chronic painless diarrhea were included; basal and stimulated concentrations of pancreatic polypeptide and fasting levels of motilin were increased. In patients with constipation but without abdominal pain, designated as "slow transit constipation," motilin release was markedly impaired. The authors postulated that this "deficiency," in contrast to the increased levels of motilin in chronic diarrhea, may reflect the actions of motilin, a peptide known to accelerate gastric emptying and initiate MMCs. However, Borody et al.[111] reported normal release of motilin, pancreatic polypeptide, and CCK in five patients with IBS and diarrhea. Levels of circulating immunoreactive somatostatin were exaggerated postprandially in IBS patients.[123] Thus, there is no consistent profile of gut peptides in IBS; however, when categorized according to symptoms, alterations observed in some patient groups may be worth further pursuit.

Of all gastrointestinal peptides, CCK has been most implicated in the pathogenesis of symptoms in functional bowel disease.[5,124,125] An exaggerated motor response to intravenous CCK was found in the sigmoid colon in IBS and this was most pronounced in eight patients who regularly complained of attacks of postprandial pain.[124] However, the peptide was administered in pharmacological doses and it was impure, almost certainly containing contaminants such as motilin. Despite these caveats, further support for the involvement of CCK's actions on the colon in IBS was provided by Snape et al.[55,126]

The response of different regions of the small intestine to CCK in health[58] and

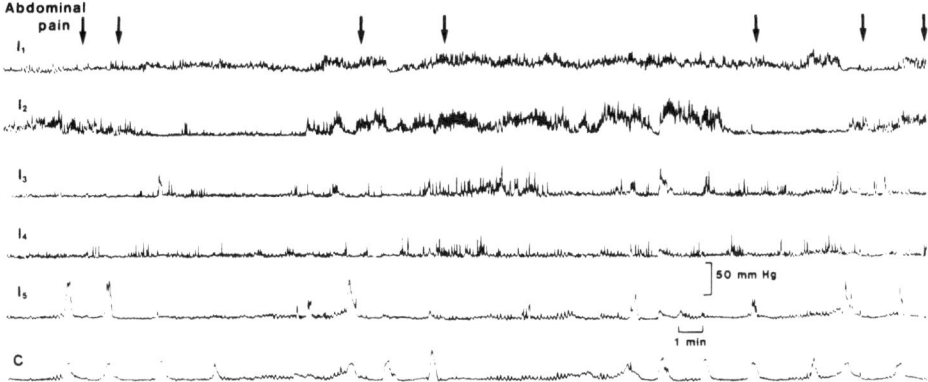

Figure 7. Multiple high-pressure, monophasic waves (PPCs) stimulated by cholecystokinin-octapeptide (CCK-OP) in a patient with irritable bowel syndrome. The dose of CCK-OP was considered within the "physiological range" (see Refs. 58, 95, 125).

IBS[125] has been reported; intravenous doses of CCK-OP were designed to span a sub-physiological to supraphysiological range. The "physiological effects" of infused doses were assessed by monitoring gallbladder contraction at the same time, using ultrasonography. At doses corresponding to a 50% contraction of the gallbladder, a response elicited by a test meal, small bowel motility was greater in IBS than in controls. These effects were most pronounced in the ileum, and in patients with predominant diarrhea. Similar findings were observed at pharmacological doses, corresponding to a 90% contraction of the gallbladder. Multiple PPCs occurred in the ileum of eight IBS patients but in only two controls; PPCs coincided with abdominal pain in six of the patients (Fig. 7). The authors concluded that CCK-OP may be useful in "unmasking" dysmotility of the small bowel in IBS.

4.2.5. Other Provocative Stimuli

Other challenges, notably cholinergic agonists and mechanical distension of the bowel, may be similarly provocative. These were applied systematically to the small intestine of patients with IBS.[125] Neostigmine increased motor activity of the jejunum and ileum, but there were no quantitative differences among IBS and controls. Neostigmine did, however, provoke PPCs in all IBS patients and in four controls; most of these ileal peristaltic waves were symptomatic. Bursts of DCCs were also recorded from the jejunum within several minutes of administration of the drug in eight IBS patients but in only one control. This motor pattern was also related in time to episodes of abdominal discomfort.

Distension of the bowel (Fig. 8) was another stimulus to which patients with IBS were more sensitive. A small balloon positioned in the ileum provoked abdominal pain more often, and at lower volumes, in IBS patients than in controls.[125] One other study has reported symptomatic responses to ileal distension in IBS; though uncontrolled, the anatomical referral of abdominal pain provoked by distension had a wide distribution.[6] Patients with IBS also show increased sensitivity to distension of the distal colon.[127]

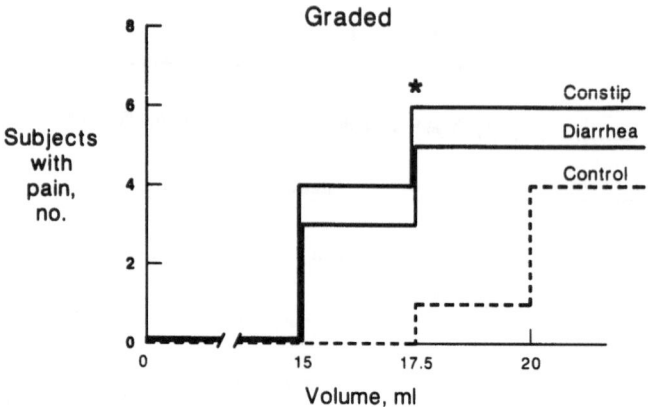

Figure 8. Response of three groups (IBS with constipation, IBS with diarrhea, healthy controls, all $n = 8$) to graded distension of the ileum with a balloon. At 17.5 ml, differences between IBS and controls were significant. From Kellow et al.[125] with permission.

These findings raise the possibility of IBS being an abnormal sensory perception of normal intestinal events; this could arise from abnormalities at the central or end-organ level. Thus, altered sensory perception to distension perhaps contributes to the abdominal pain experienced during the occurrence of specific motor patterns. An abnormally low pain threshold was suggested for the esophagus, an organ which appears to be involved in some patients with IBS.[128–130] In patients with intermittent, nonorganic dysphagia, discomfort was produced by inflating a balloon to diameters that were consistently smaller than those needed for equivalent pain in normals or in patients with reflux esophagitis.[130] A lower pain threshold to balloon distension has also been noted in patients with recurrent noncardiac chest pain.[131] However, IBS does not appear to be a manifestation of a more generalized hyperalgesia. Cook et al.[132] quantified responses to electrocutaneous stimulation in IBS patients with predominant constipation and in age-matched controls. Patients were less sensitive to low-intensity, nonpainful stimuli, and had a higher threshold for pain than did normal controls. They concluded that IBS patients do not select themselves from the general population by virtue of a generalized reduction in pain tolerance; it follows possibly that symptoms are indeed due to stimuli arising as a result of altered gut function.

Lasser et al.[133] determined the gas content of the bowel in a small number of patients with prominent symptoms of bloating and flatulence. The amount and composition of intestinal gas in IBS patients were the same as in controls. An inert gas was then infused into the duodenum and, in these patients, it refluxed back into the stomach and the symptoms experienced during gaseous distension were much greater than in controls.

4.2.6. Influence of Psychological Stress

Only one study has reported small intestinal motor activity in IBS patients during a period of controlled psychological stress.[110] Motor activity of the proximal small bowel was recorded in 22 patients with IBS (predominantly with diarrhea), 10 healthy volunteers, and 5 patients with inflammatory bowel disease. Subjects underwent prolonged periods of three intermittent mental stresses, playing an amusement arcade game, driving in heavy traffic, and undergoing delayed auditory feedback. One or more motor abnormalities occurred in 19 IBS patients but in only 1 control. The abnormalities included total abolition of MMCs and abnormal contractile activity during phase II.

4.3. Altered Absorption and Secretion

In contrast to the recent attention given to intestinal dysmotility in functional disorders, there are few reports of electrolyte transport in the small intestines of such patients. However, especially in the group with diarrhea, disorders of electrolyte and water transport are certainly possible. Krag et al.[134,135] studied fluid transport in the small bowel of patients with IBS and those with diarrhea after vagotomy and pyloroplasty. In IBS, the ileum secreted fluid and was also more sensitive to the additional secretory effects of bile acids; similar but lesser changes were noted in the jejunum.[134] These observations do not appear to have been followed up and no other information is known to us on patients with abdominal pain and loose stools, those who would fit the conventional criteria for IBS. Postvagotomy patients who had diarrhea also had fluid secretion in the ileum, but secretion was augmented little by perfusion with bile acids.[135]

More attention has been given to the syndromes of watery diarrhea,[136,137] but these patients rarely have pain as a major feature and many believe that painless diarrhea should be categorized separately from IBS. This group of patients also merges into those with laxative abuse, diarrhea as a side effect of overt or surreptitious use of other drugs,[136] and those with nonadenomatous hypersecretion of diarrheogenic peptides. These issues are beyond the present charge.

In the context of altered fluid transport in IBS, secretory peptides and the prostaglandins have been implicated. Specific food intolerances were reported in a high proportion of patients with IBS and found to be associated with elevated levels of PGE_2 in dialysates of rectal fluid.[138] However, in another report, food intolerance was confirmed in only a small proportion of such patients.[139]

It is now well established that lactose intolerance is responsible for symptoms in only a few patients who present as IBS.[140,141] The initial descriptions of lactase deficiency have raised the possibility of this abnormality explaining many examples of IBS. However, it is now better appreciated that most adults (e.g., 70–90% of the black and Oriental races) normally lack lactase activity in the brush border. On the other hand, incomplete absorption of fructose and sugar alcohols (such as sorbitol) are well recognized as causes of symptoms in otherwise healthy subjects.[72,74,142] Poorly absorbed oligosaccharides can be ingested unknowingly in amounts sufficient to cause frequent, loose stools especially among dietary faddists. Specific gas-forming foods such as beans and the propensity for high-fiber diets to provoke gaseous distension in some persons should also be appreciated.

Some patients with functional diarrhea are thought to have a primary malabsorption of bile acids as the basis of their symptoms.[143,144] It has been suggested that this results from an underlying motor or absorptive defect in the ileum,[145] and a histological abnormality, which may be immunologically mediated,[146] has even been proposed.

5. SUMMARY AND INTERIM SPECULATIONS

The functional bowel disorders still need to be considered as a heterogeneous collection of symptom complexes. Some would add that they are inadequately defined, poorly investigated, and possess no unifying concepts; also, a common nomenclature is not even available. This objective, albeit negative, view holds that when syndromes are defined solely by vague symptoms, any attempts to classify further (or perhaps even to investigate) are unjustified.

On a more positive note, the possibility that several rather more discrete syndromes exist is suggested by the greater consistency found among results when patients are categorized by their major symptoms. In the group in which abdominal pain and altered bowel habit are major features, there are even differences among those in whom diarrhea predominates as against those with constipation as a major complaint. In these groups, disorders of motor function can be demonstrated in the small as well as the large bowel. Indeed, in some patients evidence to incriminate the small bowel, though less extensive, is perhaps just as persuasive as that which focuses on dysmotility of the colon. Most exciting are the descriptions of abnormalities of the smooth muscle in multiple organs, the small bowel, colon, gallbladder, and urinary bladder.

In some patients, therefore, IBS may be a multisystem disorder. The common factor is dysfunction of smooth muscle of diverse tissues. It is attractive to speculate that ENS control of epithelial function (absorption and secretion) might also be disturbed; but, as described above, these elements remain virtually unexplored. However, we can speculate that one subgroup of patients expresses the underlying pathophysiology by dysfunction of the small bowel whereas in others the symptoms may be mainly colonic, esophageal, or gastroduodenal. Among the IBS criteria of Manning et al.,[87] several might reasonably be attributable to the small bowel; specifically these are distension, abdominal pain, altered bowel habit, and relief of pain following a loose bowel movement. How can these features be related to what we know of small bowel dysfunction in IBS?

Distension is not due to excessive amounts of gas in the bowel,[133] but the complaint is so common and usually so intense that other explanations need be sought. An exaggerated response to balloon distension of the small bowel has been reported consistently[125,133]; thus, it is logical to propose that in IBS the "sensor" for stretch is set at a level different from that of healthy subjects. This could be at the sensory end-organ level (mechanoreceptors), within the intraabdominal ganglia,[147,148] or even at higher levels in the CNS. With the "stat" set differentially, one could hypothesize that a normal degree of stretch would be sensed as an "overstretch" (giving the central sensation of distension) and might even account for a greater nociceptive response.

Pain related to specific patterns of dysmotility in the small bowel are particularly provocative. In the ileum, PPCs are infrequent but normal events and these powerful mechanical events are often "sensed" as abdominal discomfort, even by healthy persons. We speculate that coloileal reflux, by allowing short-chain fatty acid (SCFA) to gain access to the ileal lumen, increases the number of ileal PPCs.[30,149] The hypothesis that coloileal reflux is more frequent or severe in IBS is worth testing. The other motor patterns associated with symptoms in IBS are jejunal DCCs. In this instance, one can more logically propose a dysfunction of the ENS as its basis. In established cases of pseudoobstruction,[22] discrete bursts (equivalent to DCCs) are more frequent; moreover, pain is common in pseudoobstruction. Thus, the hypothesis here is that IBS represents minimal disease of the ENS, of a type perhaps equivalent to but less severe than some forms of pseudoobstruction!

The key message is that it is possible to demonstrate a pathophysiology within the small bowel and in IBS and that we can therefore reassure ourselves and our patients that, with an open mind and a touch of optimism, better understanding and therapies will follow.

ACKNOWLEDGMENT. Supported in part by Grants DK32121 and DK34988 from the National Institutes of Health.

REFERENCES

1. Phillips, SF: Diarrhea: A current view of the pathophysiology. Gastroenterology 63:495–518, 1972
2. Stephen AM, Haddad AC, Phillips SF: Passage of carbohydrates into the colon. Direct measurements in humans. Gastroenterology 85:589–595, 1983
3. Debongnie JC, Phillips SF: Capacity of the human colon to absorb fluid. Gastroenterology 74:698–703, 1978
4. Phillips SF, Gaginella TS: Intestinal secretion as a mechanism in diarrheal disease, in Glass GBJ (ed): Progress in Gastroenterology. New York, Grune & Stratton, 1977, Vol III, 481–504
5. Kellow JE, Phillips SF: Altered small bowel motility in irritable bowel syndrome is correlated with symptoms. Gastroenterology 92:1885–1893, 1987
6. Moriaty KJ, Dawson AM: Functional abdominal pain: Further evidence that whole gut is affected. Br Med J 284:1670–1672, 1982
7. Weisbrodt NW: Motility of the small intestine, in Johnson LR (ed): Physiology of the Gastrointestinal Tract. New York, Raven Press, 1987, pp 631–663
8. Szurszewski JH: A migrating electric complex of the canine small intestine. Am J Physiol 217:1757–1763, 1969
9. Kerlin P, Phillips SF: Variability of motility of the ileum and jejunum in healthy humans. Gastroenterology 82:694–700, 1982
10. Vantrappen G, Janssens J, Hellemans J, et al: The interdigestive motor complex in normal subjects and patients with bacterial overgrowth of the small intestine. J Clin Invest 59:1158–1166, 1977
11. Quigley EMM, Borody TJ, Phillips SF, et al: Motility of the terminal ileum and ileocecal sphincter in healthy humans. Gastroenterology 87:857–866, 1984
12. Kellow JE, Borody TJ, Phillips SF, et al: Human interdigestive motility: Variations in patterns from oesophagus to colon. Gastroenterology 91:386–395, 1986
13. Rayner V, Weeks TEC, Bruce JB: Insulin and myoelectric activity of the small intestine of the pig. Dig Dis Sci 26:33–41, 1981
14. Scott LD, Cahall DL: Influence of the interdigestive myoelectric complex on enteric flora in the rat. Gastroenterology 82:737–745, 1982
15. Quigley EMM, Phillips SF, Dent J: Distinctive patterns of interdigestive motility at the canine ileocolonic junction. Gastroenterology 87:836–844, 1984
16. Siegle M-L, Ehrlein H-J: Interdigestive contractile patterns of the ileum in dogs. Am J Physiol 16:G452–G460, 1987
17. Arndorfer RC, Stef JJ, Dodds WJ, et al: Improved infusion system for intraluminal oesophageal manometry. Gastroenterology 23:23–27, 1977
18. Thompson DG, Wingate DL, Archer L, et al: Normal patterns of human upper small bowel motor activity recorded by prolonged radiotelemetry. Gut 21:500–506, 1980
19. Kumar D, Wingate DL, Ruckebusch Y: Circadian variation in the propagation velocity of the migrating motor complex. Gastroenterology 91:926–930, 1986
20. Gill RC, Kellow JE, Wingate DL: The migrating motor complex (MMC) at home. Gastroenterology 92:1405, 1987 (abstr)

21. Malagelada J-R, Camilleri M, Stanghellini V: Manometric Diagnosis of Gastrointestinal Motility Disorders. New York, Thieme, 1986
22. Summers RW, Anuras S, Green J: Jejunal manometry patterns in health, partial intestinal obstruction and pseudo-obstruction. Gastroenterology 85:1290–1300, 1983
23. Fleckenstein P, Oigaard A: Electrical spike activity in the human small intestine. A multiple electrode study of fasting diurnal variations. Dig Dis Sci 23:776–780, 1978
24. Fleckenstein P: Migrating electrical spike activity in the fasting human small intestine. Am J Dig Dis 23:769–775, 1978
25. Fleckenstein P, Bueno L, Fioramonti J, et al: Minute rhythm of electrical spike bursts of the small intestine in different species. Am J Physiol 242:G654–G659, 1982
26. Kellow JE, Gill RC, Wingate DL: Proximal gut motor activity in irritable bowel syndrome (IBS) patients at home and at work. Gastroenterology 92:1463, 1987 (abstr)
27. Code CF, Rogers AG, Schlegel J, et al: Motility patterns in the terminal ileum: Studies on two patients with ulcerative colitis and ileal stomas. Gastroenterology 32:651–665, 1957
28. Heppell J, Pemberton JH, Kelly KA, et al: Ileal motility after endorectal ileo-anal anastomosis. Surg Gastroenterol 1:123–127, 1982
29. Kruis W, Azpiroz F, Phillips SF: Contractile patterns and transit of fluid in canine terminal ileum. Am J Physiol 249:G264–G270, 1985
30. Kamath PS, Hoepfner MT, Phillips SF: Short-chain fatty acids stimulate motility of the canine ileum. Am J Physiol 253:G427–G433, 1987
31. Helm JD, Kramer P, MacDonald M, et al: Changes in motility of the human small intestine during sleep. Gastroenterology 10:135–137, 1948
32. Ritchie HD, Thompson DG, Wingate DL: Diurnal variation in human jejunal fasting motor activity. J Physiol (London) 305:54P, 1980 (abstr)
33. Evans DF, Foster GE, Hardcastle JD: The motility of the human antrum and jejunum during the day and during sleep: An investigation using a radiotelemetry system, in Wienbeck M (ed): Motility of the Digestive Tract. New York, Raven Press, 1982, pp 185–192
34. Frexinos J, Bueno L, Fioramonti J: Diurnal changes in myoelectric spiking activity of the human colon. Gastroenterology 88:1104–1110, 1985
35. Code CF, Marlett JA: The interdigestive myoelectric complex of the stomach and small bowel of dogs. J Physiol (London) 246:289–309, 1975
36. De Weever I, Eeckhout C, Vantrappen G, et al: How does oil disrupt the interdigestive myoelectric complex? Gastroenterology 76:1120, 1979 (abstr)
37. Sillin LF, Schulte WJ, Woods JH, et al: Electromotor feeding responses of primate ileum and colon. Am J Surg 137:99–105, 1979
38. Douglas DM, Mann FC: The gastroileac reflex: Further experimental observations. Am J Dig Dis 7:53–57, 1940
39. Thompson DG, Archer L, Green WJ, et al: Fasting motor activity occurs during a day of normal meals in healthy subjects. Gut 22:489–492, 1981
40. Schemann M, Ehrlein H-J: Mechanical characteristics of phase II and phase III of the interdigestive migrating motor complex in dogs. Gastroenterology 91:117–123, 1986
41. Read NW, Al-Janabi MN, Edwards CA, et al: Relationships between postprandial motor activity in the human small intestine and the gastrointestinal transit of food. Gastroenterology 86:721–727, 1984
42. Wood JD: Physiology of the enteric nervous system, in Johnson LR (ed): Physiology of the Gastrointestinal Tract, ed 2. New York, Raven Press, 1987, pp 67–109
43. Hall KE, El-Sharkawy TY, Diamant NE: Vagal control of migrating motor complex in the dog. Am J Physiol 243:G276–G284, 1982
44. Bueno L, Praddaude F, Ruckebusch Y: Propagation of electrical spiking activity along the small intestine: Intrinsic versus extrinsic neural influences. J Physiol (London) 292:15–26, 1979
45. Gregory PC, Rayner DV, Wenham G: Initiation of migrating myoelectric complex in sheep by duodenal acidification and hyperosmolality: Role of vagus nerves. J Physiol (London) 355:509–521, 1984
46. Whitehead WE, Schuster MM: Irritable bowel syndrome: Physiological and psychological mechanisms, in Gastrointestinal Disorders: Behavioral and Psychological Basis for Treatment, Whitehead WE, Schuster MM (eds), New York, Academic Press, 1985, pp 179–210
47. McRae S, Younger K, Thompson DG, et al: Sustained mental stress alters human jejunal motor activity. Gut 23:404–409, 1982

48. Valori RM, Kumar D, Wingate DL: Effects of different types of stress and of "prokinetic" drugs on the control of the fasting motor complex in humans. Gastroenterology 90:1890–1900, 1986

49. Marik F, Code CF: Control of the interdigestive myoelectric activity in dogs by the vagus nerve and pentagastrin. Gastroenterology 69:387–395, 1975

50. Mukhopadhyay AK, Thor PJ, Copeland EM, et al: Effect of cholecystokinin on myoelectric activity of small bowel of the dog. Am J Physiol 232:E44–E47, 1977

51. Wingate DL, Pearce EA, Hutton M, et al: Quantitative comparison of the effects of cholecystokinin, secretin and pentagastrin on gastrointestinal myoelectric activity in the conscious fasted dog. Gut 19:593–601, 1978

52. Thor K, Rosell S, Rokaeus A, et al: (Gln^4)-neurotensin changes the motility pattern of the duodenum and proximal jejunum from a fasting-type to a fed-type. Gastroenterology 83:569–574, 1982

53. Schang J-C, Kelly KA: Inhibition of canine interdigestive proximal gastric motility by cholecystokinin-octapeptide. Am J Physiol 240:G217–G220, 1981

54. Harvey RF: The irritable bowel syndrome: Hormonal influences. Clin Gastroenterology 6:631–641, 1977

55. Snape WJ, Carlson GM, Matarazzo SA, et al: Evidence that abnormal myoelectrical activity produces colonic motor dysfunction in the irritable bowel syndrome. Gastroenterology 72:383–387, 1977

56. Yamagishi T, Debas HT: Cholecystokinin inhibits gastric emptying by acting on both proximal stomach and pylorus. Am J Physiol 234:E375–E378, 1978

57. Rehfeld JF: how to measure cholecystokinin in plasma? Gastroenterology 87:434–438, 1984

58. Kellow JE, Miller LJ, Phillips SF, et al: Sensitivities of human jejunum, ileum, proximal colon and gallbladder to cholecystokinin octapeptide. Am J Physiol 252:G345–G356, 1987

59. Anuras S, Cooke AR, Christensen J: An inhibitory innervation at the gastroduodenal junction. J Clin Invest 54:529–535, 1974

60. Persson CGA, Ekman M: Effect of morphine, cholecystokinin and sympathomimetics on the sphincter of Oddi and intraluminal pressure in cat duodenum. Scand J Gastroenterol 7:345–351, 1972

61. Weems WA, Weisbrodt NW: Ileal and colonic propulsive behaviour: Contribution of enteric neural circuits. Am J Physiol 250:G653–G659, 1986

62. Ruckebusch Y, Bueno L: Migrating myoelectrical complex of the small intestine: An intrinsic activity mediated by the vagus. Gastroenterology 73:1309–1314, 1977

63. Chung SA, Diamant NE: Small intestinal motility in the fasted and postprandial states: Effect of transient vagosympathetic blockade. Am J Physiol 252:G301–G308, 1987

64. Fielding JF: The irritable bowel syndrome: Clinical spectrum. Clin Gastroenterol 6:709–722, 1977

65. Cann PA, Read NW, Cammack J, et al: Psychological stress and the passage of a standard meal through the stomach and small intestine in man. Gut 24:236–240, 1983

66. O'Brien J, Thompson DG, Burnham WR, et al: Action of centrally mediated autonomic stimulation on human upper gastrointestinal transit: A comparative study of two stimuli. Gut 28:960–969, 1987

67. Turnberg LA, Fordtran JS, Carter NW, et al: Mechanism of bicarbonate absorption and its relation to sodium transport in the human jejunum. J Clin Invest 49:548–556, 1970

68. Turnberg LA, Bieberdorf FA, Morawski SG, et al: Interrelationships of chloride, bicarbonate, sodium and hydrogen transport in the human ileum. J Clin Invest 49:557–567, 1970

69. Field M: Secretion of electrolytes and water by mammalian small intestine, in Johnson LR (ed), Physiology of the Gastrointestinal Tract. New York, Raven Press, 1981, pp 963–982

70. Anderson IH, Levine AS, Levitt MD: Incomplete absorption of the carbohydrate in all purpose wheat flour. N Engl J Med 304:891–892, 1981

71. Kerlin P, Wong L, Harris B, et al: Rice flour, breath hydrogen, and malabsorption. Gastroenterology 87:578–585, 1984

72. Ravich WJ, Bayless TM, Thomas M: Fructose: Incomplete intestinal absorption in humans. Gastroenterology 84:26–29, 1983

73. Bond JH, Levitt MD, Prentiss R: Investigation of small bowel transit time in man utilising pulmonary hydrogen (H_2) measurements. J Lab Clin Med 85:546–555, 1975

74. Hyams JS: Sorbitol intolerance: An unappreciated cause of functional gastrointestinal complaints. Gastroenterology 84:30–33, 1983

75. Read NW, McFarlane A, Kinsman RI, et al: Effect of infusion of nutrient solutions into the ileum on gastrointestinal transit and plasma levels of neurotensin and enteroglucagon. Gastroenterology 86:274–280, 1984

76. Spiller RC, Trotman IF, Higgins BE, et al: The ileal brake—Inhibition of jejunal motility after ileal fat perfusion in man. Gut 25:365–374, 1984
77. Kinsman RI, Read NW: Effect of naloxone on feedback regulation of small bowel transit by fat. Gastroenterology 87:335–337, 1984
78. Morris AI, Turnberg LA: Influence of a parasympathetic agonist and antagonist on human intestinal transport in vivo. Gastroenterology 89:861–866, 1980
79. Morris AI, Turnberg LA: Influence of isoproterenol and propranolol on human intestinal transport in vivo. Gastroenterology 81:1076–1079, 1981
80. Isaacs PET, Whitehead JS, Kim YS: Muscarinic acetylcholine receptors of the small intestine and pancreas of the rat: Distribution and the effect of vagotomy. Clin Sci 62:203–207, 1982
81. Chang EB, Field M, Miller RJ: Enterocyte α-2-adrenergic receptors: Yohimbine and p-aminoclonidine binding relative to ion transport. Am J Physiol 244:G76–G82, 1983
82. Barclay GR, Turnberg LA: Effect of psychological stress on salt and water transport in the human jejunum. Gastroenterology 93:91–97, 1987
83. Read NW, Cooper K, Fordtran JS: Effect of modified sham feeding on jejunal transport and pancreatic and biliary secretion in man. Am J Physiol 234:E417–E420, 1978
84. Powell DW: Intestinal water and electrolyte transport, in Johnson LR (ed): Physiology of the Gastrointestinal Tract, ed 2. New York, Raven Press, 1987, pp 1267–1306
85. Bukhave K, Rask-Madsen J: Saturation kinetics applied to in vitro effects of low prostaglandin E_2 and $F_{2\alpha}$ concentrations on ion transport across human jejunal mucosa. Gastroenterology 78:32–42, 1980
86. Woodmansey P, Bates TE, Read NW: Effect of psychological stress on fluid and electrolyte transport in the human jejunum. Gut 24:A991, 1983 (abstr)
87. Manning AP, Thompson WD, Heaton KW, et al: Towards positive diagnosis in the irritable bowel syndrome. Br Med J 2:653–654, 1978
88. Thompson WG, Heaton KW: Functional bowel disorders in apparently healthy people. Gastroenterology 79:283–288, 1980
89. Chaudhary NA, Truelove SC: The irritable colon syndrome. Q J Med 31:307–322, 1962
90. Chaudhary NA, Truelove SC: Human colonic motility: A comparative study of normal subjects, patients with ulcerative colitis and patients with irritable colon syndrome. I. Resting patterns of motility. Gastroenterology 40:1–17, 1961
91. Chaudhary NA, Truelove SC: Human colonic motility: A comparative study of normal subjects, patients with ulcerative colitis and patients with irritable colon syndrome. II. The effect of prostigmin. Gastroenterology 40:18–26, 1961
92. Talley NJ, Phillips SF: Non-ulcer dyspepsia: Potential causes and pathophysiology. Ann Intern Med 108:865–879, 1988
93. Thompson WG: The irritable bowel syndrome. Gut 25:1089–1092, 1984
94. Kruis W, Thieme CH, Weinzierl M, et al: A diagnostic score for the irritable bowel syndrome. Its value in the exclusion of organic disease. Gastroenterology 87:1–7, 1984
95. Kellow JE, Miller LJ, Phillips SF, et al: Altered sensitivity of the gallbladder to cholecystokinin octapeptide in irritable bowel syndrome. Am J Physiol 253:G650–G655, 1987
96. Talley NJ, Piper DW: The association between non-ulcer dyspepsia and other gastrointestinal disorders. Scand J Gastroenterol 20:896–900, 1985
97. Whorwell PJ, McCallum M, Creed FH, et al: Non-colonic features of irritable bowel syndrome. Gut 27:37–40, 1986.
98. Whorwell PJ, Lupton EW, Erduran D, et al: Bladder smooth muscle dysfunction in patients with irritable bowel syndrome. Gut 27:1014–1017, 1986
99. Braverman DZ: Gallbladder contraction in patients with irritable bowel syndrome. Isr J Med Sci 23:181–184, 1987
100. Collins S: Irritable bowel syndrome—the asthma of the gut? Gastroenterology 94:494, 1988 (abstr)
101. Horowitz L, Farrar JT: Intraluminal small intestinal pressures in normal patients and in patients with functional gastrointestinal disorders. Gastroenterology 42:455–464, 1962
102. Holdstock DJ, Misiewicz JJ, Waller SL: Observations on the mechanism of abdominal pain. Gut 10:19–31, 1969
103. Connell AM, Jones FA, Rowlands EN: Motility of the pelvic colon: Pain associated with colonic hypermotility after meals. Gut 6:105–112, 1965

104. Ritchie JA, Salem SN: Upper intestinal motility in ulcerative colitis, idiopathic steatorrhea and the irritable colon syndrome. Gut 6:325–337, 1965
105. Thompson DG, Laidlow JM, Wingate DL: Abnormal small bowel motility demonstrated by radiotelemetry in a patient with irritable colon. Lancet 2:1321–1322, 1979
106. Foster GE, Arden-Jones J, Beattie A, et al: Disordered small bowel motility in gastrointestinal disease. Gastroenterology 82:1059, 1982 (abstr)
107. Kingham JGC, Bown R, Colson R, et al: Jejunal motility in patients with functional abdominal pain. Gut 25:375–380, 1984
108. Mathias JR, Carlson GM, Di Marino AJ, et al: Intestinal myoelectric activity in response to live Vibrio cholerae and cholera enterotoxin. J Clin Invest 58:91–96, 1976
109. Mathias JR, Martin JL, Burns TW, et al: Ricinoleic acid effects on the electrical activity of the small intestine in rabbits. J Clin Invest 61:640–644, 1978
110. Kumar D, Wingate DL: The irritable bowel syndrome: A paroxysmal motor disorder. Lancet 2:973–977, 1985
111. Borody TJ, Byrnes D, Bell D, et al: The migrating motor complex: Its return to circulating CCK, motilin and pancreatic polypeptide in irritable bowel patients and in controls. Clin Res 32:23A, 1984 (abstr)
112. Cann PA, Read NW, Brown C, et al: Irritable bowel syndrome: Relationship of disorders in the transit of a single solid meal to symptom patterns. Gut 24:405–411, 1983
113. Jian R, Najean Y, Bernier JJ: Measurment of intestinal progression of a meal and its residues in normal subjects and patients with functional diarrhoea by a dual isotope technique. Gut 25:728–731, 1984
114. Corbett CL, Thomas S, Read NW, et al: Electromechanical detector for breath hydrogen determination: Measurement of small bowel transit time in normal subjects and patients with the irritable bowel syndrome. Gut 22:836–840, 1981
115. Youle MS, Read NW: Effect of painless rectal distension on gastrointestinal transit of solid meal. Dig Dis Sci 29:902–906, 1984
116. Kellow JE, Gill RC, Wingate DL: Modulation of human upper gastrointestinal motility by rectal distension. Gut 28:864–868, 1987
117. Trotman IF, Price CC: Bloated irritable bowel syndrome defined by dynamic ^{99m}Tc bran scan. Lancet 2:364–366, 1986
118. Hardy JG, Wood E, Clark AG, et al: Whole bowel transit in patients with the irritable bowel syndrome. Eur J Nucl Med 11:393–396, 1986
119. Hardy JG, Wilson CG, Wood E: Drug delivery to the proximal colon. J Pharm Pharmacol 37:874–877, 1985
120. Besterman HS, Sarson DL, Rambard JC, et al: Gut hormone responses in the irritable bowel syndrome. Digestion 21:219–224, 1981
121. Geoghegan J, Fielding JF: Serum gastrin and irritable bowel syndrome. Ir J Med Sci 147:156, 1978 (abstr)
122. Preston DM, Adrian TE, Christofides ND, et al: positive correlation between symptoms and circulating motilin, pancreatic polypeptide and gastrin concentrations in functional bowel disorders. Gut 26:1059–1064, 1985
123. Binimelis J, Webb SM, Mones J, et al: Circulating immunoreactive somatostatin in gastrointestinal diseases. Scand J Gastroenterol 22:931–937, 1987
124. Harvey RF, Read AE: Effect of cholecystokinin on colonic motility and symptoms in patients with the irritable bowel syndrome. Lancet 1:1–3, 1973
125. Kellow JE, Miller LJ, Phillips SF, et al: Dysmotility of the small intestine is provoked by stimuli in irritable bowel syndrome. Gut 29:1236–1243, 1988
126. Sullivan MA, Cohen S, Snape WJ: Colonic myoelectrical activity in the irritable bowel syndrome; effect of eating and anticholinergics. N Engl J Med 298:878–883, 1978
127. Ritchie J: Pain from distension of the pelvic colon by inflating a balloon in the irritable bowel syndrome. Gut 14:125–132, 1973
128. Clouse RE, Eckert TC: Gastrointestinal symptoms of patients with oesophageal contraction abnormalities. Dig Dis Sci 31:236–240, 1986
129. Whorwell PJ, Clouter C, Smith CL: Oesophageal motility in the irritable bowel syndrome. Br Med J 1:1101–1103, 1981
130. Edwards DL: The "tender" oesophagus. Gut 25:A986, 1984 (abstr)

131. Richter JE, Barish CF, Castell DO: Abnormal sensory perception in patients with oesophageal chest pain. Gastroenterology 91:845–852, 1986

132. Cook IJ, Van Eeden A, Collins SM: Patients with irritable bowel syndrome have greater pain tolerance than normal subjects. Gastroenterology 93:727–733, 1987

133. Lasser RB, Bond JH, Levitt MD: The role of intestinal gas in functional abdominal pain. N Engl J Med 293:524–526, 1975

134. Oddsson E, Rask-Madsen J, Krag E: A secretory epithelium of the small intestine with increased sensitivity to bile acids in irritable bowel syndrome associated with diarrhea. Scand J Gastroenterol 13:409–416, 1978

135. Hempel-Sparso B, Fredricksen H-JB, Malchow-Møller A, et al: Mucosal function of the perfused ileum in patients with and without diarrhea and dumping after vagotomy and pyloroplasty. Scand J Gastroenterol 18:669–674, 1983

136. Fordtran JS, Santa Ana CA, Morawski SG, et al: Pathophysiology of choice diarrhea: Insights derived from intestinal perfusion studies in 31 patients. Clin Gastroenterol 15(3):477–490, 1986

137. Read NW: Diarrhée motrice. Clin Gastroenterol 15(3):657–688, 1986

138. Jones VA, McLaughlan P, Shorthouse M, et al: Food intolerance: A major factor in the pathogenesis of irritable bowel syndrome. Lancet 2:1115–1117, 1982

139. Bentley SJ, Pearson DJ, Rix KJB: Food hypersensitivity in irritable bowel syndrome. Lancet 2:295–297, 1983

140. Newcomer AD, McGill DB: Irritable bowel syndrome: Role of lactase deficiency. Mayo Clin Proc 58:339–341, 1983

141. Eastwood MA, Walton BA, Brydon WG, et al: Faecal weight, constituents, colonic motility, and lactose tolerance in the irritable bowel syndrome. Digestion 30:7–12, 1984

142. Rumessen JJ, Gudmand-Hoyer E: Malabsorption of fructose–sorbitol mixtures: Interactions causing abdominal distress. Scand J Gastroenterol 22:431–436, 1987

143. Thaysen EH, Pedersen L: Idiopathic bile acid catharsis. Gut 17:965–970, 1976

144. Merrick MV, Eastwood MA, Ford MJ: Is bile acid malabsorption underdiagnosed? An evaluation of accuracy of diagnosis by measurement of SEHCAT retention. Br Med J 290:665–668, 1985

145. Schiller LR, Hogan RB, Morawski SG, et al: Studies of the prevalence and significance of radiolabeled bile acid malabsorption in a group of patients with idiopathic chronic diarrhoea. Gastroenterology 92:151–160, 1987

146. Popovic OS, Kostic KM, Milovic VB, et al: Primary bile acid malabsorption: Histologic and immunologic study in three patients. Gastroenterology 92:1851–1858, 1987

147. Kreulen DL, Muir TC, Szurszewski JH: Peripheral sympathetic pathways to gastroduodenal region of the guinea pig. Am J Physiol 245:G369–G375, 1983

148. Kreulen DL, Peters S: Noncholinergic transmission in a sympathetic ganglion of the guinea pig elicited by colon distension. J Physiol (London) 374:315–334, 1986

149. Kamath PS, Phillips SF, Zinsmeister AR: Short-chain fatty acids stimulate ileal motility in man. Gastroenterology 95:1496–1502, 1988

10

Mechanisms and Management of Chronic Constipation

James C. Reynolds

1. INTRODUCTION

The mechanisms of chronic constipation are complex and vary in severity from a dietary deficiency of fiber to a diffuse systemic neuropathy. Most patients with milder degrees of constipation will respond promptly to an increase in dietary fiber.[1-3] In fact, epidemiologic studies indicate that many colonic disorders that are endemic to Western nations, including the irritable bowel syndrome (IBS), constipation, and colon cancer, occur rarely in societies that injest higher quantities of dietary fiber.[4,5] In contrast, there are increasing reports about the medical and surgical treatment of more intractable forms of constipation.[6-12] Figure 1 shows the abdominal x-rays of a patient with severe constipation due to anal sphincter dysfunction. The diagnosis went unrecognized for over a decade, and thus led to years of discomfort that could have been avoided by earlier treatment. Data from several centers suggest that in a subset of patients, constipation may be the presenting symptom of a diffuse disorder of enteric and autonomic nerves.[7,10] An increased understanding of the mechanisms of constipation will lead to a more rational approach to the diagnosis and treatment of patients suffering from this condition.

It is not clear whether the pathophysiologic mechanisms that result in severe constipation are different from the causes of milder degrees of constipation or whether they differ only in the degree of functional impairment.[3] Chronic severe constipation represents an extreme in the spectrum of a very common problem. An improved understanding of the mechanisms of chronic severe constipation may also lead to a better understanding of the basic pathophysiology and treatment of other forms of colonic dysfunction.

The incidence of severe constipation has not been defined, but several factors indicate that this is a common problem.[7-13] While it has been stated that there is no indication for the chronic use of laxatives,[14,15] clinical experience and economic indicators suggest

James C. Reynolds • Department of Medicine and Physiology, Hospital of the University of Pennsylvania, Philadelphia, Pennsylvania 19104.

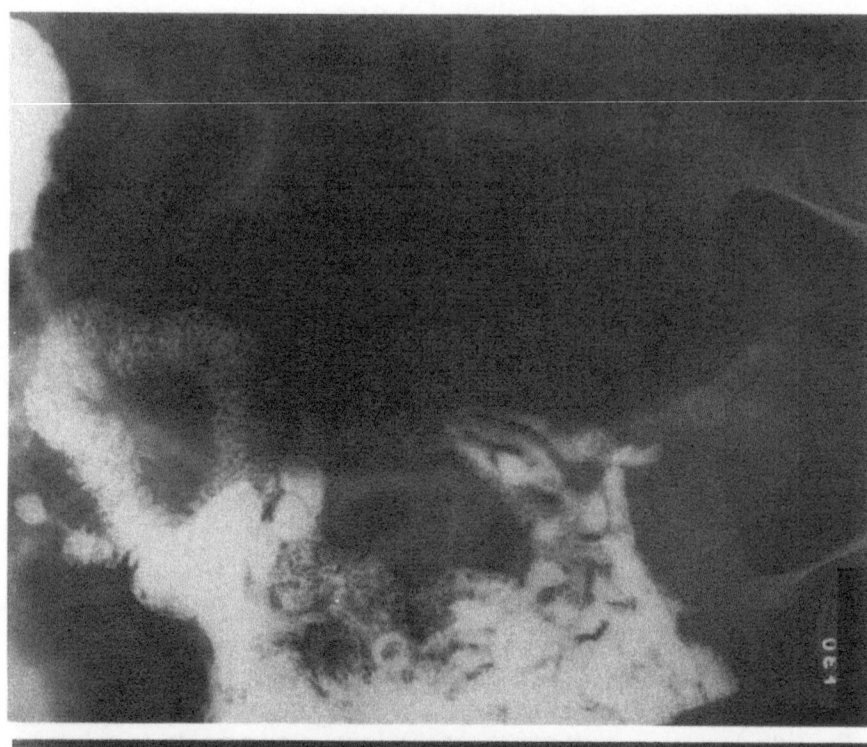
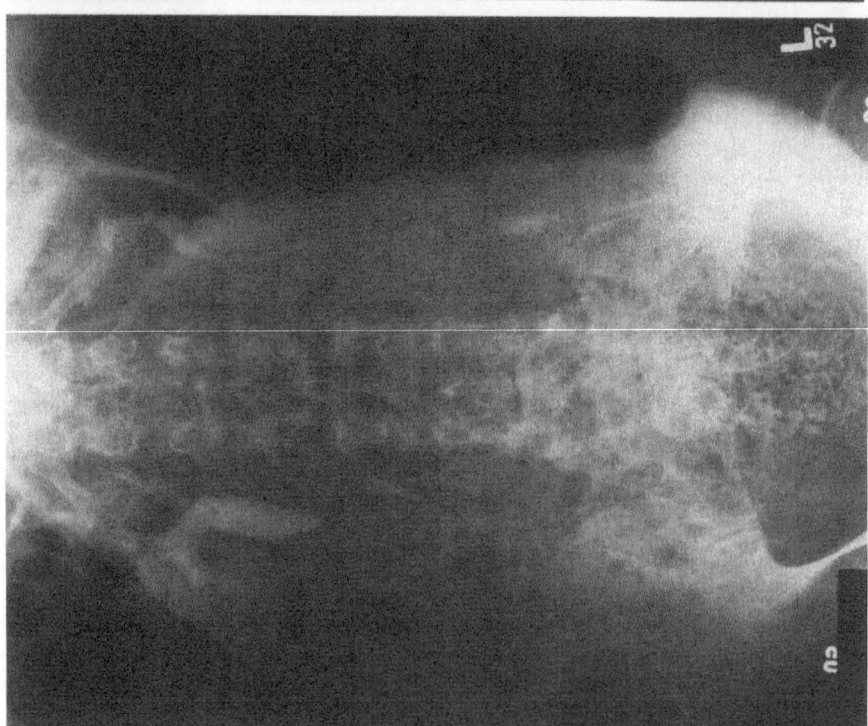

Figure 1. Massive dilatation of the sigmoid colon is shown before (left) and after (right) elimination of a huge volume of fecal impaction. The cleansing enemas resulted in a 12-pound weight loss. Further studies revealed normal colonic, gastric, and esophageal function with an absent rectal–anal inhibitory reflex.

that chronic constipation occurs more commonly than previously appreciated. Many patients admit to habitual use of laxatives. The national expenditure for laxatives approaches a half billion dollars per year. Furthermore, dozens of prescription or over-the-counter medications with a wide variability in efficacy and pharmacologic mechanisms are available to the patient and physician to treat constipation. Each year new agents are being marketed and the medical journals are replete with advertisements for these products. Finally, it is most clear to the practicing gastroenterologist that colonic dysfunction leading to constipation is a common problem that warrants a better understanding of both mechanism and treatment.

The increasing recognition of the importance of chronic constipation suggests that a review of mechanism and treatment of the disorders that lead to constipation will be valuable to practitioner and investigator alike. This chapter summarizes a rational approach to the diagnosis of constipation, its complications, causes, and management of patients with chronic severe impairment in their ability to eliminate solid waste from the body.

2. THE DIAGNOSIS OF COLONIC MOTOR DYSFUNCTION

2.1. The Initial Approach to the Patient

Once the diagnosis of constipation has been entertained, the physician should attempt to identify the mechanism of the impairment. An approach that can be used to characterize the cause of constipation into practical categories is shown in Fig. 2. It is especially

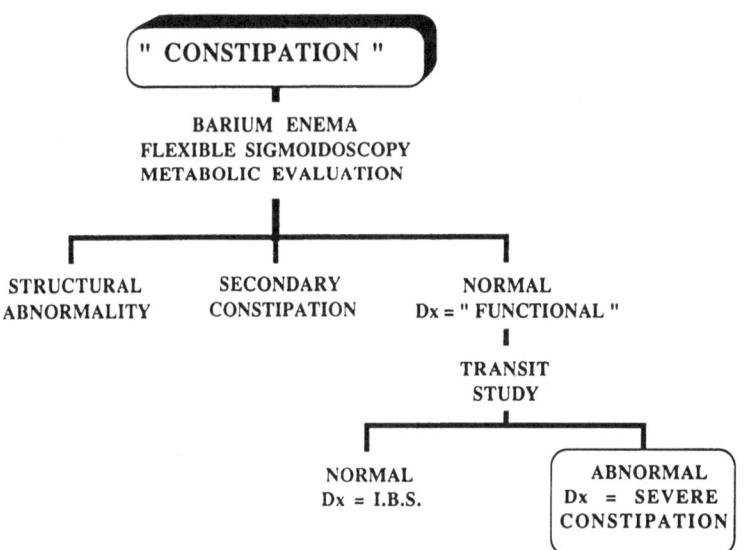

Figure 2. Every patient who presents with a chronic complaint of constipation can be readily characterized into four diagnostic categories: mechanical obstruction, secondary functional constipation, irritable bowel syndrome, and chronic severe constipation.

Table I. Mechanical Causes of Constipation

Intrinsic neoplasms
   Adenocarcinoma
   Leiomyosarcoma
   Lymphoma
Inflammatory strictures
   Diverticulosis
   Crohn's disease
   Adhesions
Intermittent lesions
   Volvulus
   Hernias
   Intussusception
Impinging lesions
   Endometriosis
   Metastatic malignancies

important to identify the presence of any secondary factors that may be the cause of the constipation or of the patient's decompensation. A thorough history, physical exam, and laboratory studies should be followed by a barium enema and proctosigmoidoscopy to exclude mechanical obstruction. Mechanical causes of constipation are listed in Table I. In addition to the obvious, intrinsic lesions of the colon, one must consider disorders that lead to intermittent mechanical obstruction and extrinsic compression.

If the patient has recently had a normal barium enema, repeating this study is rarely helpful and exposes the patient to unnecessary radiation.[16,17] In patients with severely impaired colonic transit, elimination of the barium can be very difficult, and an impediment to further diagnostic and therapeutic measures. Prudence dictates that in every patient presenting with constipation, however, the previous barium studies should be reviewed and the left colon should be thoroughly examined by flexible sigmoidoscopy before a diagnosis of functional disturbance can be entertained. Neoplasms may be identified by adhering to this approach. Once structural causes of constipation are excluded, functional ones must be considered.

A functional cause of chronic constipation is supported by a history of prolonged, intermittent abdominal pain, prolonged episodes of abdominal distension, abnormal abdominal flatplates, prolonged nausea and vomiting with viral infections, or symptoms of diffuse esophageal dysmotility such as early satiety or dysphagia. The finding of orthostatic change in blood pressure but not pulse suggests the presence of an autonomic neuropathy which is present in a minority of patients.[10] In children, a history of encopresis often accompanies constipation, but this is distinctly uncommon in adults.[18,19] In patients who have compensated colonic dysfunction, determination of an accurate estimate of the duration of the disorder may only be elicited by discussing medications, the use of enemas, and diet. When taking a medication history, the clinician must remember that many patients do not consider over-the-counter medications to be "drugs." The influence of clinical situations that may worsen or precipitate constipation should be evaluated. The most common inciting factors include: prolonged bed rest, altered diet, pregnancy, back injuries, medications that alter intestinal motility, or impaired hydration.

Once the presence of a functional disorder of the colon has been established, the physician must distinguish patients with impaired colonic transit from those with IBS.[1-3,20] Interestingly, patients with severe constipation often report that they cannot remember having had an episode of diarrhea associated with viral gastroenteritis. This is in striking contrast to the patient with IBS who typically reports alternating diarrhea and constipation. The challenging aspects of diagnosing and treating IBS are discussed in a separate chapter of this text. It has been estimated that fewer than 10% of all patients presenting to a specialist with a complaint of constipation, have objective evidence of impaired colonic transit. Within this subgroup, however, are many patients who suffer from a chronic disorder that significantly impairs their quality of life. Recognizing this fact, it is surprising to observe the degree of continuing confusion that surrounds the definition of constipation.

2.2. The Need for an Objective Definition of Constipation

Determination of the incidence, causes, and treatment of constipation depends on establishing a clear understanding of what patients, physicians, and investigators mean by this term. While a diagnosis of chronic constipation may be apparent by the history and the abdominal x-ray, specific criteria are needed to establish an objective definition of colonic dysfunction and to accurately assess the value of therapy or the need for surgical intervention. Greater uniformity in the definition of constipation must be reached before comparisons can be made between studies or before the practicing physician can apply published data to predict the response or prognosis of an individual patient.

2.3. Subjective Definitions of Constipation

Patients may use the term *constipation* to describe the consistency, size, or frequency of the bowel movement. Others are referring to the difficulty associated with its passage or their dissatisfaction with the completeness of the evacuation. Regrettably, the use of subjective or arbitrary definitions of constipation also extends to the medical literature and makes it difficult to interpret the few objective studies that have been reported.[10,15,18,21] The use of these subjective definitions leads to the arbitrary inclusion of patients for analysis and treatment. This leads to further confusion about the management of patients who have more significant disorders of colonic dysfunction.

Consistency and ease of passage vary as a function of diet and hydration. Such subjective criteria should be discarded due to their lack of interpretive value. Factors such as ease of passage, completeness of evacuation, bloating, and the subjective reporting of bowel consistency may be useful in depicting the patient's illness but have limited utility in the evaluation of mechanisms of disease or the response to treatment.[20] More importantly, these are intrinsically subjective factors that defy reliable experimental analysis.

2.4. Objective Variables of Colonic Function

Confusion surrounding the definition of constipation also results from the wide variability in the objective parameters used to define constipation in healthy subjects.[22-24] This variability extends both between subjects and in the same individual when examined from day to day.[4,24,25] Three factors used to objectively appraise colonic function are: stool frequency, weight and volume, and colonic transit time.[4,22-35]

Colonic function is more frequently defined in terms of stooling frequency.[22-25] In Western countries, the frequency of defecation in normal subjects varies from three times per day to once every 3 days.[22,23] Clearly, the patient's retrospective reporting of frequency is unreliable. It is influenced by memory and a complex array of psychological and social bias. Daily diaries attempt to avoid these pitfalls with variable success. The patient's reporting of frequency can both over- and underestimate the severity of impaired colonic transit. A dependence on frequency alone can be particularly misleading if volume is not considered. This is most obviously the case in patients who pass small amounts of hard stools or in patients who take laxatives that impair continence, such as mineral oil. Patients can present with a considerable fecal impaction while passing frequent small, liquid bowel movements. This presentation, known as "paradoxical diarrhea," results from the seepage of liquid around impacted stool.

Stool weight and volume are two other objective parameters used to define the completeness of elimination, which are also highly variable from day to day and between normal subjects.[24] Normal values for stool weight vary considerably with the quantity of calories, fluid, and fiber ingested.[4,25,30] Fiber content of the diet may be the most important determinant of these variables and varies greatly in different cultures.[4,5,30] Surprisingly, the weight of stool output also varies for a given individual over time even when the intake of calories and fiber is controlled.[25] Bacteria are known to make up nearly 50% of stool bulk and may account for these intrapersonal variations. Water-soluble fiber, particularly pectin, may increase stool weight by providing a substrate for bacteria since it cannot be recovered after passage through the intestine. In this regard, it should be noted that while pectin increases stool weight, it does not decrease colonic transit time[31] as would be expected by studies with other fibers that show an inverse relationship between stool weight and intestinal transit time. This inverse relationship between weight and transit rate is also less consistent with men than women, and may not be present for fecal weights greater than 150 g.[25,32,36] The impracticality of controlling diet and fluid intake; collecting, storing, and analyzing stool over prolonged periods; and accounting for differences in the contribution of bacteria and water in the content of stool limits the utility of this test.

Variability in these subjective and objective variables that suggest the presence of disordered elimination demands the establishment of widely acceptable criteria to be used to establish a practical definition of impaired colonic transit.

2.5. A Working Definition of Slowed Transit Constipation

Colonic transit time is an objective measure that can be reliably compared from patient to patient and from one time to another. Scintigraphic techniques have recently been introduced to assess colonic function.[34,35] While holding great promise to clarify our understanding of the complexities of colonic function, the need to intubate the ileocecal sphincter is likely to limit this test to the research laboratory.

Colonic transit can be estimated without enteral intubations by measuring whole gut transit time. While small intestinal transit varies from 2 to 4 hr, 2 to 5 days is normally required for materials to move through the colon. A variety of techniques have been used including radioactive fiber, radiotelemetry capsules, and dyes.[26–29,33] The use of radio-telemetry capsules has been limited by additional cost and equipment that is needed.[33] These capsules also have a much greater specific gravity than normal fecal contents, and may not represent a physiologic marker.

Hinton et al. first described the use of inert radioopaque plastic rings to measure whole gut transit time.[26] This technique offers several advantages.[22,26,28,37] The rings are safe, easily swallowed, inexpensive, and can be made in the office or hospital by sectioning a radioopaque nasogastric tube into 1.5-mm-thick rings. The widespread use of these markers has resulted in a clear definition of normal. They can be assessed by x-raying the stool after it has been collected in plastic bags[26] or by x-raying the patient on alternate days.[22] in normal subjects, 80% of markers should be expelled by day 5 and all markers should be expelled by day 7. More recently, a simplified variation of this technique has been reported from the Mayo Clinic.[28]

Occasionally, the markers will collect in one bowel segment, indicating a specific region of functional obstruction.[37] This is most often the case in patients with anal sphincter or rectal dysfunction, described as "anorectal outlet obstruction."[7] Caution must be used, however, in employing these markers to diagnose or exclude specific areas of regional dysfunction because of the normal reflux of materials from the left to the right colon.[38] In the exceptional patient, these rings may produce diarrhea. This observation has been confirmed experimentally in the pig,[31] and suggests that the presence of delayed transit will occasionally be missed (false negative) by this test.

Thus, a practical definition of chronic constipation based on these observations includes the following criteria: (1) continuous symptoms for more than 1 year, (2) absence of mechanical obstruction by barium enema and flexible sigmoidoscopy, and (3) objective evidence of colonic dysfunction with the presence of a prolonged colonic transit time.

3. MECHANISMS OF CHRONIC CONSTIPATION

3.1. Normal Colonic Function

An extensive discussion of the basic control mechanisms of colonic and anal sphincter motor function has appeared elsewhere, and is beyond the scope of this review.[39,40] The role of the colon in health and the mechanisms of defecation will be briefly reviewed to introduce the events that may be responsible for impaired elimination of solid waste from the body.

Approximately 1 to 1.5 liters of liquid chyme passes through the ileocecal sphincter into the cecum daily. Undigested solids are transported to the cecum from the stomach and upper intestinal tract to the colon by phase III of the interdigestive migrating motor complex (MMC). This mixture of solid and liquid is retained within the colon to permit the active transport of sodium, water, and other electrolytes by the colonic epithelium against incredible concentration gradients. This exchange occurs under the influence of aldosterone and other hormones. Intraluminal contents are actively biotransformed by colonic bacteria which add significantly to the fecal bulk. In humans, the absorption of nutrients by the colonic epithelium is minimal except for vitamin K and short-chain fatty acids which are an important source of energy for the colonic epithelium. The function of

Table II. Defecation Reflex

Delivery
   Transit of colonic contents
      Mass action
      Propagating contractions
   Sigmoid emptying into rectum
Detection
   Accommodation
   Sensory innervation
Decreased resistance
   Rectoanal inhibitory reflex
   Opening of anorectal angle
      Hip flexure
      Relaxation of puborectalis and pubococcygeus
   Perineal descent
   Relaxation of the EAS
Discharge
   Valsalva
   Contraction of rectum
   Sigmoid peristalsis

---

the colonic motor apparatus therefore is to retain this liquid chyme to maximize the exposure of the intraluminal contents to the surface epithelium until this reclamation process is complete, resulting in the daily production of less than 200 ml of solid and liquid waste.

3.2. Mechanisms of Defecation

The four phases of the normal defecation process (Table II) are briefly described below. In general, the chyme and solid materials emptied from the ileum are slowly delivered to the sigmoid colon, then the rectum. When the rectum is distended, the presence of material to be eliminated is detected and a series of reflexes are initiated which constitute the defecation reflex. These reflexes decrease the resistance of structures responsible for maintaining continence, permitting the discharge of rectal contents.

3.2.1. Delivery

The factors that influence the rate at which intraluminal contents are delivered to the rectum therefore include an increase in propulsive forces and a reduction in resistance forces as shown in Fig. 3. Factors that enhance the net propagating forces would promote the movement of cecal contents toward the rectum. These forces include short contractile sequences and a propagating burst of contractions that travel from the right to the left colon, known as "mass action." These forward forces are opposed by: (1) segmenting contractions, which have a mixing function, (2) the retrograde movement of material that occurs as a consequence of retrograde peristaltic events; and (3) a gradient of colonic slow wave frequencies that favors orad movement of materials. Delivery of material to the

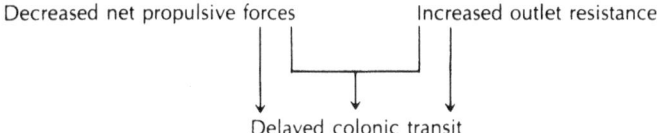

Figure 3. Slowed colonic transit will result from either a decrease in the sum of all propulsive forces or an increase in outlet resistance. The net propulsive force is the consequence of events that move the luminal contents in an aborad direction: mass action and short peristaltic sequences, and contractions that retard this effect such as the segmenting contractions and the net left-to-right gradient in colonic slow waves.

rectum occurs over a prolonged period, therefore, because of the relative infrequency of peristaltic events compared to the influence of resistance factors, primarily the segmenting contractions within the colon itself.

3.2.2. Detection

The detection of material delivered to the rectum results in a series of both voluntary and involuntary reflexes that ultimately result in defecation. The detection of rectal contents is a consequence of sensory innervation to the muscularis propria and the accommodation of these muscles to stretch. The importance of stretch receptors in the muscularis in initiating the final events of defecation has been shown in the laboratory and demonstrated clinically by the presence of a normal rectoanal inhibitory reflex after resection of the rectal mucosa in patients with polyposis syndromes and ulcerative colitis.

3.2.3. Decreased Resistance

Defecation cannot occur unless the normal resistance factors that maintain continence are decreased. The rectoanal inhibitory reflex is the best studied of these events.[6,12,16,39,41,42] This reflex arc includes the stretch receptors in the muscularis, an afferent spinal reflex arc, inhibitory nerves to the smooth muscle of the internal anal sphincter, and excitatory nerves to the external anal sphincter.[39] The relaxation of the internal anal sphincter is mediated by nonadrenergic, noncholinergic inhibitory nerves that probably contain vasoactive intestinal peptide (VIP).[43]

Tonic resistance of the anal canal is also imparted by the striated muscles of the pelvic floor, primarily the puborectalis and pubococcygeus, which interdigitate with the muscles of the anal sphincter. Relaxation of these muscles results in perineal descent. Further opening of the rectoanal angle is accomplished by hip flexure as occurs in the sitting or squatting position. The final resistance to the elimination of rectal contents is the external anal sphincter, which is striated muscle and must be relaxed by nerves from the corticospinal tract.

3.2.4. Discharge

The final discharge of rectal contents is produced by rectal contraction and increased intraabdominal pressure in response to a Valsalva maneuver. Subsequent contractions of the sigmoid colon may also be an important means of delivering more material to the rectum. The viscous properties of stool rich in undigested fiber may also be important in producing a formed movement that is discharged by a single elimination.

Therefore, an impairment in defecation may occur as a result of disorders of over a dozen separate events that are responsible for the normal motor functions of the colon. Understanding the complexities of normal colonic function makes it unlikely that any single defect is responsible for impaired colonic function in all or even most of the patients who present with objective evidence of constipation. It is hoped that through an enhanced understanding of the mechanisms of normal and abnormal colonic function, we can identify specific, treatable causes of constipation. Normal colonic function can be impaired as a consequence of factors primary to the gastrointestinal tract or secondary to unrelated processes.

3.3. Secondary Causes of Constipation

Chronic constipation may occur secondary to iatrogenic factors, trauma, or a systemic neurologic or metabolic disease.[44-50] An exhaustive review of the secondary causes of constipation is beyond the scope of this chapter. Medications are an important iatrogenic cause of constipation. The most important of these medications are listed in Table III. Other secondary causes of chronic constipation are shown in Table IV. These diseases are similar to those that result in disordered motility in other organs of the gastrointestinal tract and to chronic intestinal motility in other organs of the gastrointestinal tract and to chronic intestinal pseudoobstruction.[49-53] In many patients, making a distinction between a primary intestinal motility disorder and a secondary complication of a systemic disease can be difficult. Watier et al. reported that constipation may be a symptom of a more widespread disorder.[10] Many of their patients had orthostatic hypotension, urologic dysfunction, and a high incidence of positive antinuclear antibodies. We have seen several patients with chronic constipation who also had depression of thyroid

Table III. Constipating Medications

Cation-containing agents
Iron supplements
Calcium supplements
Aluminum (antacids, sulcralfate)
Barium sulfate
Anticholinergic agents
Antispasmodics
Antidepressants
Antipsychotics
Other neurally active agents
Opiates
Antiseizure
Antihypertensives
Calcium channel blockers
Ganglionic blockers

Table IV. Secondary Causes of Functional Constipation

Metabolic disorders
  Hypo- or hyperthyroidism
  Disorders of calcium metabolism
    Hypo- or hyperparathyroidism
    Hypercalcemia associated with malignancy
  Porphyria
Neuropathic conditions
  Diabetes mellitus
  Multiple sclerosis
  Spinal cord damage secondary to disc or tumor or trauma
  Heavy metal intoxication
Collagen vascular diseases
  Scleroderma
  Amyloidosis
  Mixed connective tissue disease
Parneoplastic syndromes: Ogilvie's syndrome
Inherited neural or muscular disorders
  Familial visceral myopathy
  Familial autonomic neuropathy
  Neurofibromatosis
Infectious diseases: Chagas's disease
Immobility
Pregnancy

function, in whom the constipation persisted long after correction of the thyroid deficiency.

The suspicion that the constipation results from a metabolic problem should be heightened when specific motility abnormalities cannot be identified.[6] While systemic diseases may cause widespread dysfunction, they usually do so after the diagnosis has been well established for years.[44–46] When a secondary cause is identified, every effort should be made to improve this condition and to restrict sophisticated motility testing to those patients who do not respond to treatment. The identification of specific systemic disorders that cause constipation is particularly important, however, because these systemic disorders can be potentially life threatening, while constipation can be managed with little or no risk to the patient's overall health in all but the most unusual patient.[47,52]

Less frequent secondary causes of constipation include: scleroderma, hypothyroidism, diabetes, and diseases affecting the spinal cord including multiple sclerosis and trauma.[44–48] A thorough history, physical and neurologic examination, and directed laboratory evaluation will reveal a contributing systemic condition in up to 20% of patients with intractable constipation.[6] This observation emphasizes the need to take several detailed histories and appropriate laboratory studies to exclude secondary causes of constipation. A detailed physical and neurologic examination should be performed for every patient. Every patient should also have a complete biochemical profile including electrolytes, glucose and renal function studies, and evaluation of thyroid function. Other tests which may be valuable in selected patients include: protein electrophoresis and a rectal biopsy to exclude amyloidosis and 24-hr urine collection to screen for porphyria or heavy metal toxicity.

Familial or acquired disorders of the smooth muscle or enteric nerves can produce profound constipation and diffuse gastrointestinal dysfunction that progresses to widespread pseudoobstruction.[49-51] Familial hollow visceral myopathy is a myopathic disorder with an autosomal dominant pattern of inheritance that typically presents with symptoms of chronic obstruction of the gastrointestinal and/or urinary tracts.[49,50] Familial visceral neuropathy is characterized by an inherited, widespread dysfunction of both central and peripheral nerves.[51] Acquired forms of degenerative neuropathy have been reported as paraneoplastic syndromes.[47,52]

3.4. Patterns of Chronic Constipation

Idiopathic constipation can result from a net decrease in propulsive forces or functional outlet obstruction at the level of the rectum or anus. At any level, colonic dysfunction can result from dysfunction of intrinsic or extrinsic neural reflexes or of the hormones controlling normal colonic function. Colonic dysfunction can occur as an isolated finding, or as part of a widespread gastrointestinal motility disorder.[6,10] Of 25 consecutive patients who met rigid criteria for the diagnosis of chronic severe constipation, the site of dysfunction as defined by specific motility studies was used to identify the clinical patterns of motility abnormalities.[6] No specific motility disorder could be documented in 8 patients. Seventeen patients were found to have significant motility abnormalities that fit into three specific patterns: 5 had an isolated anal sphincter dysfunction, 6 had isolated colonic dysfunction, and 6 had a generalized gastrointestinal motor dysfunction. The subsequent discussion of the mechanisms of constipation will be based on these three clinical groups.

In our experience with severely constipated adults, the patient's age (36.5 ± 2.5 years), duration of illness (mean 13.0 ± 2.5 years), and the severity of the illness based on either the number of days between spontaneous bowel movements (mean 11.3 ± 1.8 days) or the number of hospital admissions (3.0 to 7.5 admissions) was not helpful in understanding the mechanisms of constipation.[6] Thus, specific motility studies, but not historical features, provided a valuable mans of identifying specific patterns of colonic or sphincteric dysfunction. These patterns furthermore may provide a mechanism for the logical management of the patient with medical or surgical treatment.

3.5. Colonic Outlet Obstruction

A functional obstruction of the rectum can occur at the level of the internal anal sphincter or of the muscles in the pelvic floor. The latter has been described as the "spastic pelvic floor syndrome."[54,55] Disorders of internal anal sphincter relaxation can be identified by anal manometric studies that evaluate the inhibitory response of the internal anal sphincter to balloon rectal distension.[6,16,41,42]

3.5.1. Impaired Rectoanal Inhibitory Reflex

The importance of disorders of rectal outlet in producing severe constipation is exemplified by Hirschsprung's syndrome.[56] This syndrome is characterized by: (1) the presence of an aganglionic segment of rectum that may extend for a variable length from the anal verge, (2) absence of the rectoanal inhibitory reflex, and (3) a resultant mega-colon. Studies in the piebald mouse model of Hirschsprung's disease suggest that this congenital disease results from an impaired migration of ganglion cell precursors into the distalmost colon and rectum.[57] Variations of this disorder have been reported related to the length of the aganglionic segment. Adults who present with severe constipation and an absent rectoanal inhibitory reflex may have a normal full thickness biopsy despite the presence of indistinguishable manometric findings.[6,51] Thus, the presence of ganglion cells should not preclude the diagnosis of isolated anal sphincter dysfunction. The terms *short* or *ultrashort segment Hirschsprung's disease* have been used to describe these patients[6,41,58] with the implication that some length of the sphincter mechanism is aganglionic, despite the presence of normal numbers of ganglia on the biopsy. It seems equally plausible, however, that this is a separate syndrome that results from a dysfunc-tion of sphincteric neurons despite the presence of normal numbers of ganglia.

Of adult patients presenting with severe constipation, approximately 8–10% will have an impaired rectoanal inhibitory reflex.[6,7] We previously referred to these patients as having a variant of Hirschsprung's disease. Several factors, however, distinguish im-paired rectoanal inhibitory reflex in adults from classic Hirschsprung's disease. First, adults rarely present with an aganglionic segment that can be diagnosed by full thickness biopsy. Second, in adults with anal sphincter dysfunction, the diagnosis is rarely sug-gested by barium enema while this is frequently possible in infants and young children with the classic syndrome. Finally, adults will invariably respond to a posterior anal sphincter myomectomy and do not require the more involved anal pull-through procedures described by Duhamel and Swensen.[6,7,41,58,59] Further studies will be needed to deter-mine if these differences result from a short length of aganglionic sphincter or from partial impairment of the neural control of the entire sphincter.

Because disorders of the internal anal sphincter can be readily diagnosed and effec-tively treated, every patient with chronic severe constipation should have an anal sphincter manometric exam to exclude the presence of an isolated dysfunction of the rectoanal inhibitory reflex. The exam must be performed by experts who are able to recognize factors that may lead to a false-positive test. These factors include: chronic, uncorrected rectal distension by fecal impaction; an insufficient distension stimulus; recent rectal intubation; and insensitive recording instruments. Other manometric studies should also be performed to exclude a widespread motility disorder since these patients are not likely to respond to anal myomectomy alone. While the indiscriminate use of anal myomectomy will lead to an unacceptable incidence of fecal incontinence,[7] the appropriate selection of patients for this procedure will lead to very satisfactory results. Often the patient will become free of the need for further therapy after a period of bowel retraining and the ingestion of a high-fiber diet. While the diagnosis of isolated anal sphincter dysfunction rests on the identification of a specific manometric disturbance, the presence of this disorder may be suggested by a disproportionate distension of the rectum or by the persistence of markers in the rectosigmoid region when performing a whole gut transit time study.[7,37]

3.5.2. Spastic Pelvic Floor Syndrome

Functional rectal obstruction may also occur at the level of the pelvic floor. Several disorders that have been suggested to result in the "spastic pelvic floor syndrome" or "anismus" include: spasticity of the levator ani, abnormal angulation of the recto-anal axis, failure of perineal descent, impaired neural relaxation of the puborectalis muscle, or to a combination of these related factors.[11,12,54,55] Significant differences in the anorectal angle have been shown in constipated patients compared to normals.[12] This angle is measured by performing dynamic cine fluoroscopy of the patients as they sit upright and attempt to defecate. The importance of obtaining this measurement is clouded by the fact that the abnormal rectoanal angulation has been reported to be both excessively acute and obtuse in patients with constipation compared to normals.[12,60] Furthermore, there is considerable overlap in the change in rectoanal angle during defeca-tion in normal and constipated subjects. Roe et al. studied 64 subjects and found the same degree of angle opening in two groups of constipated patients as there was in healthy controls.[61] Furthermore, efforts to correct this disorder by surgical ablation of the rectal sling have been disappointing. It has also been suggested that abnormalities of anorectal angle may be the consequence of nerve entrapment during straining and therefore not the primary cause of constipation. Further studies are under way to clarify the clinical impor-tance of pelvic floor dysfunction and to determine the optimal method of diagnosing this disorder.

3.5.3. Abnormalities in Rectal Sensation

Impaired relaxation of either the internal anal sphincter or the pelvic floor may be the consequence of impaired rectal sensation. In a study of 144 children with severe constipa-tion, 65% had significant impairment of sensation.[42] In contrast, adults studied by the same investigators invariably had normal rectal sensation if studied several weeks after removal of any rectal impaction. Other studies have indicated that patients with chronic severe constipation have abnormal rectoanal afferent innervation.[11,12,29,62] This was most commonly manifested by a decreased motor response to chemical or balloon stim-ulation and a decrease in the urge to defecate. The patients did not, however, have abnormalities in more objective measures of sensation such as the threshold volume needed to perceive distension or in the volume needed to induce the rectoanal inhibitory reflex.[12] While impaired sensation has been reported in adults, this seems to be an infrequent finding if sufficient time is allotted prior to the study to permit rectal accom-modation to normalize as the muscularis propria regains its normal tone. The subjective nature of asking the patients to describe when they have the urge to defecate and vari-abilities in the design of the balloon may also contribute to the conflicting results of the importance of rectal sensation.

3.6. Impaired Colonic Transit

It is apparent that chronic constipation most commonly results from impaired colonic transit. Delayed transit can result from dysfunction of specific colonic segments, the entire colon, or as just one of several dysfunctions in a diffuse gastrointestinal disorder.

Recent advances in the use of long catheters that are capable of recording from various levels in the colon have been used to examine healthy subjects and patients with IBS.[62,63] It may be possible to define specific abnormalities in the frequency or force of propulsive contractions in specific regions of the colon. The presence of such limited disorders of motor function has been supported by Wald's studies using radioopaque transit markers.[37] As discussed above, however, the normal to-and-fro movement of materials within the colon may severely limit the value of such observations.[38] Disappointing results from limited surgical resections of the colon in patients with constipation also raise a note of concern over making the diagnosis of a selected regional dysfunction within the colon.[65]

Devroede has used the term *colonic inertia* to describe patients with chronic constipation due to an isolated dysfunction of the propulsive forces of the colon.[10] The hallmark of this diagnosis is the persistence of radioopaque markers in a scattered distribution throughout both the left and right colon[5-7] days after ingestion. Esophageal manometry, gastric emptying, and anal manometric studies will be normal. While this is the only group of patients that we consider for subtotal colectomy, the majority of these patients respond to less invasive measures.[6]

Twenty to fifty percent of patients who present with chronic constipation will be found to have a generalized gastrointestinal motility disorder.[6,10] These generalized abnormalities typically include: disordered esophageal peristalsis, incomplete relaxation of a normal or hypertonic lower esophageal sphincter, and delayed gastric emptying. Small bowel involvement may be manifested by the presence of megaduodenum, reduced MMCs, intestinal stasis, and bacterial overgrowth. Patients with more severe motility disorders may also present with small intestinal bacterial overgrowth, orthostatic hypotension, neurogenic bladder, megaureter, and megaduodenum.[10] These patients are the most difficult to manage medically but surgical intervention may have an even more disastrous outcome because of the similarities of this widespread disorder to pseudo-obstruction.

3.6.1. Smooth Muscle Disorders Impair Colonic Transit

Impaired transit can result from smooth muscle dysfunction or of the factors that regulate normal motility patterns. Dysfunction at the level of the smooth muscle could impair excitation–contraction coupling or alter the normal basal electric rhythm (slow waves) that serves to coordinate contractions. Abnormalities in the systems that regulate colonic motility may include enteric hormones or extrinsic and intrinsic nerves.

An abnormality of slow-wave frequency has been reported to characterize the colonic dysfunction associated with IBS.[6,29] Several subsequent studies have confirmed the presence of an increased frequency of 3 cpm slow waves in constipated patients with spastic colon. A further discussion of the physiologic abnormalities in patients with IBS is found elsewhere in this volume. The importance of irregularities of the basal electric rhythm of the colon in causing constipation is unclear.

In patients who have known disorders of the smooth muscle such as familial myopathy, contraction amplitudes are low, and constipation may result. Patients with scleroderma and diabetes have a markedly reduced rectosigmoid contractile response to a meal (gastrocolic reflex).[44,45] In patients with early scleroderma, the muscle contracted normally to direct stimulation of smooth muscle but had a reduced response to agents whose response was dependent on neural input. Patients with advanced scleroderma have severe impairment of the contractile response both to directly acting stimulants and indirectly to induce contractions. These studies suggest that disorders of smooth muscle can result in constipation by reducing the amplitude of contractions but that abnormalities in the regulatory systems predominate in earlier stages of the disease.

3.6.2. Disordered Regulatory Mechanisms Cause Constipation

Further evidence of the importance of disorders of the regulatory systems in producing constipation is the prevalence of increased, not decreased contractile force in patients with constipation. While colonic contraction amplitudes in patients with myopathy and scleroderma are decreased, most studies of patients with idiopathic constipation have found an increase in both basal and stimulated motor activity.[11,66-69] Connell described this increased response as the "paradoxical increase in motility in constipation and a decrease in contractile activity during diarrhea."[67] In a comparison of 33 patients with severe constipation and 17 patients with diarrhea, constipated patients had significantly more contractile activity. The increase in contractile activity was most significant in constipated patients less than 40 years of age. This paradoxical increase in contractile activity was recently confirmed in a sophisticated study of right and left colonic contractile activity by Sasaki et al.[69] Presumably the increased contractility is in the form of segmenting, nonpropulsive contractions.[11] Opioid antidiarrheal agents also reduce bowel movement frequency by increasing the incidence of segmenting contractions. Unfortunately, while it is inviting to hypothesize that impaired colonic transit is due to an increase in segmenting contractions, this observation has not been uniformly seen.[8,29]

The possibility that a hormone imbalance could be responsible for chronic constipation has received little attention. Motilin concentrations were found to be reduced in some patients with constipation.[70] Pituitary hypothalamic function has been observed in patients with constipation.[10] Elegant studies by Narducci et al have demonstrated remarkable diurnal variation in colonic contractility.[63] It is unclear if this marked decrease in nocturnal motor activity results from diurnal variations in hormones or a decrease in CNS activation.

Constipation could result from abnormalities of extrinsic or intrinsic neural input to the colon. Chronic constipation in multiple sclerosis is the consequence of both local and spinocortical neuraxis.[46] Abnormalities in cortical somatosensory evoked potentials were consistent with visceral CNS dysfunction in these patients.

Pathologic examination of the colonic myenteric ganglia of patients with chronic constipation may show an increase in Schwan cells, granuloma, or ballooning ganglial cells. Occasionally, there may be thickening of the colonic circular muscle layer. More often, however, a detailed light microscopic examination of the colon will be normal, even when the pathologist pays particular attention to the intermuscular neural plexus.

The lack of gross or light microscopic abnormalities in the number of ganglia or the morphology of the ganglial cells has led investigators to examine the relative concentrations of specific transmitters in the colonic smooth muscle. A dense innervation of VIP is present in tissues from patients with intractable constipation. The content of VIP and peptide histidine isoleucine in the colonic muscle was, however, recently reported to be decreased when compared to normal.[72] Further studies are needed to more completely examine the neural circuitry of the colon in health and disease.

3.7. Other Factors Contributing to Delayed Colonic Transit

3.7.1. Female Gender

Women far outnumber men in every series of patients with chronic severe constipation. The percentage of women in published series varies from 72 to 100%.[6,11,12] The reason for this striking female predominance is unclear. Possible contributing factors include the inhibitory effect progestins have on intestinal smooth muscle, pelvic damage related to childbirth, differences in socialization, psychologic influences, or learned behavioral factors. Factors that suggest that hormonal influences are the most likely cause for this striking sex difference include the observation that patients with severe constipation most commonly present in childbearing years and that there is no prevalence of females in series of constipated children.[18,19,42] Two observations suggest that hormonal differences are not the only factors increasing the risk for women to develop severe constipation: (1) females also predominate in series of constipated geriatric patients,[73] and (2) whole gut transit times are not altered by the time of the menstrual cycle.

3.7.2. Psychosocial Factors

The importance of psychosocial factors in the etiology of chronic constipation is unclear. Our understanding of the causes of colonic dysfunction is biased by factors that influence the selection of patients who will seek professional help and who will undergo studies. The patient's pursuit of medical evaluation is based more on preconceived notions of normalcy, psychosocial, economic, and learned factors than on objective definitions of disease. In this regard, the inclusion of some patients in studies of constipation who have habits within the range of normal may result from the severity of their complaints rather than the severity of their motility disorder.[20] The identification of the psychosocial factors that influence the patient's perception of disease and result in either the inappropriate denial of intestinal disease or the excessive emphasis of insignificant symptoms will be helpful in the overall management of these patients.[2,3]

While patients with IBS often perseverate about their inability to effect a daily movement, patients with more severe forms of constipation typically present only after they become unable to cope with a progressively disabling situation. Many of these patients have quietly endured years of discomfort without evaluation for fear of ostracization or a physician's diagnosis of psychopathology. They present only when their usual coping mechanisms decompensate such as may result from intercurrent illnesses, unrelated surgery, or changes in activity, diet, or medications. The paucity of the psychologic overtones, the persistent and chronic nature, and the severity of the problem distinguish patients with chronic severe constipation from the more commonly seen patients with IBS[1−3] and make it less likely that psychologic factors play an important role in the cause of more chronic, severe forms of constipation.

Several authors have suggested that the spastic pelvic floor syndrome results, at least in part, from the patient's inability to relax. This may be due to unrecognized phobias, malingering, or high-anxiety states. Biofeedback and hypnosis have thus been suggested to be potentially effective treatments for this disorder. The value of these techniques in altering objective parameters of colonic function will need more discriminative evaluation in double-blind studies.

3.7.3. Additional Nonspecific Factors

A dietary deficiency of crude fiber is an important cause of the development of chronic constipation. Constipation and other colonic disorders occur very rarely in societies that consume large quantities of fiber in their diet.[4,5] The implications of these observations are discussed below in regard to treatment.

The report of an increased incidence of antinuclear antibodies in patients with chronic severe constipation raises the intriguing possibility that immunologic factors may also be present.

Age alone, in the absence of systemic disease, does not predispose to severe constipation, although as a group, transit may be somewhat prolonged.[9,27,33]

4. COMPLICATIONS OF CHRONIC CONSTIPATION

Patients with chronic severe constipation may develop complications, some of which may be life-threatening.[74-76] When the diagnosis of severe constipation or its causes is delayed, the patient may undergo unnecessary surgery or develop a spontaneous complication. Perhaps the most dramatic case of chronic severe constipation reported in the literature is that of a 29-year-old man found dead in a water closet in 1902 with severe idiopathic megacolon.[4] Constipation, which began in infancy, was unexplained despite an exploratory laparotomy 2 years before his death and a detailed pathologic evaluation at autopsy. Stercoral ulcers typically present with abdominal pain which progressively worsens as the ulcer grows. Impacted stool induces persistent trauma and pressure-induced local ischemia which may lead to free perforation.[76] Most stercoral ulcers occur in elderly patients in the rectosigmoid region, but can occur anywhere in the colon. While usually single, they can be multiple in more severe cases.

Solitary ulcers typically occur on the anterior wall of the rectum, perhaps a result of mucosal prolapse and local ischemia.[77] pathologically, solitary rectal ulcers can be distinguished from stercoral ulcers by the presence of reactive hyperplasia resulting in a localized colitis cystica profunda or a villous configuration. A fibrous obliteration of the lamina propria also occurs commonly. Both medical and surgical treatment are frequently unsatisfactory.

Colonic perforation rarely occurs as the consequence of an acute tear following a forceful attempt to eliminate inspissated stool. The history of pain is much more acute in patients with longitudinal tear and the pathologic exam reveals no chronic inflammation.

Bleeding rarely occurs in patients with chronic constipation from colonic tears or a stercoral ulcer. Much more commonly, hemorrhoids are the cause of bleeding in chronic constipation. The excessive straining at stool associated with constipation; the impingement on venous structures by the hard, impacted stool; and the local trauma experienced in passing this type of movement contribute to the development of the hemorrhoids. While typically large and chronic, they will invariably respond to medical therapy if the chronic constipation can be improved.

Rectal prolapse may also complicate severe constipation, particularly in the patient who habitually strains at stooling. Multiparous women are particularly predisposed to this complication. It has been suggested that frequent straining may also damage extrinsic nerves as they impinge on the pelvic floor. Thus, if straining leads to nerve compression, a viscous cycle can develop with increased rectal sensation, impaired reflex responses, further impairment of defecation, and a resultant increase in straining.

5. TREATMENT

The development of clear understanding of the mechanisms causing constipation will lead to the development of effective treatments for this common disorder. In the individual patient with chronic severe constipation, the physician must also understand the factors contributing to the decompensation in the condition; the mechanisms, safety, and efficacy of therapeutic options; and the degree to which the patient's quality of life is impaired. Therapy may include alterations of diet, medications, and life-style; laxatives and cathartics; enemas or surgery in selected cases. The regimen selected may vary with the individual's severity of symptoms and extent of physiologic impairment but in every case should be tailored to emphasize safety and efficacy over a prolonged period.

Before considering the addition of any therapeutic agents, several readily correctable disorders must be excluded. Most patients will have significant improvement by simply adding bulk to their fiber-deficient diet.[4,30,79] A detailed history of medications should be taken that includes both prescriptions and over-the-counter agents. The most common offending agents are shown in Table III. When possible, these drugs should be discontinued or the dose reduced. Nonsteroidal anti-inflammatory drugs can often be effectively substituted for narcotic analgesics. The serotonin antagonist trazodone is less constipating than are tricyclic antidepressants. Magnesium-containing antacids or an H_2 antagonist should be substituted for aluminum-containing antacids or sulcralfate. Metabolic disorders should be excluded by appropriate testing and treatment. The addition of an exercise program appropriate for the patient's age and cardiovascular status can be recommended both to improve intestinal motility and to enhance the patient's feeling of well-being. A recommendation to reduce excessive stress, establish a time of the day to relax and be quiet, and gently attempting a movement on a daily or alternative day regimen can be recommended on an intuitive but not scientific basis. The presence of isolated anal sphincter dysfunction should be excluded in every patient by anal sphincter manometry performed by experts before proceeding with any therapy.

5.1. Therapeutic Agents and Their Mechanisms of Action

Because the list of agents available to treat chronic constipation continues to grow, the choice of a proper medical agent may seem unnecessarily confusing. In addition to promoting the emptying of colonic contents, the ideal therapy should: (1) be useful for chronic symptoms and acute decompensation, (2) promote the return of normal bowel function and reduce the dependency on further treatment, (3) reduce the bloating and pain that accompany this motility disorder, (4) have a high safety profile, and (5) have a cost that would not be prohibitive for chronic use. For the patient with minimal symptoms, withholding ineffective and potentially harmful agents may be the most desirable approach.

Dozens of products, with several distinct mechanisms of action, have been used alone or in combination to treat individuals with chronic constipation.[15] The selection of a specific type of therapy can be enhanced by understanding its mechanisms of action and tailoring the therapy to the individual's needs. Agents which are occasionally helpful in the treatment of the irritable colon, such as those containing phenobarbital and anticholinergics, do not have a defined role in the treatment of severe constipation and may be contraindicated. Therapeutic agents can be separated into three broad categories: (1) dietary fiber and bulk-forming agents, (2) laxatives and cathartics, and (3) prokinetic agents.

5.2. Dietary Fiber

Several epidemiologic studies have suggested that a major cause of colonic pathology, including constipation, occurs in industrialized nations as a result of an inadequate intake of dietary fiber.[4,5] Burkitt and colleagues have shown that colon cancer, diverticulosis, and other disorders endemic to the United States occur very rarely in people living in countries whose high dietary fiber intake results in up to 500 g of stool daily compared to 100 g per day in Western countries. Individuals in these countries often excrete several large bowel movements a day and constipation is exceedingly rare. The incidence of dimethylhydrazine-induced colonic neoplasm was reduced by the addition of fiber to the animals' chow.[36,80] Several studies have demonstrated that the addition of fiber to the diet of patients with milder forms of constipation increases bulk and frequency of stooling and may decrease the incidence of pain.[5,30,31,36,79] Many patients presenting with constipation can be corrected by the addition of 10 to 15 g of fiber to their diet either in the form of supplements or by increasing the intake of high-fiber foods. This regimen may be used chronically without adverse reaction. The patient should be led to understand that the ingested fiber is not a medication but rather a natural substance which their diet is deficient in. A high-fiber diet thus should be initiated in every patient with constipation.[36,79] It is important to note that a high-fiber diet should not be initiated until the colon has been cleansed of solid waste and should be withheld whenever obstructive symptoms are present. Fiber should be given with caution to the patient with a diffuse gastrointestinal motility disorder that is accompanied by severe gastroparesis and/or an absence of MMCs. Bezoars have been rarely reported to occur in this situation.

5.3. Laxatives and Cathartics

A classification of laxatives and cathartics by mechanism of action is shown in Table V. A detailed explanation of the mechanism of action of these agents is beyond the scope of this chapter and has been reviewed elsewhere.[15] The effect of most of these agents is to promote a net increase in the water content of the stool and to promote propagating contractions. The water content of the stool is increased by osmotic trapping of solute, by inhibiting absorption, stimulating secretion, or by adsorption to hydrophilic substances. Contact laxatives may increase the stool water content by increasing the mucosal permeability, perhaps through direct damage to the epithelium or intercellular junctions.[81] The increase in endothelial permeability produced by irritant laxatives may explain the formation of melanosis coli in patients who chronically use anthraquinone cathartics.[81] Motility is enhanced by: the direct irritation of intramural sensory nerves; reflex-induced contractions in responding to stretch receptors in the presence of increased bulk; and promoting the frequency of mass movements that propel intraluminal contents form the right colon. Transit may also be increased through laxative-induced increase of substances that increase gut motility such as cholecystokinin, prostaglandins, VIP, and cAMP. The ability to design the most effective therapies will be enhanced by a greater insight into the specific mechanisms by which these agents work.

While laxatives are still among the most potent agents available to treat constipation, the routine daily use of these agents is to be strongly discouraged and should be considered to be potentially harmful. Patients with impactions and severe obstipation may have

Table V. Pharmacologic Therapy of Chronic Constipation

General class	Mechanisms of action	Subclass	Example
Laxatives and cathartics			
Saline cathartics	Osmotic water retention	Magnesium salts	Mg^{2+} citrate
		Sodium phosphates	Na^+ phosphate enemas
		Polyethylene glycol–saline solutions	GolYtely
Osmotic laxatives	Same	Lactulose	Lactulose
Contact cathartics	Net water secretion via:	Diphenylmethane derivatives	Phenolphthalein
	Damage to enterocytes		Biscodyl
	Weakening intercellular junctions	Anthraquinones	Senna
	Stimulating PG, cAMP, perhaps CCK, VIP		Cascara
	May also stimulate motility		Danthron
		Ricinoleic acid	Castor oil
Stool softeners			
Mineral oil	Emollient, softener		Mineral oils
Dulcosates	Result in net secretion (may cause mucosal damage similar to the contact cathartics)	Dioctyl sulfosuccinate	Sodium salt
			Calcium salt
Agents effecting neurotransmission			
Cholinomimetics	Stimulate cholinergic receptors, predominantly muscarinics	Cholinergic agents	Bethanechol
		Cholinesterase inhibitors	Neostigmine
Prokinetic agents	Facilitate the release of Ach and antagonize DA receptors		Metoclopramide
	Only facilitate neurotransmitter release in periphery		Cisapride
Opioid antagonists	Selective inhibition of peripheral opioid receptors		Naloxone (available for i.v. only)

severe pain induced by potent laxatives whose mode of action develops a head of pressure proximal to a point of relative obstruction. Available data suggest that the safety of these agents must be questioned when used on a long-term basis for a condition that is a chronic, daily problem. Melanosis coli, a striking black discoloration of the colonic mucosa, has been correlated to the chronic use of anthraquinone cathartics.[81] The long-term health implications of this lesion are not certain, but the discoloration can persist for years after discontinuation of the laxative. Histologic data from animals and humans suggest that the chronic use of some laxatives may also result in damage to the intrinsic neural innervation of the colon.[72] These and other observations have led to the following warning in the package insert of several popular irritant laxatives. "Frequent or prolonged use of this or any other laxative may result in dependence on laxatives."

The term *cathartic colon* has been coined to describe the colonic dysfunction that is associated with the chronic use of laxatives with the implication that there is a causal relationship between the use of laxatives and the colonic disturbance.[14,72,83] Since most patients suffered from constipation prior to the use of laxatives, the causal relationship of laxative use and constipation has been questioned. Laxatives have been used inappropriately, however, by patients with a normal frequency of bowel movements to reduce caloric intake and control weight. This variant of bulemia has resulted in marked disruption of the previously normal bowel habit.[82] Patients with these eating disorders may also develop gastroparesis, when laxative abuse is absent. The contribution of malnutrition, thyroid disturbances, and fiber deprivation to the acquisition of motility disorders by these patients cannot be overlooked.

Available data indicating adverse effects from the chronic use of irritant laxatives strongly suggest that additional studies are needed to further evaluate the safety and efficacy of these agents when used for prolonged periods. The possibility that the physician may be recommending a treatment that could worsen the underlying condition conflicts with the first dictum of medicine, to "do no harm." Until the safety of these agents is established, the use of irritant laxatives should be restricted to patients with acute symptoms. It is recommended that the judicious use of a cathartic or purgative once every 2–3 weeks will avoid the development of impactions and reduce the intraluminal diameter to a degree that will permit the circular muscle to generate more effective contractions. Alternating these agents reduces the likelihood of developing potential adverse side effects that could accompany the use of a single agent over prolonged periods. Newly developed polyethylene glycol-containing saline purgatives are particularly effective, and well tolerated for this function.

Other agents that are effective in the acute setting must also be used with caution in patients with chronic disease. Mineral oil can bind to fat-soluble vitamins and inhibit their absorption. This and other oils taken at bedtime may be aspirated and result in lipoid pneumonia. Mineral oil is not infrequently complicated by encopresis. The chronic use of magnesium-containing laxatives, particularly in the presence of renal insufficiency, can lead to hypermagnesemia. When the magnesium level approaches 4.0, the patient may experience muscle weakness, sedation, confusion, and ECG changes.

While the safety of more potent laxatives is unclear, the efficacy of many milder agents, such as stool softeners, is even less certain. Docusate sodium and related surface-acting compounds are thought to act by increasing the water content of the stool. While the mechanisms of action were evaluated in animal models many years ago, this extremely popular agent was evaluated in a double-bind controlled study in humans only recently. Two studies were unable to demonstrate any improvement in stool water content, colonic transit time, or any other objective measure of efficacy by dulcosate in currently recommended doses compared to placebo.[73,83]

5.4. Agents That Promote Neurally Mediated Propulsive Colonic Contractions

The use of agents that enhance the normal propulsive action of the bowel is intuitively more appealing than the use of agents whose efficacy is the result of irritation of local nerves or that alter the integrity of the mucosal barrier. Toward this aim, agents that promote bowel contractility have been used in the treatment of constipation. Cholinomimetics, such as bethanechol chloride, have been used for this purpose for many years with variable success. The stimulation of muscarinic receptors would be expected to enhance contractile amplitude and reduce the stimulus threshold for peristaltic reflexes. Cholinesterase inhibitors, such as neostigmine, have been recommended for the same reasons, and are often associated with fewer systemic side effects.[84]

The newest class of agents that enhance the intrinsic motor functions of the gut have been classified as the prokinetic agents. Metoclopramide, the first prokinetic agent, is extremely useful in the treatment of gastroparesis and gastroesophageal reflux disease. Motility is enhanced by promoting the release of acetylcholine in enteric nerves, and blocking of dopamine receptors. Although metoclopramide does induce colonic contractions, it is rarely useful in the treatment of constipated patients except when upper intestinal symptoms predominate. Metoclopramide is also limited because athetoid movements, tremors, or sedation are seen in up to 20% of patients. Second- and third-generation prokinetic agents, such as domperidone and cisapride,[62] promise to have fewer side effects. In preliminary studies, we have found cisapride to be effective in treating the majority of patients who were intractable to other treatments.

Endogenous opioid compounds have been shown to be among the most abundant neurotransmitters in the gut and contribute to the mechanisms that initiate the gastrocolic reflex. Kreek et al. were able to reverse chronic severe constipation in two patients by the intravenous infusion of a specific opioid antagonist, naloxone.[85] Oral opioid antagonists are under development.

5.5. The Use of Enemas

Enemas containing a variety of agents have been effective in the treatment of chronic constipation. Tap water enemas, slightly warm, administered as a retention enema are the safest and easiest to use. While normal patients often obtain an effective elimination with an enema volume of 250 ml, chronically constipated patients often require four times this volume. Reassurance must be given to the patient who becomes anxious when they are unable to eliminate the enema fluid. This is a hallmark of the patient with severe disease and is a strong argument against the use of more irritant laxative mixtures such as soapsuds. The latter has rarely been reported to cause a chemically induced colitis. Mineral oil enemas are messy but may be necessary for the patient with a particularly inspissated stool. When all else fails, a milk and molasses enema is almost always effective and is surprisingly well tolerated by the patient (if not the nurse).

Colonic irrigations continue to be given by some health spas and related, nonprofessional entrepreneurs. The long-term effect of this therapy is not known. Reports of inadvertent perforations and the passage of infectious agents from one client to another are well documented.[86] This practice should be emphatically discouraged because of the potential risks from trauma and infection, particularly as long as hepatitis B and AIDS remain a major health risk.

5.6. Surgery in the Treatment of Chronic Constipation

Treatment of the patient with chronic severe constipation who is found to have an abundant rectoanal inhibitory reflex by anal myotomy can lead to extremely satisfying result.[6,7,56,58,59,87] This approach can be so helpful that one group treated all patients with chronic severe constipation with this procedure for a time.[7] When myomectomy was performed indiscriminately in this manner, however, only one third of patients received an objective benefit and another third experienced complications including incontinence of stool. In our experience, when objective evidence of anal sphincter dysfunction is present, with or without aganglionosis, the vast majority of patients will be freed of the need for laxatives with a limited posterior myotomy and a high-fiber diet. Similar results have been reported by others.[58,59,87] More extensive procedures such as the Soave or Duhamel procedures that are performed in children with classic Hirschsprung's disease are rarely if ever needed in adults or in children after age ten.[56,58,59,87]

The role for colectomy is not clear for the patients who present with chronic severe constipation. Through the early modern era, colectomy was performed for fatigue, "auto-intoxication," and other vague indications at a time when the procedure was associated with a high mortality.[89] Some consensus of opinion has been reached regarding the futility of a limited resection of the colon in the absence of mechanical obstruction.[65,89] This procedure results in both unsatisfactory results and a high rate of anastomotic leaks. A subtotal colectomy with ileorectal anastomosis is the procedure of choice for the patient with incapacitating constipation. In the patient whose physiologic studies establish the presence of normal esophageal, gastric, and small bowel function, this procedure can be accompanied by excellent results and minimal diarrhea that often clears in 3–6 months. Published reports indicate that the mortality associated with this procedure is 2% and the complication rate $> 20\%$.[65,90] When extreme care is taken to cleanse the colon pre-operatively with enemas and several gallons of a polyethylene glycol purgative (Go-Lytely), a lower morbidity and mortality can be expected in well-selected patients. Patients who have evidence of widespread motility disorders, such as esophageal spasm, LES dysfunction, gastroparesis, or megaduodenum, are analogous to patients with chronic idiopathic intestinal pseudoobstruction.[53] These patients would be anticipated to have a less satisfactory result,[65] although no large series have been published where this distinction was made.

In summary, the development of a logical diagnostic plan can often lead to a clear understanding of the mechanisms of chronic constipation and to the initiation of a treatment program that can be successful in the majority of patients. All patients should be placed on a high-fiber diet with a high fluid intake. A concerted but judicious use of enemas, laxatives, and purgatives is often also needed intermittently. Novel therapeutic approaches are being developed to treat this problem including the use of nonabsorbable saline cathartics, third-generation prokinetic agents and oral opioid antagonists. Surgery can produce dramatic and effective results when reserved for selected patients.

REFERENCES

1. Manning AP, Thompson WG, Heaton KW, et al: Towards positive diagnosis of the irritable bowel. Br Med J suppl 2:653–654, 1978
2. Whitehead WE, Engel BT, Schuster MM: Irritable bowel syndrome. Dig Dis Sci 25:404, 1980
3. Drossman DA, Powell DW, Sessions JT: The irritable bowel syndrome. Gastroenterology 73:811, 1977
4. Burkitt DP, Walker ARP, Painter NS: Effect of dietary fibre on stools and transit-times, and its role in the causation of disease. Lancet 2:1408, 1972
5. Burkitt D: Fiber as protective against gastrointestinal diseases. Gastroenterology 79:249, 1984

6. Reynolds JC, Ouyang A, Lee CA, et al: Chronic severe constipation: Prospective motility studies in twenty-five consecutive patients. Gastroenterology 92:414–420, 1987

7. Martelli H, Devroede G, Arhan P, et al: Mechanisms of idiopathic constipation: Outlet obstruction. Gastroenterology 75:623, 1978

8. Muenier P, Rochas A, Lambert R: Motor activity of the sigmoid colon in chronic constipation: Comparative study with normal subjects. Gut 20:1095, 1979

9. Corazziari E, Bausano G, Torsoli A, et al: Italian cooperative study on chronic constipation, in Wienbeck M (ed): Motility of the Digestive Tract. New York, Raven Press, 1982, p 523

10. Watier A, Devroede G, Duranceau A, et al: Constipation with colonic inertia: A manifestation of systemic disease? Dig Dis Sci 28:1025, 1983

11. Preston DM, Lennard-Jones JE: Pelvic motility and response to intraluminal bisacodyl in slow-transit constipation. Dig Dis Sci 30:289, 1985

12. Read NE, Timms JM, Barfield LJ, et al: Impairment of defecation in young women with severe constipation. Gastroenterology 90:53, 1986

13. Lennar-Jones JE: Functional gastrointestinal disorders. N Engl J Med 308:431–435, 1983

14. Plum GE, Weber HM, Sauer WG: Prolonged cathartic abuse resulting in roentgen evidence suggestive of enterocolitis. Roentgenology 83:919, 1960

15. Fingl E: Laxatives and cathartics, in Gillman AG, Goodman LS, Gilman A (eds): The Pharmacological Basis of Therapeutics, ed 6. New York, Macmillan Co, 1980, p 1002

16. Mahboubl S, Schnaufer L: The barium-enema examination and rectal manometry in Hirschsprung's disease. Radiology 130:643, 1979

17. Patriquin H, Martelli H, Devroede G: Barium enema in chronic constipation: Is it meaningful? Gastroenterology 75:619, 1978

18. Loening-Baucke VA, Younoszai MK: Effect of treatment on rectal and sigmoid motility in chronically constipated children. Pediatrics 73:199, 1984

19. Liebman WM: Disorders of defecation in children. Postgrad Med 66:105, 1979

20. Schuster MM: Motions without emotion. Gastroenterology 75:744, 1978

21. Kirwan WO, Smith AN: Colonic propulsion in diverticular disease, idiopathic constipation and the irritable colon syndrome. Scand J Gastroenterol 12:331, 1977

22. Martelli H, Devroede G, Arhan P, et al: Some parameters of large bowel motility in normal man. Gastroenterology 75:612, 1978

23. Drossman DA, Sandler RS, McKee DC, et al: Bowel patterns among subjects not seeking health care: Use of a questionnaire to identify a population with bowel dysfunction. Gastroenterology 83:529, 1982

24. Connell AM, Hilton C, Irvine G, et al: Variation of bowel habit in 2 population samples. Br Med J 2:1095, 1965

25. Wyman JB, Heaton KW, Manning AP, et al: Variability of colonic function in healthy subjects. Gut 19:146, 1978

26. Hinton JM, Lennard-Jones, JE, Young AC: A new method for studying gut transit times using radio-opaque markers. Gut 10:842, 1969

27. Melkersson M, Andersson H, Bosaeus I, et al: Intestinal transit time in constipated and nonconstipated geriatric patients. Scand J Gastroenterol 18:593, 1983

28. Metcalfe AM, Phillips SF, Zinmeister, et al: Simplified assessment of segmental colonic transit. Gastroenterology 92:40–47, 1987

29. Frieri G, Parisi F, Corazziari, et al: Colonic electromyography in chronic constipation. Gastroenterology 84:737, 1983

30. Tucker DM, Sandstead HH, Logan GM Jr, et al: Dietary fiber and personality factors as determinants of stool output. Gastroenterology 81:879, 1981

31. Bueno L, Praddaude F, Fioramonte J, et al: Effect of dietary fiber on gastrointestinal and jejunal transit time in dogs. Gastroenterology 80:701, 1981

32. Spiller GA: Can fecal weight be used to establish a recommendation intake of dietary fiber? Am J Clin Nutr 30:659, 1977

33. Becker U, Elsborg L: A new method for the determination of gastrointestinal transit times. Scand J Gastroenterol 14:355, 1979

34. Krevsky B, Malmud L, D'Ercole F, et al: Colonic transit scintigraphy, a physiologic approach to the quantitative measurement of colonic transit in humans. Gastroenterology 91:1102–1112, 1986

35. Krevsky B, Malmud L, Somers MB, et al: Patterns of colonic transit in chronic idiopathic constipation. Gastroenterology 90:1503A, 1986
36. Slavin JL, Levine AS: Dietary fiber and gastrointestinal disease. Part 1. What is fiber and how much should you take? Part 2. How to use fiber to treat disease. Pract Gastroenterol May/June, Vol X, 1986, pp 19–56
37. Wald A: Colonic transit and anorectal manometry in chronic idiopathic constipation. Arch Intern Med 146:1713–1716, 1986
38. Likongo Y, Devroede G, Schang J-C, et al: Hindgut dysgenesis as a cause of constipation with delayed colonic transit. Dig Dis Sci 31:993–1003, 1986
39. Burleigh DE, D'Mello A: Neural and pharmacologic factors affecting motility of the internal anal sphincter. Gastroenterology 84:409, 1983
40. Huizinga JD, Daniel EE: Control of human colonic motor dysfunction. Dig Dis Sci 31:865, 1986
41. Todd IP: Adult Hirschsprung's disease. Br J Surg 64:311, 1977
42. Meunier P, Marechal JM, DeBeaujeu J: Rectoanal pressures and rectal sensitivity studies in chronic childhood constipation. Gastroenterology 77:330, 1979
43. Biancani P, Walsh J, Behar J: Vasoactive intestinal peptide: A neurotransmitter for relaxation of the rabbit internal anal sphincter. Gastroenterology 89:867–874, 1985
44. Battle WM, Snape WJ Jr, Alavi A, et al: Colonic dysfunction in diabetes mellitus. Gastroenterology 79:1217, 1980
45. Battle WM, Snape WJ Jr, Wright S, et al: Abnormal colonic motility in progressive systemic sclerosis. Ann Intern Med 94:749, 1981
46. Glick ME, Meshkinpour H, Haldeman S, et al: Colonic dysfunction in multiple sclerosis. Gastroenterology 83:1002, 1982
47. Ahmed MN, Carpenter S: Autonomic neuropathy and carcinoma of the lung. CMA J 113:410, 1975
48. Devroede G, Arhan P, Duguay C, et al: Traumatic constipation. Gastroenterology 77:1258, 1979
49. Faulk DL, Anuras S, Gardner GD, et al: A familial visceral myopathy. Ann Intern Med 89(pt 1):600, 1978
50. Anuras S, Mitros FA, Nowak TV, et al: A familial visceral myopathy with external ophthalmoplegia and autosomal recessive transmission. Gastroenterology 84:346, 1983
51. Schuffler MD, Bird TD, Sumi SM, et al: A familial neuronal disease presenting as intestinal pseudo-obstruction. Gastroenterology 75:889, 1978
52. Schuffler MD, Baird HW, Fleming CR, et al: Intestinal pseudo-obstruction as the presenting manifestation of small-cell carcinoma of the lung. Ann Intern Med 98:129, 1983
53. Schuffler MD, Rohrmann CA, Chaffee RG, et al: Chronic intestinal pseudo-obstruction: A report of 27 cases and review of the literature. Medicine 60:173, 1981
54. Bleijenberg G, Kuijpers HC: Treatment of the spastic pelvis floor syndrome with biofeedback. Dis Colon Rectum 30:108–111, 1987
55. Preston DM, Lennard-Jones JE: Pelvis motility and response to intraluminal bisacodyl in slow-transit constipation. Dig Dis Sci 30:289–294, 1985
56. Harrison MW, Deitz DM, Campbell JR, et al: Diagnosis and management of Hirschsprung's disease. Am J Surg 152:49–56, 1986
57. Webster W: Embryogenesis of the enteric ganglia in normal mice and in mice that develop congenital aganglionic megacolon. J Embryol Exp Morphol 30:573–585, 1973
58. Udassin R, Nissan S, Lernau O, et al: The mild form of Hirschsprung's disease (short segment). Ann Surg 3:767, 1981
59. McCready RA, Beart RW: Adult Hirschsprung's disease: Results of surgical treatment at Mayo Clinic. Dis Colon Rectum 23:401, 1980
60. Bartolo DC, Read NW, Jarret JA, et al: Differences in anal sphincter function and clinical presentation in patients with pelvic floor descent. Gastroenterology 85:68–75, 1983
61. Roe AM, Bartolo DCC, Read NW, et al: Diagnosis and surgical management of intractable constipation. Br J Surg 73:854–861, 1986
62. Reboa G, Arnulfo G, Frascio M, et al: Colonic motility and colon-anal reflexes in chronic idiopathic constipation. Effects of a novel enterokinetic agent cisapride. Eur J Clin Pharmacol 26:745, 1984
63. Narducci F, Gassotti G, Gaburri M, et al: Twenty-five hour manometric recording of colonic motor activity in healthy man. Gut 28:17–25, 1987
64. Belliveau P, Goldberg SM, Rothenberger DA, et al: Idiopathic acquired megacolon: The value of subtotal colectomy. Dis Colon Rectum 25:118, 1982

65. Sullivan MA, Cohen S, Snape WJ Jr: Colonic myoelectrical activity in irritable bowel syndrome. N Engl J Med 298:878, 1978
66. Chaudhury NA, Phil D, Truelove S: Human colonic motility: A comparative study of normal subjects, patients with ulcerative colitis and patients with the irritable colon syndrome. Gastroenterology 40:1, 1960
67. Connell AM: The motility of the pelvic colon. (part II). Paradoxical motility in diarrhoea and constipation. Gut 3:342, 1962
68. Waller SL, Misiewicz JJ, Kiley N: Effect of eating on motility of the pelvic colon in constipation or diarrhoea. Gut 13:805, 1972
69. Sasaki D, Kido A, Yoshida Y: An endoscopic method to study the relationship between bowel habit and motility of the ascending and sigmoid colon. Gastro Endoscopy 32:185-189, 1986
70. Sjolung KE, Ekman R, Akre F, et al: Motilin in chronic idiopathic constipation. Scand J Gastroenterol 21:914-918, 1986
71. Smith B: Effect of irritant purgatives on the myenteric plexus in man and the mouse. Gut 9:139, 1968
72. Koch TR, Carney JA, Go L, et al: Idiopathic chronic constipation is associated with decreased colonic vasoactive intestinal peptide. Gastroenterology 94:300-310, 1988
73. Fain AM, Susat R, Herring M, et al: Treatment of constipation in geriatric and chronically ill patients: A comparison. South Med J 71:677, 1978
74. Formad HF: A case of giant growth of the colon, causing coprostasis or habitual constipation. University of Pennsylvania Medical Magazine, June 1892, pp 1-9
75. Munnings DB, Gardiner GW, Colapinto ND: Stercoral perforation in a patient with adult Hirschsprung's disease. Dis Colon Rectum 24:526, 1981
76. Gekas P, Schuster MM: Stercoral perforation of the colon: Case report and review of the literature. Gastroenterology 80:1054, 1981
77. Ford MJ, Anderson JR, Gilmore HM, et al: Clinical spectrum of "solitary ulcer" of the rectum. Gastroenterology 84:1533, 1983
78. Graham DY, Mose SE, Estes MK, et al: The effect of bran on bowel function in constipation. Gastroenterology 77:599, 1982
79. Freeman HJ, Spiller GA, Kim YS: A double blind study on the effect of purified cellulose dietary fiber on 1,1 dimethyl hydrazine-induced rat colonic neoplasia. Cancer Res 38:2912, 1978
80. Morehouse JL, Specian RD, Stewart JJ, et al: Translocation of indigenous bacteria from the gastrointestinal tract of mice after oral ricinoleic acid treatment. Gastroenterology 91:673, 1986
81. Balzs M: Melanosis coli: Ultrastructural study of 45 patients. Dis Colon Rectum 29:839-844, 1986
82. Harris RT: Bulimarexia and related serious eating disorders with medical complication. Ann Intern Med 99:800, 1983
83. Chapman RW, Sillery J, Fontana DD, et al: Effect of oral dioctyl sodium sulfosuccinate on intake-output studies of human small and large intestine. Gastroenterology 89:489, 1985
84. Glick ME, Meshkinpour A, Haldeman S, et al: Colonic dysfunction in patients with thoracic spinal cord injury. Gastroenterology 86:287-294, 1984
85. Kreek MC, Hahn EF, Schaefer RA, et al: Naloxone: A specific opioid antagonist, reverses chronic idiopathic constipation. Lancet 1:261, 1983
86. Istre GR, Kreiss K, Hopkins RS: An outbreak of amebiasis spread by colonic irrigation at a chiropractic clinic. N Engl J Med 307:339, 1982
87. Orr JD, Anderson JR, Scobie WG: The treatment of Hirschsprung's disease. J R Coll Surg 26:153, 1981
88. Smith JL: Arbuthnot Lane, chronic intestinal stasis and autotoxication. Ann Intern Med 96:365, 1982
89. McCready RA, Beart RJ Jr: The surgical treatment of incapacitating constipation associated with idiopathic megacolon. Mayo Clin Proc 54:779, 1979

11

Irritable Colon Syndrome

William J. Snape, Jr.

1. EPIDEMIOLOGY

The irritable colon syndrome is a common cause of visits to a physicians's office and time lost from work in the United States. The number of such patients who present to a physician appears to be the tip of the iceberg, since approximately a third of otherwise healthy persons have similar symptoms.[1,2] The subgroup of patients who present to a physician may be selected by factors other than their symptoms. These patients have increased numbers of negative life events which may alter their psychologic makeup and their ability to cope with their symptoms.[3,4] There is also evidence that during their childhood, many of these many of these patients received positive reinforcement for their symptoms.[5] This explains why patients with increased bowel complaints in childhood may have similar complaints as adults.[6,7] However, it is unclear if there is a genetic predisposition to the irritable colon, or if the symptoms are learned behavior.

Patients generally begin recognizing their symptoms in their 20s and seek medical advise in their 30s.[8] There does not appear to be an ethnic or racial predisposition to the irritable bowel syndrome.[1,2] The increased prevalence of the irritable bowel syndrome in Western society may reflect the increased resources available for the care of nonlethal diseases.

2. CLINICAL SYMPTOMS

Functional colon disease consists of a group of diseases which are associated with symptoms of colonic dysfunction in the absence of a structural alteration of the gastrointestinal tract. The major symptoms of functional colonic disease are abdominal pain, an alteration in bowel habit (diarrhea and/or constipation), the perception of abdominal distension, and increased amounts of mucus in the stool. The symptoms are often tem-

William J. Snape, Jr. • Inflammatory Bowel Disease Center, Harbor–UCLA Medical Center, Torrance, California 90502; and Department of Medicine, University of California–Los Angeles, Los Angeles, California 90073.

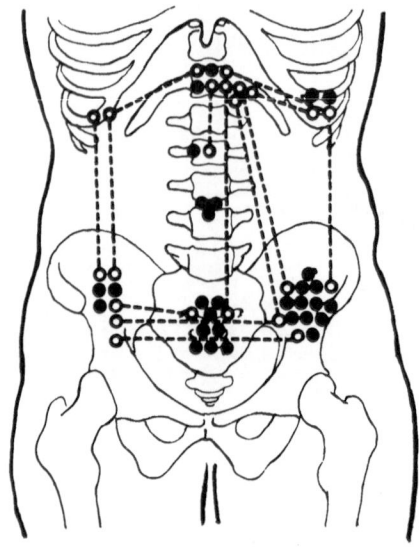

Figure 1. Distribution of sites of abdominal pain. O---O, multiple sites of pain in the same patient. Reprinted by permission from Lancet 2:753–756, 1969.

porally related to eating. The majority of patients will have the irritable colon syndrome[1,2]; however, symptoms of functional bowel disease can occur secondary to other systemic diseases, such as diabetes mellitus.[9,10]

The abdominal pain is crampy and most often in the lower abdominal quadrants. However, the pain is not always in the usual location; it may be anywhere over the anatomic distribution of the colon (Fig. 1).[8,11] A minority of patients may have pain in a location seemingly far removed from the colon, such as in the back or in the left chest. In these patients the colonic origin of the pain is demonstrated by pain relief after passing flatus or a bowel movement.[12] The pain also may be intensified by stimuli which increase colonic motor function including eating a high-fat meal or emotional stress. Although the colon is the major cause of symptoms in the irritable bowel syndrome, symptoms may also originate from other parts of the gastrointestinal tract (see Kellow and Phillips, this volume).

Patients with the irritable colon syndrome commonly have an alteration of their bowel habit which includes constipation, diarrhea, or alternation between the two. It is important to exactly define the bowel habit in each patient in order to successfully treat the symptoms. The symptoms of constipation may include the daily passage of hard, pelletal stools, or a bowel movement less than three times a week. Patients with diarrhea may not have an increased daily volume of stool, but rather may have an increase in the frequency of small mucous stools.[13] Some patients pass an increased volume and increased number of stools. The exacerbation of diarrhea by eating meals that do not have an osmotic load suggests a motility disorder. However, if the diarrhea is exacerbated by lactose or other osmotic products, a dietary cause of the diarrhea must be sought with an exclusion diet. If the diarrhea is present in the absence of eating, a primary secretory diarrhea must be considered.

Commonly the patients complain of increasing abdominal girth, which is felt to be due to abdominal distension. However, flat plate x-rays of the abdomen do not show an increase in the amount of bowel gas in these patients.[14] The perception of increased abdominal girth appears to be caused by increased afferent signals from the gut at normal levels of gut distension.

3. DIAGNOSIS

3.1. Differential Diagnosis

Care must be taken to ensure that another disease which resembles the irritable colon and requires different treatment is not overlooked. An exhaustive review of the differential diagnosis is beyond the scope of this chapter.

Although the irritable bowel syndrome occurs predominantly in young females,[1,2,8] carcinoma of the colon must still be considered in the diagnosis,[15] especially in older patients. If a younger patient does not respond to therapy promptly, studies to exclude colonic carcinoma must be initiated. Diverticular disease of the colon may have a presentation similar to that of the irritable colon syndrome. Inflammatory bowel disease, especially Crohn's disease, may imitate the irritable bowel syndrome.

Since females are predominantly affected by the irritable bowel syndrome, gynecologic disorders may present with lower abdominal discomfort. Bowel disturbances also may be altered by the menstrual cycle.[16,17]

Deficiency of the intestinal enzyme lactase occurs in most of the world's populations after adolescence.[18] Lactose intolerance is associated with diarrhea and abdominal bloating which are symptoms that are similar to the irritable bowel syndrome.[19]

3.2. Diagnostic Studies

The history and physical examination do not definitively suggest the diagnosis of the irritable bowel syndrome. However, if a young patient has increased frequency of loose bowel movements associated with the abdominal pain, there is a high probability that the symptoms are due to the irritable bowel syndrome.[1,2,20,21] A positive history of symptoms associated with milk ingestion will suggest that lactase deficiency is present which may be confirmed by a lactose tolerance test.

The stool should be tested for occult blood and fecal leukocytes. If there is blood or white blood cells in the stool, the patient (no matter what age) should have further studies to investigate the cause of the symptoms. Either colonoscopy or a barium enema can be used to visualize the colon and exclude mucosal disease. In patients in whom diarrhea is a component of the symptom complex, a small bowel follow-through x-ray should be performed to exclude small intestinal mucosal disease. Inflammatory bowel disease (especially Crohn's disease) must be carefully considered in these patients, because it is a common disease which affects a similar age group.

In order to exclude a gynecologic contribution to the symptoms, a careful menstrual history should be taken. Correlation of the symptom pattern with the menstrual cycle suggests a hormonal cause of the colonic symptoms. In some patients a thorough gynecologic examination is necessary to exclude pathology including endometriosis.

The pseudoobstruction syndrome may also cause symptoms which are similar to the irritable bowel syndrome. History of autonomic involvement in diabetes mellitus or symptoms and signs of progressive systemic sclerosis should be sought. Visceral distention on flat plate will suggest pseudoobstruction, since there is generally no increase in bowel gas in the irritable colon syndrome.[14]

4. GENERAL PATHOPHYSIOLOGY

The pathophysiology of functional colon syndrome cannot necessarily be predicted from the clinical history.[22] The symptoms of functional colonic disease are caused in part by a disturbance in the transit of contents through the colon. The direction and speed of transit are determined by coordination of the smooth muscle contraction which is controlled by multiple sites including the central nervous system (CNS), the enteric nervous system (ENS), and humoral agents (Fig. 2). The transit of contents through the colon is also affected by changes in the absorption of fluid and electrolytes. The colonic mucosa will absorb more if the contact time is increased due to uncoordinated contraction of the colon or anal sphincter.[23]

Recent studies have suggested that two basic motor patterns control transit of intraluminal colonic contents. Segmenting contractions are responsible for the usual movement of intraluminal contents. In the cat retrograde contractions maintain the luminal contents in prolonged contact with the mucosa of the proximal colon.[24] In humans there also is an increase in segmenting contractile activity in the descending colon compared to the transverse colon and sigmoid colon (Fig. 3). The increased pressure in the descending colon moves intraluminal contents from the descending colon back into the transverse colon and forward into the sigmoid colon.[25] The retrograde movement of colonic intraluminal contents explains the comingling of markers that have been ingested on different days.[26] In healthy subjects, propagating contractions occur 60–90 min after eating. These contractions rapidly transport intraluminal contents from the transverse colon to the descending colon.

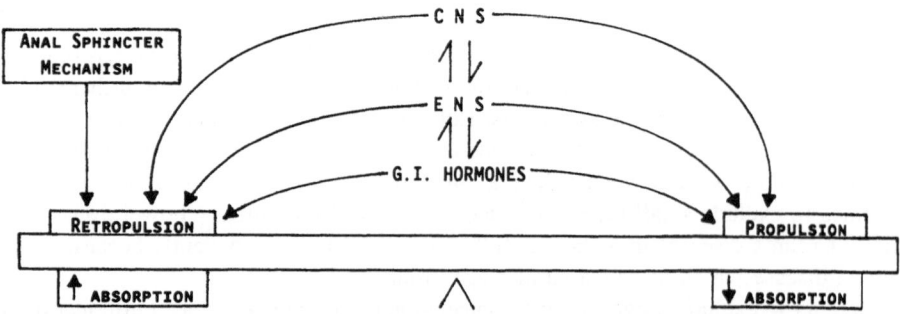

Figure 2. Interaction between different forces which control bowel habit in patients. The speed of transit is inversely related to the absorption within the colon. The central nervous system, the enteric nervous system, and the circulating hormones control the colonic motility and transit.

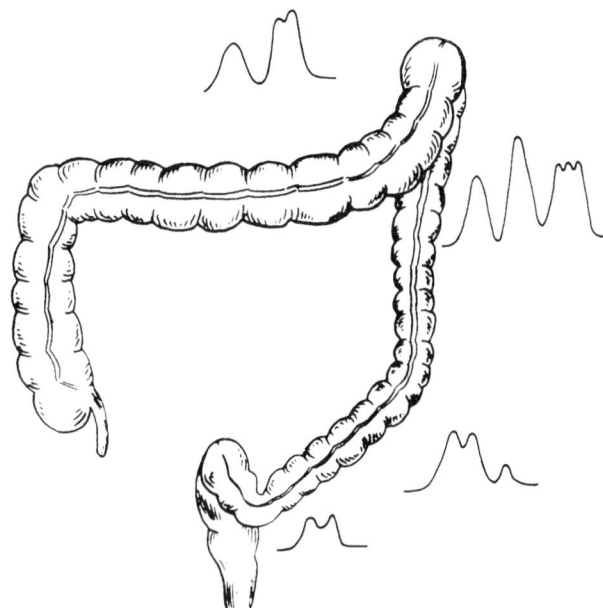

Figure 3. Schematic diagram showing the increase in colonic motility
that occurs in the descending colon,
compared to the transverse and sigmoid colon, which is responsible for
the movement of the luminal contents
from the descending colon to the
transverse colon.

The frequency of propagating contractions is increased in patients with diarrhea and decreased in patients with constipation.[25] Patients with constipation also may have disturbances over different segments of the colon. In some patients there is an isolated abnormality of the transit in the proximal or distal colon.[27] Associated abnormalities in the relaxation of the anal sphincter may contribute to slow flow through the distal colon. The poor relaxation of the anal sphincter suggests that the neural control of the colon is disturbed.

The limited number of studies show that there are multiple disturbances in the transit of luminal contents through the colon which may account for the patient's symptoms. The contribution of the different components of the colon to the altered transit will be discussed below.

4.1. Myogenic

In addition to the coordination between neighboring segments of colonic muscle, the transit of colonic contents depends on the amplitude and frequency of contraction of the muscle. The pattern and frequency of smooth muscle contractions are controlled by cyclical changes in the smooth muscle membrane potential. In the circular muscle these potentials appear to be classical slow waves, whereas in the longitudinal muscle oscillatory potentials appear to be the predominant electrical event.[24,28] In humans the synchronization of slow waves is less than in other species.[29]

The cyclical slow-wave activity sets the rhythm, while spike potentials initiate the contraction. The spike potentials are associated with an influx of Ca^{2+}.[30] The amplitude of the contractions depends on the intracellular Ca^{2+} concentration, quantity and speed of actin—myosin crossbridge formation, and extracellular matrix surrounding the muscle cells.[31—33] The increase in calcium can come from either extracellular sources or intracellular stores.[34]

Recent studies have shown an abnormal pattern of slow waves in patients with the constipation-predominant irritable colon syndrome.[35—37] In these patients there is an increase in the frequency of slow waves with a frequency of 3 cycles/min compared to healthy subjects who have a slow-wave frequency of approximately 6 cycles/min.[38—41] When colonic motility is stimulated in these patients, the colonic contractions also occur at 3 cycles/min.[36] The 3 cycle/min contractions have been associated with segmenting contractions.[42,43] Patients with constipation tend to have increased segmenting contractions, which may cause a functional partial obstruction and symptoms of abdominal pain.[44]

4.2. Neural

Neural control of colonic motility comprises three components: (1) the enteric and splanchnic nervous systems, (2) the CNS, and (3) the afferent nervous system.

The earliest description of the irritable colon syndrome recognized the importance of the CNS in causing the symptoms of the irritable colon syndrome.[13] Psychoneurosis is associated with an altered slow-wave pattern that is similar to the irritable colon syndrome.[45] Emotional stress increases intestinal motility in healthy subjects.[46—48] The CNS can transport its signal through connections in the autonomic nervous system (Fig. 4). Different emotional stimuli have been shown to provoke a different response in the human colon. Weeping associated with emotional distress is associated with decreased colonic motility.[49,50] In contrast, anger, emotional stress associated with competition, or pain is associated with increased colonic motility.[51]

Patients with the irritable bowel syndrome have a similar magnitude of increase in colonic motility in response to stress as do healthy subjects.[46] However, patients with constipation-predominant symptoms respond with an increase in segmenting nonpropulsive contractions in the rectosigmoid.[35—38] The absence of propagating peristaltic contractions, which transport the luminal contents from the transverse colon to the sigmoid colon, may exacerbate the constipation. Therefore, the increase in colonic motility that occurs after common stimuli may cause symptoms in constipated patients, but not in healthy subjects.

The ENS receives input from both the splanchnic ganglia and the CNS. The enteric neurons contain different neurotransmitters, including acetylcholine and neuropeptides. The large number of peptides within the enteric neurons can either excite or inhibit colonic motility.[52]

Although there are many putative excitatory neuropeptides, substance P may be the most important. The neuropeptides may interact with acetylcholine to stimulate colonic contractions. Substance P stimulates the muscle directly and also releases acetylcholine from the enteric neurons.[53] Electrical field stimulation of the human colonic circular muscle results in an on- and off-contraction.[54] In the rabbit the on-contraction is mediated by acetylcholine. However, the off-contraction is mediated by both acetylcholine and substance P.[55] The humoral mediators for colonic motility in humans are presently unclear.

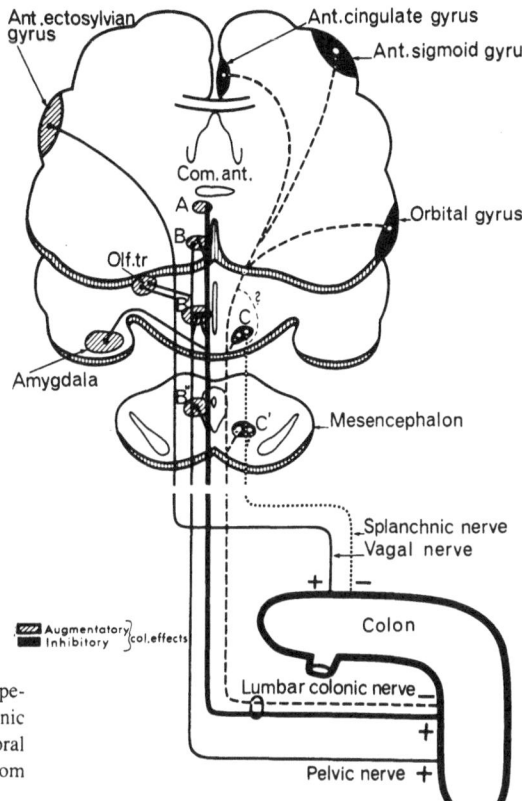

Figure 4. Schematic drawing showing the peripheral pathways mediating the effects on colonic motility induced by stimulation of various cerebral areas in the cat. Reprinted with permission from Acta Physiol Scand 89:155–168, 1973.

There is evidence that inhibitory peptides are important modulators of colonic motility. Vasoactive intestinal polypeptide (VIP) is important in the control of the internal anal sphincter[56,57] and may have some role in the control of colonic motility also. Calcitonin gene-related peptide (CGRP) may also inhibit colonic motility.[58] There is also evidence that the purinergic nervous system may contribute a component to the inhibitory control of the colon. The neuropeptides, especially somatostatin, may work by inhibiting release of acetylcholine.[59,60] The importance of this mechanism is unclear, since VIP stimulates acetylcholine release under certain conditions.[61] The adrenergic neurons from the mesenteric ganglia can both inhibit acetylcholine release from the enteric plexus (α-receptor)[62] and inhibit the muscle contraction directly (β-receptor).[63] The importance of a balance between excitation and inhibition is highlighted by the severe diarrhea that occurs after sympathetic ganglionectomy in dogs.[64]

The importance of the enteric and splanchnic nervous system in humans can be demonstrated by symptoms of functional bowel disease that are associated with pathologic abnormalities in either the enteric neurons or the sympathetic ganglia.[64–66] Severe constipation may require colectomy due to damage of the colonic enteric neurons.[65] It is unclear if the pathologic changes in the neurons are primary or if long standing laxative use harms the neurons.[67]

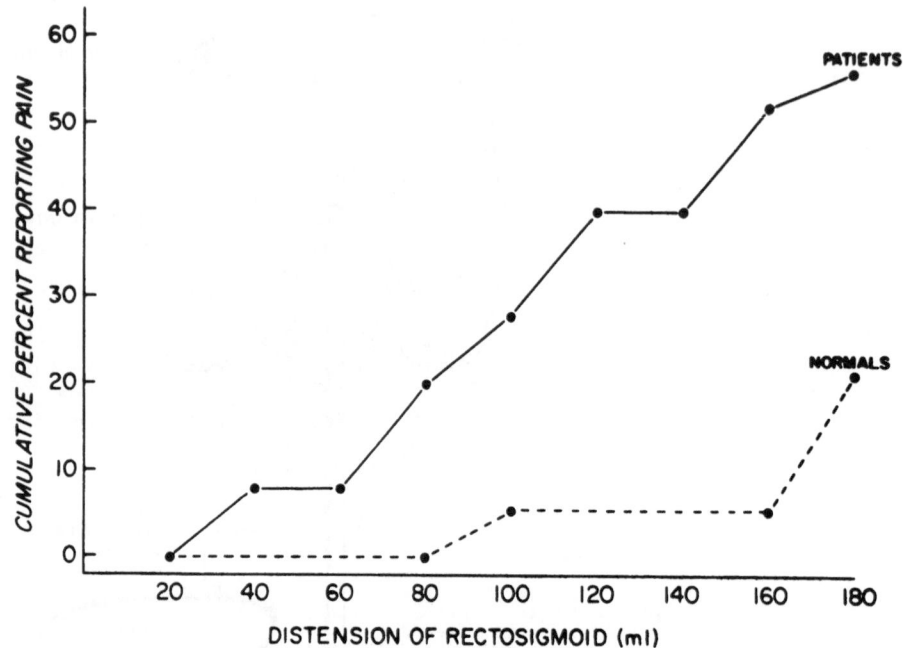

Figure 5. Effect of rectal distension on pain recognition in patients with the irritable bowel compared to healthy subjects. Reprinted with permission from Dig Dis Sci 25:404–413, 1980.

Afferent signals are relayed from different parts of the colon through the superior and inferior mesenteric ganglia to the brain and other parts of the colon.[68] These ganglia integrate signals that come from the brain with afferent signals from the colon. There is also local integration of afferent signals so that distension of either the proximal or the distal colon will inhibit contractions in the opposite side of the colon.[68]

The perception of abdominal discomfort is an important component of most gastrointestinal diseases. Patients with the irritable colon syndrome have increased sensation of visceral pain an distension of the small intestine and colon compared to healthy subjects.[69–71] However, the threshold for recognition of sensation is similar to healthy subjects.[71] Although patients with the irritable colon and healthy subjects recognize the presence of a distended balloon in the rectum equally, the patients with irritable bowel syndrome report pain in lower levels of distension (Fig. 5). The altered afferent recognition of pain leads to symptoms of abdominal pain and the sensation of abdominal distension that are common in patients with the irritable colon syndrome. Despite the sensation of abdominal distension, these patients do not have an increase in the amount of gas in their intestine.[14]

4.3. Humoral

Circulating neuropeptides may contribute to the control of colonic motility. Exogenous administration of gastrin, cholecystokinin, or neurotensin stimulates colonic smooth muscle.[72,73] Eating stimulates an increase in the plasma concentration of these peptides which may contribute to the physiologic stimulation of the colon postprandially.[73,74] Gastrin and CCK alter the slow-wave rhythm as well as stimulate smooth muscle contraction.[75,76] Neurotensin, like bethanechol, stimulates smooth muscle contraction without altering the slow-wave rhythm.[77] The maximal increase in the plasma concentration of these peptides does not correlate with the maximal increase in colonic motor activity, but these peptides may be important ancillary stimulants of the postprandial increase in colonic motility.[73,74] In patients with the irritable colon syndrome, circulating peptides may contribute to the abnormal motility response.[78] However, the importance of the circulating peptide to the normal physiologic control of colonic motility is suspect. The increase in plasma concentrations of the peptides occurs 45–60 min after eating, whereas the increase in colonic motility occurs immediately after eating.[73,74] The increase in neurotensin plasma levels has a similar time course as the increase in colonic motility.[70]

It is possible that a major inhibitory control of colonic motility is humoral. Both intraluminal and intravenous administration of amino acids inhibit the postprandial increase in colonic motility.[80,81] The amino acids may inhibit colonic motility by releasing another circulating inhibitory peptide such as enteroglucagon[82] which inhibits colonic smooth muscle.[83] Amino acids by themselves stimulate an increase in colonic contractility in vitro.[84]

4.4. Gastrocolonic Response

Eating stimulates an immediate increase in colonic motility in all regions of the colon in healthy subjects.[25,85] This response is mediated in large part through a neural reflex. Figure 6 shows the interaction between the CNS and ENS in mediating the gastrocolonic response. Dietary fat is the major stimulant in the diet that stimulates colonic motility.[85] Inhibition of mucosal afferent receptors in the gastroduodenal mucosa with procaine inhibits the gastrocolonic response.[86] Sham eating of the meal does not increase colonic motility, although emotional stress does stimulate an increase in motility.[46] Therefore, some, but not all, stimuli from the brain can initiate colonic motility in humans as in cats.[87]

The spinal cord is necessary for the gastrocolonic response, because patients with spinal cord lesions do not have a postprandial increase in colonic motility.[88,89] The final mediator of the gastrocolonic response is still unclear.

Substance P and neurotensin are possible excitatory neurotransmitters. Figure 7 shows that acetylcholine and opioids appear to be major mediators of the response, since atropine and naloxone inhibit the gastrocolonic response.[86,90] CCK interacts with the opioid receptor in other tissues. Naloxone inhibits CCK stimulation of colonic motility.[91] Therefore, we must still consider that CCK may have a physiologic role in the control of postprandial colonic motility.

The gastrocolonic response is altered in different functional disease states. In patients with the irritable bowel syndrome, the increase in the gastrocolonic response is delayed, occurring 60 min after eating the meal.[90] The mechanism for this delay in the gastrocolonic response is unclear. Gastric emptying is normal in these patients.[92] Other studies also have shown little correlations between the timing of the postprandial increase in colonic motility and gastric emptying.[9]

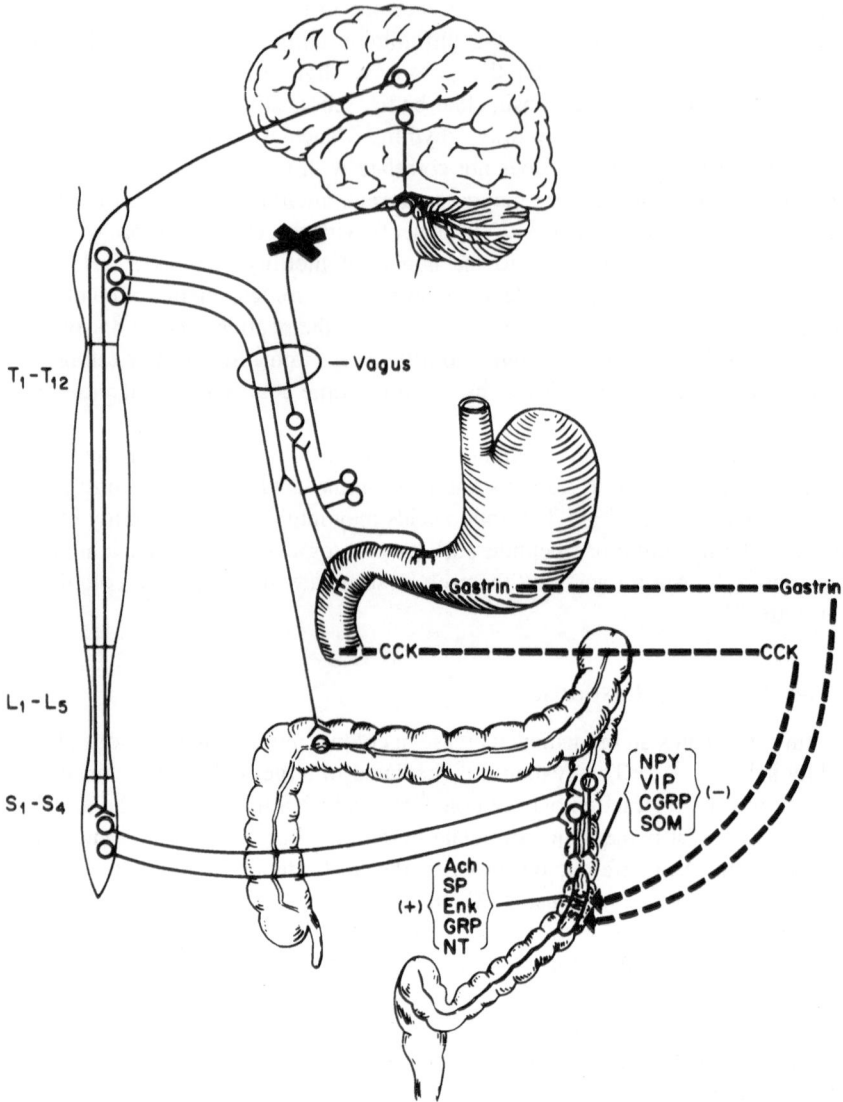

Figure 6. Schematic diagram of the regulation of the gastrocolonic response in healthy subjects. There is integration of the central nervous system, the enteric nervous system, and the release of gastrointestinal hormones.

In patients with the irritable colon syndrome there may be an abnormality in the local neural control of colonic motility, since atropine inhibits the delayed gastrocolonic response in patients with the irritable colon syndrome.[90] Peptides delivered as hormones may contribute to the abnormal gastrocolonic response. Patients with postprandial abdominal pain have an exaggerated increase in the postprandial gastrocolonic response.[93] A delayed release of CCK into the plasma may be an important stimulus to colonic contraction in patients with the irritable bowel syndrome.

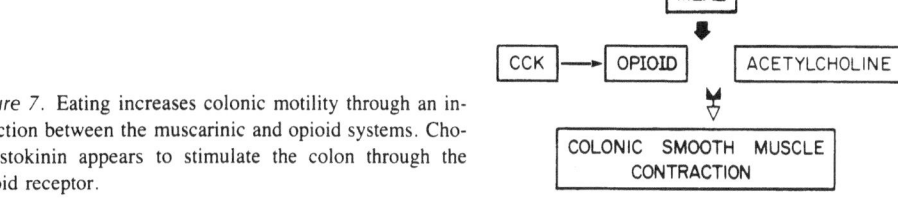

Figure 7. Eating increases colonic motility through an interaction between the muscarinic and opioid systems. Cholecystokinin appears to stimulate the colon through the opioid receptor.

The argument for disordered neuromuscular control in the irritable colon syndrome is strengthened by the abnormal bowel habit that occurs in patients with more defined defects in the gastrointestinal nerves and muscle. Constipation in patients with insulin-requiring diabetes mellitus is associated with an absent gastrocolonic response.[9] There is a defect in the neural excitation of the distal colonic smooth muscle, since the muscle can be stimulated normally with metoclopramide or bethanechol. Patients with neuropathic pseudoobstruction have a similar pattern of postprandial colonic motility.[94,95] Patients with visceral myopathy will not respond to the administration of stimulants. Patients with progressive systemic sclerosis (PSS) (scleroderma) also have an absent gastrocolonic response; however, if their muscle can be stimulated with exogenous drugs, they generally do not have any symptoms.[96] Only the PSS patients with smooth muscle replacement with collagen have gastrointestinal symptoms. Although diverticular disease of the colon is associated with abnormalities in colonic motility[97] and may be an extension of the irritable bowel syndrome,[98] the pattern of the slow waves and the gastrocolonic response differs from that in the irritable colon syndrome.[97,99,100]

5. PATHOPHYSIOLOGY OF SPECIFIC CONDITION

5.1. Constipation

Early studies by Connell suggested that constipation could be caused by increased or decreased colonic motility.[44] Increased segmenting contractions impeded the forward movement of colonic contents and caused a stepwise movement of the colonic contents.[101] Patients with the irritable bowel syndrome have increased occurrence of slow waves at a frequency of 3 cycles/min which are associated with segmenting contractions.[44] Other patients with constipation have decreased postprandial colonic motility.[25,102] In these patients the colon does not move the luminal contents backward and the luminal contents remain stationary. The propagating contraction is absent in all patients with constipation independent of the presence of increased or decreased colonic motility.

It is hard to differentiate the patients with constipation associated with increased or decreased motility from their subjective symptoms. However, patients with increased segmenting contractions are more likely to have cramping colonic pain compared to the symptoms of abdominal distension and more generalized abdominal discomfort than occurs in the patients with colonic inertia. These differences in the colonic response to a physiologic stimulus suggest that a different therapy will be needed in the various functional syndromes associated with constipation.

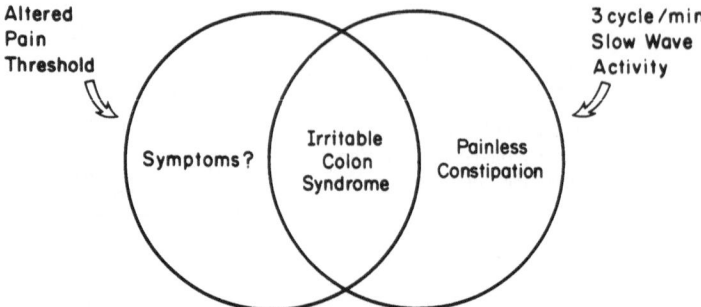

Figure 8. The irritable colon is caused by combination of an alteration of the pain threshold and the pattern of smooth muscle contraction. When both of these variables are present, the patient has the symptom pattern of the irritable colon syndrome.

5.2. Spastic Irritable Colon Syndrome

Abdominal pain and the perception of abdominal distension are important symptom patterns of the spastic variety of irritable colon. Figure 8 is a conceptual representation of symptom patterns that comprise the spastic irritable colon syndrome. The abnormalities in bowel habit and in afferent abdominal pain recognition may be independent phenomena. If they occur simultaneously, patients present with the classical symptoms of the irritable colon syndrome. Several studies have suggested that the altered slow-wave pattern can occur in subjects who have no symptoms at the time of the study response. In order for the complete syndrome to be present, the patient must have a proclivity for abdominal pain. The increased sensitivity to pain is not generalized, since there is no increase in cutaneous pain sensation.[103]

It is possible that the group of patients with painless constipation may have an abnormal slow-wave rhythm without having the increased abdominal pain sensitivity.[39] However, in some of these patients, there is an abnormality of the myenteric plexus.[65] This alteration in the myenteric plexus is not associated with a familial incidence of pseudoobstruction and is not associated with abnormalities in the motility of other parts of the gastrointestinal tract.

5.3. Painless Diarrhea

Several studies have suggested that patients with diarrhea have a decreased amount of postprandial colonic motility.[71,104,105] However, these patients also have an increased frequency of propagating contractions from the transverse colon into the rectosigmoid colon.[25] The pathogenesis of the abnormal increase in propagating contractions is unknown. Distension of the transverse colon can initiate propagating contractions.[106]

An idiopathic increase in fecal bile salts also may be a pathogenic factor in functional diarrhea,[107,108] although not all studies have shown an increase in bile salts in the irritable colon.[109] Studies in the rabbit showed that bile salts cause propagating contractions.[110] It is possible that the increase in propagating contractions in painless diarrhea may be secondary to increased fecal concentrations of bile salts, but this has not been studied.

Patients with either primary or secondary pseudoobstruction may present with painless diarrhea. The diarrhea in these patients is most often secondary to poor transit through the small intestine with ensuing development of bacterial overgrowth causing the diarrhea. In general, these patients have dilated loops of small bowel which can be identified on an abdominal flat plate.

6. TREATMENT

In many patients an alteration in bowel habit and other symptoms of functional colon disease have been difficult to successfully treat. In the United States a great deal of money is spent on drugs to treat diarrhea and constipation. Successful treatment is often elusive. Newer diagnostic techniques have improved the classification of the different components of functional colonic disease. Hopefully in the near future these advances will be translated into improved treatment.

6.1. Constipation Associated with Increased Motility

Segmenting colonic contractions can be decreased by blocking the stimuli that reach the muscle or by inhibiting the smooth muscle contractile response. Table I shows the potential therapies for the irritable colon associated with increased colonic motility.

Alteration of the diet can decrease the colonic motor response. Colonic motility can be reduced by decreasing the fat in the diet. Increasing the amino acids in the diet will decrease the postprandial colonic response.[80,81] The effective intraluminal pressure may be decreased by increasing the diameter of the colon (Laplace's theorem). The decrease in the effect of the segmenting contractions will reduce the impediment to the forward flow of luminal contents and lessen the functional obstruction.[110] Increasing the fiber content of the stool will enlarge the colonic luminal diameter.[112,113] Increasing the fiber content of the stool by increasing the fiber content of the diet has improved symptoms of the irritable colon,[114,115] but it has not been universally successful.[116] In studies in which there were no decrease in the symptoms, there was also no increase in the frequency or volume of the stool.[112] Complete endorsement of the fiber hypothesis of symptoms must await resolution of the inconsistencies in studies that have evaluated the role of increased fiber in the treatment of the irritable colon syndrome.

Table I. Therapy to Decrease Colonic
Contractions

Diet
CCK antagonist
Papaverine
Peppermint oil
Mood alteration
Calcium channel blockers
Nitrates
Opioid antagonists

Blockade of stimulatory receptors on the colonic smooth muscle cell may be useful to decrease colonic smooth muscle contraction. Acetylcholine is one of the major stimulatory neurotransmitters for the colon. Anticholinergic drugs decrease the gastrocolonic response.[90] The anticholinergic effect appears to be mediated systemically since intravenous and orally administered anticholinergics inhibit the gastrocolonic response. Not all studies have shown a positive response to anticholinergic drugs.[117]

CCK also may be an important mediator of the gastrocolonic response, especially in the patient with the irritable colon syndrome.[93] Blockade of the CCK receptor with the antagonist proglumide[118] has not been evaluated as a potential therapeutic regimen. New pharmacologic agents are being developed which are specific antagonists of the CCK receptor.[119] Clinical trials of these drugs are just beginning, but they have shown pharmacologic efficacy in humans.[120] Naloxone, an opioid antagonist, inhibits CCK stimulation of colonic motility.[91] This compound may interact with the CCK receptor, preventing the effect of CCK.[121] Naloxone has been used successfully to treat the spastic component of the irritable colon syndrome.[122]

Reduction in colonic motility can also be mediated by decreasing the smooth muscle response to physiologic stimuli. Colonic smooth muscle contraction results from stimuli which increase the intracellular concentration of calcium. The latter can be increased by influx of calcium from extracellular sources or by release from intracellular stores. Complete discussion of the control of intracellular calcium is beyond the scope of this chapter and is discussed in other reviews.[123,124] Since changes in intracellular calcium are important, therapy to reduce the colonic motility can be based on reducing the calcium available for initiating and maintaining a contraction. The voltage-dependent calcium channel is important for calcium influx into the muscle cell which has been stimulated by agents which depolarize the muscle membrane (e.g., acetylcholine).[125] The dihydropyridine class of organic channel blockers seem to have the greatest effect on gastrointestinal smooth muscle, although most studies have been performed in the esophagus.[126] Presently, studies are ongoing to evaluate the effect of the calcium channel blockers on the symptoms of the irritable bowel syndrome.

Nitrates increase the intracellular concentration of cGMP.[127,128] This compound decreases the calcium influx into the cell through receptor-operated calcium channels. Nitrates have not been demonstrated to be useful in the colon, but they decrease motility in esophageal motor diseases.[129,130]

Papaverine can decrease colonic smooth muscle contraction, by increasing intracellular cAMP levels or by decreasing intracellular calcium concentrations.[131] There has been no trial of papaverine, but the drug may be effective in treating the irritable colon syndrome. Peppermint oil also decreases colonic motility and improves symptoms in the irritable colon syndrome,[132,133] although it has not been successful in all studies.[134]

A great deal of attention has been focused on treating the symptoms of the irritable colon syndrome through reducing the effect of stress. Stress increases colonic motility. Treatment of patients with mild tranquilizers reduces the effect of external stressors on the colon[46] and decreases symptoms in the irritable colon.[135] Psychotherapy has been shown to improve the symptoms of the irritable colon syndrome and their psychologic profile.[136,137] Recent studies have begun to explore the use of biofeedback as therapy in the irritable colon syndrome.[138] Identification of pathophysiologic responses will advance the use of this technique.

Recent studies suggest constipation is secondary to an absence of propagating contractions in addition to the increase in segmenting contractions. Agents which can increase propagating contractions may be expected to improve the bowel habit. The laxative bisacodyl stimulates an increased number of propagating contractions in the colon upon direct contact.[139] Increased bile salts also stimulate migrating spike bursts in rabbits, which are associated with a propagating contraction.[110] Studies in humans showed that increased intraluminal bile salts will treat constipation[140] and the increased concentrations of intraluminal bile salts will cause diarrhea.[107,109]

6.2. Constipation Associated with Decreased Motility

Cholinomimetics have been used to stimulate motility and improve function in other parts of the gastrointestinal tract.[86,87] In the stomach, bethanechol is a major stimulatory drug.[142,143] Neostigmine may have a theoretical advantage over the direct stimulation by bethanechol. Inhibition of acetylcholinesterase may allow the gastrointestinal tract's normal integrative function, since neostigmine increases the availability of the acetylcholine that is normally released.

In patients with decreased colonic motility associated with constipation, the bowel habit is improved when colonic motility is improved. Table II shows the prokinetic drugs with potential use in stimulating colonic motility. Metoclopramide stimulates an increase in colonic motility in healthy subjects and in patients with diabetes mellitus.[9] Metoclopramide also improved the bowel habit in a group of patients with insulin-requiring diabetes mellitus.[9] Metoclopramide did not improve a group of patients with idiopathic pseudoobstruction.[141] Possibly the lack of an effect is secondary to the involvement of the colonic smooth muscle in many of these patients. Domperidone has not been successful in the treatment of the irritable colon syndrome.

Cisapride is a recently developed compound which also has a stimulatory effect on gastrointestinal smooth muscle.[144] There has been some suggestion that cisapride stimulates release of acetylcholine from the myenteric plexus[145]; however, this does not occur in all tissues.[146] Cisapride could work through serotonin receptor antagonism.[147] Studies are under way to evaluate if this compound has an effect in patients with poor colonic contractions. Cisapride has been shown to coordinate contractions in the stomach and duodenum.[144] It is possible that there is altered coordination of motility between different

Table II. Therapy to Increase Colonic Contractions

Cholinergic agonists
   Bethanechol
   Acetylcholinesterase inhibitors
Dopamine antagonists
   Metoclopramide
   Domperidone
Release of acetylcholine
   Cisapride

regions of the colon. Therefore this drug may have an effect in improving this coordination and improving symptom in that way.

The stimulatory drugs should have the greatest effect in those patients with a decreased colonic motility pattern. Certain patients with idiopathic constipation (colonic pseudoobstruction), PSS, or diabetes all have decreased colonic motor response to physiologic stimuli. The drugs have shown some effect in certain patients. Patients with PSS and smooth muscle replacement with collagen have no improvement in their bowel habit after stimulation with these drugs. Patients with diabetes do have an improvement in the bowel habit.[9] There have not been enough studies on patients with colonic pseudoobstruction to determine if there will be a response to therapy.

6.3. Diarrhea

This review will discuss only therapy of diarrhea secondary to colonic disease. The most consistent abnormality described for patients with diarrhea is decreased contractions.[45] Therefore, agents which increase the colonic segmenting contractions should have a beneficial effect on the diarrhea. Loperamide slows intestinal transit[148] and stimulates anal sphincter contractions.[149]

In patients with bacterial overgrowth the treatment involves eradication of the small intestinal bacteria. Therapy with a broad-spectrum antibiotic will ameliorate the diarrhea. The secretory stimulus of the unconjugated bile salts, which results from the bacterial overgrowth, can be diminished with cholestyramine which binds the bile salts and prevents their action on the mucosa. β-Adrenergic inhibitors also may be useful in the treatment of bile salt diarrhea.[150]

7. CONCLUSION

There has been a large increase in interest in the irritable colon over the last 25 years. This interest has increased our knowledge of the pathogenesis of this elusive syndrome, and begun to allow therapy to be tailored to the individual patient. It is still too early to know if this approach will be successful.

REFERENCES

1. Drossman DA, Powell DW, Sessions JT Jr: The irritable bowel syndrome. Gastroenterology 73:811–822, 1977
2. Thompson WG, Heaton KW: Functional bowel disorders in apparently healthy people. Gastroenterology 79:283–288, 1980
3. Drossman DA, McKee DC, Sandler RS, et al: Psychosocial factors in the irritable bowel syndrome: A multivariate study of patients and non-patients with irritable bowel syndrome. Gastroenterology 95:701–708, 1988
4. Whitehead WE, Bosmajian L, Zonderman AB, et al: Symptoms of psychological distress associated with irritable bowel syndrome: Comparison of communities and medical clinic samples. Gastroenterology 95:709–714, 1988
5. Whitehead WE, Winget C, Fedoravicius AS, et al: Learned illness behavior in patients with irritable bowel syndrome and peptic ulcer. Dig Dis Sci 27:202–208, 1982

6. Apley J, Hale B: Children with recurrent abdominal pain: How do they grow up? Br Med J 3:7–9, 1973
7. Davidson M, Wasserman R: The irritable colon of childhood (chronic nonspecific diarrhea syndrome). J Pediatr 69:1027–1038, 1966
8. Waller SL, Misiewicz JJ: Prognosis in the irritable-bowel syndrome. Lancet ii:753–756, 1969
9. Battle WM, Snape WJ Jr, Alavi A, et al: Colonic dysfunction in diabetes mellitus. Gastroenterology 79:1217–1221, 1980
10. Feldman M, Schiller LR: Disorders of gastrointestinal motility associated with diabetes mellitus. Ann Intern Med 98:378–384, 1983
11. Kingham JGC, Dawson AM: Origin of chronic right upper quadrant pain. Gut 26:783–788, 1985
12. Editorial (anonymous): The irritable bowel. Lancet 112–114, 1969
13. White BV, Jones CM: Mucous colitis: A delineation of the syndrome with certain observations on its mechanism and on the role of emotional tension as a precipitating factor. Ann Intern Med 14:854–872, 1940
14. Lasser RB, Bond JH, Levitt MD: The role of intestinal gas in functional abdominal pain. N Engl J Med 293:524–526, 1975
15. Rao BN, Pratt CB, Flemming ID, et al: Colon carcinoma in children and adolescents. Cancer 55:1322–1326, 1985
16. Ryan JP, Bhojwani A: Colonic transit in rats: Effect of ovariectomy, sex steroid hormones, and pregnancy. Am J Physiol 251:G46–G50, 1986
17. Gill RC, Bowes KL, Kingma YJ: Effect of progesterone on canine colonic smooth muscle. Gastroenterology 88:1941–1947, 1985
18. McMichael HB, Webb J, Dawson AM: Lactase deficiency in adults. Lancet 1:718–720, 1965
19. Weser E, Rubin W, Ross L, et al: Lactase deficiency in patients with the "irritable-colon syndrome." N Engl J Med 273:1070–1075, 1965
20. Manning AP, Thompson WG, Heaton KW, et al: Towards positive diagnosis of the irritable bowel. Br Med J 2:653–654, 1978
21. Kruis W, Weinzierl M, Schussler P, et al: A diagnostic score for the irritable bowel syndrome. Gastroenterology 87:1–7, 1984
22. Oettle GJ, Heaton KW: Is there a relationship between symptoms of the irritable bowel syndrome and objective measurements of large bowel function? A longitudinal study. Gut 28:146–149, 1987
23. Devroede G, Soffie M: Colonic absorption in idiopathic constipation. Gastroenterology 64:552–561, 1973
24. Christensen J: Myoelectric control of the colon. Gastroenterology 68:601–609, 1975
25. Bazzocchi G, Ellis J, Meyer J, et al: Colonic scintigraphy and manometry in constipation, diarrhea and inflammatory bowel disease. Gastroenterology 94: A29, 1988
26. Cummings, JH, Wiggins HS: Transit through the gut measured by analysis of a single stool. Gut 17:219–223, 1976
27. Arhan P, Devroede G, Jehannin B, et al: Segmental colonic transit time. Dis Colon Rectum 24:6255–6259, 1981
28. Huizinga JD, Stern HS, Edwin C, et al: Electrophysiologic control of motility in the human colon. Gastroenterology 88:500–511, 1985
29. Huizinga JD, Waterfall WE: Electrical correlate of colonic circular muscle. Gut 29:10–16, 1988
30. Snape WJ Jr, Tan ST: Role of sodium or calcium in electrical depolarization of feline colonic smooth muscle. Am J Physiol 249:G66–G72, 1985
31. Dillon PF, Murphy RA (VA Claes): Tonic force maintenance with reduced shortening velocity in arterial smooth muscle. Am J Physiol 242:C102–C108, 1982
32. Moreland RS, Murphy RA: Determinants of Ca^{2+}-dependent stress maintenance in skinned swine carotid media. Am J Physiol 251:C892–C903, 1986
33. Cooke P: Organization of contractile fiber in smooth muscle. Cell Muscle Motil 3:57–77, 1983
34. Bitar KN, Burgess GM, Putney WJ Jr, et al: Source of activator calcium in isolated guinea pig and human gastric muscle cells. Am J Physiol 250:G280–G286, 1986
35. Snape WJ Jr, Carlson GM, Cohen S: Colonic myoelectric activity in the irritable bowel syndrome. Gastroenterology 70:326–330, 1976
36. Snape WJ Jr, Carlson GM, Matarazzo SA, et al: Evidence that abnormal myoelectric activity produces colonic motor dysfunction in the irritable bowel syndrome. Gastroenterology 72:383–387, 1977
37. Taylor I, Darby C, Hammond P: Comparison of rectosigmoid myoelectrical activity in the irritable bowel syndrome during relapses and remissions. Gut 19:923–929, 1978

38. Taylor I, Darby C, Hammond P, et al: Is there a myoelectrical abnormality in the irritable colon syndrome? Gut 19:391–395, 1978

39. Frieri G, Parisi F, Corazziar E, et al: Colonic electromyography in chronic constipation. Gastroenterology 84:737–740, 1983

40. Parker R, Whitehead WE, Schuster MM: Pattern recognition program for analysis of colon myoelectric and pressure data. Dig Dis Sci 32:953–961, 1982

41. Sarna S, Latimer P, Campbell D, et al: Electrical and contractile activities of the human rectosigmoid. Gut 23:698–705, 1982

42. Code CF, Hightower NC, Morlock CG: Motility of the alimentary canal in man. Am J Med 13:328–351, 1952

43. Sun EA, Bower R, Snape WJ Jr, et al: Use of video-taped barium enema for studying colonic motility. Gastroenterology 80:1297, 1981

44. Connell AM: The motility of the pelvic colon. Part II. Paradoxical motility in diarrhea and constipation. Gut 3:342–348, 1962

45. Latimer P, Sarna S, Campbell D, et al: Colonic motor and myoelectrical activity: A comparative study of normal subjects, psycho-neurotic patients, and patients with the irritable bowel syndrome. Gastroenterology 80:893–901, 1981

46. Narducci F, Snape WJ Jr, Battle WM, et al: Increased colonic motility during exposure to a stressful situation. Dig Dis Sci 30:40–44, 1985

47. Welgan P, Meshkinpour H, Hoehler F: The effect of stress on colon motor and electrical activity in irritable bowel syndrome. Psychosom Med 47:139–149, 1985

48. Kumar D, Wingate DL: The irritable bowel syndrome: A paroxysmal motor disorder. Lancet ii:973–977, 1985

49. Almy TP, Tulin M: Alterations in colonic function in human under stress: Experimental production of changes stimulating the "irritable colon." Gastroenterology 8:616–626, 1947

50. Almy TP, Abbot FK, Hinkle LE Jr: Alterations in colonic function in man under stress. IV. Hypomotility of the sigmoid colon, and its relationship to the mechanism of functional diarrhea. Gastroenterology 15:95–103, 1950

51. Almy TP, Hinkle LE Jr, Berle B, et al: Alterations in colonic function in man under stress. III. Experimental production of sigmoid spasm in patients with spastic constipation. Gastroenterology 12:437–449, 1949

52. Furness JB, Costa M: Types of nerves in the enteric nervous system. Neuroscience 5:1–20, 1980

53. Koelbel CBM, Mayer EA, Reeve JR Jr, et al: Evidence for the involvement of substance P in non-cholinergic excitation of rabbit colonic muscle. Am J Physiol 256:G246–G253, 1989

54. Snape WJ Jr, Mayer EA, Koelbel C, et al: Different response of smooth muscle from different regions of the human colon. Gastroenterology 94:A434, 1988

55. Snape WJ Jr, Kim BH, Willenbucher R, et al: The response of proximal and distal rabbit colonic muscle after electrical field stimulation. Gastroenterology 96: 321–326, 1989

56. Biancani P, Walsh J, Behar J: Vasoactive intestinal peptide: A neurotransmitter for relaxation of the rabbit internal anal sphincter. Gastroenterology 89:867–874, 1985

57. Nuko S, Rattan S: Role of vasoactive intestinal polypeptide in the internal anal sphincter relaxation of the opossum. J Clin Invest 81:1146–1153, 1988

58. Koelbel CBM, Mayer EA, Snape WJ Jr, et al: Dual effect of capsaicin on rabbit colonic muscle. Gastroenterology 94:A233, 1988

59. Teitelbaum DH, O'Dorisio TM, Perkins WE, et al: Somatostatin modulation of peptide-induced acetylcholine release in guinea pig ileum. Am J Physiol 246:G509–G514, 1984

60. Guillemin R: Somatostatin inhibits the release of acetylcholine induced electrically in the myenteric plexus. Endocrinology 99:1653–1654, 1976

61. Kusunoki M, Tsai LH, Taniyama K, et al: Vasoactive intestinal polypeptide provokes acetylcholine release from the myenteric plexus. Am J Physiol 251:G51–G55, 1986

62. Wiley J, Owyang C: Neuropeptide Y inhibits cholinergic transmission in the isolated guinea pig colon: Mediation through α-adrenergic receptors. Proc Natl Acad Sci USA 84:2047–2051, 1987

63. Lyrenas E: Beta adrenergic influence on esophageal and colonic motility in man. Scand J Gastroenterol Suppl 116:1–48, 1985

64. Martlett JA, Code CF: Effects of celiac and superior mesenteric ganglionectomy on interdigestive myoelectric complex in dogs. Am J Physiol 237:E432–E436, 1979

65. Krishnamurthy S, Schuffler MD, Rohrmann CA, et al: Severe idiopathic constipation is associated with a distinctive abnormality of the colonic myenteric plexus. Gastroenterology 88:26–34, 1985
66. Devroede G, Lamarch J: Functional importance of extrinsic parasympathetic innervation to the distal colon and rectum in man. Gastroenterology 66:273–280, 1974
67. Smith B: Effect of irritant purgatives on the myenteric pexus in man and the mouse. Gut 9:139–143, 1968
68. Kreulen DL, Szurszewski JH: Reflex pathways in the abdominal prevertebral ganglia: Evidence for a colocolonic inhibitory reflex. J Physiol (London) 295:21–32, 1979
69. Ritchie J: Pain from distension of the pelvic colon by inflating a balloon in the irritable colon syndrome. Gut 14:124–132, 1973
70. Moriarty KJ, Dawson AM: Functional abdominal pain: Further evidence that whole gut is affected. Br Med J 284:1670–1672, 1982
71. Whitehead WE, Engel BT, Schuster MM: Irritable bowel syndrome/physiological and psychological differences between diarrhea-predominant and constipation-predominant patients. Dig Dis Sci 25:404–413, 1980
72. Thor K, Rosell S: Neurotensin increased colonic motility. Gastroenterology 90:27–31, 1986
73. Snape WJ Jr, Matarazzo SA, Cohen S: Effect of eating and gastrointestinal hormones on human colonic myoelectrical and motor activity. Gastroenterology 75:373–378, 1978
74. Walsh JH, Lamers CB, Valenzuela JE: Cholecystokinin-octapeptidelike immunoreactivity in human plasma. Gastroenterology 82:438–444, 1982
75. Snape WJ Jr, Cohen S: Effect of bethanechol, gastrin I, or cholecystokinin on myoelectrical activity. Am J Physiol 246:E458–E463, 1979
76. Huizinga JD, Chang G, Diamant NE, et al: The effects of cholecystokinin-octapeptide and pentagastrin on electrical and motor activities of canine colonic circular muscle. Can J Physiol Pharmacol 62:1440–1447, 1984
77. Snape WJ Jr, Tan ST, Kao HW, et al: Mechanisms of neurotensin depolarization of rabbit colonic smooth muscle. Regul Peptide 18:287–297, 1987
78. Preston DM, Adrian TE, Christofides ND, et al: Positive correlation between symptoms and circulating motilin, pancreatic polypeptide and gastrin concentrations in functional bowel disorders. Gut 26:1059–1064, 1985
79. Rosell S, Rikoeusm A: The effect of ingestion of amino acids, glucose and fat in circulating neurotensin-like immunoreactivity (NTLI) in man. Acta Physiol Scand 107:263–267, 1979
80. Battle WM, Cohen S, Snape WJ Jr: Inhibition of postprandial colonic motility after ingestion of an amino acid mixture. Dig Dis Sci 25:647–652, 1980
81. Levinson S, Bhasker M, Gibson TR, et al: A comparison of intraluminal and intravenous mediator of colonic response to eating. Dig Dis Sci 30:33–39, 1985
82. Ohneda AE, Parada EA, Eisentront AM, et al: Characterization of response of circulating glucagon to intraduodenal and intravenous administration of amino acid. J Clin Invest 47:2305–2322, 1968
83. Taylor I, Duthie HL, Cumberland DC, et al: Glucagon and the colon. Gut 16:973–978, 1975
84. Snape WJ Jr, Yoo S: Effect of amino acids on isolated colonic smooth muscle from the rabbit. J Pharmacol Exp Ther 235:690–695, 1985
85. Wright SH, Snape WJ Jr, Battle W, et al: Effect of dietary components on gastrocolonic response. Am J Physiol 238:G228–G232, 1980
86. Sun EA, Snape WJ Jr, Cohen S, et al: The role of opiate receptors and cholinergic neurons in the gastrocolonic response. Gastroenterology 82:689–693, 1982
87. Rostad H: Colonic motility in the cat. IV. Peripheral pathways mediating the effects induced by hypothalamic and mesencephalic stimulation. Acta Physiol Scand 89:154–168, 1973
88. Glick ME, Meshkinpour H, Haldeman S, et al: Colonic dysfunction in patients with thoracic spinal cord injury. Gastroenterology 86:287–294, 1984
89. Connell AM, Frankel H, Guttmann L: The motility of the pelvic colon following complete lesions of the spinal cord. Paraplegia 1:98–115, 1963
90. Sullivan MA, Cohen S, Snape WJ Jr: Colonic myoelectrical activity in irritable-bowel syndrome. N Engl J Med 298:878–883, 1978
91. Renny A, Snape WJ Jr, Sun EA, et al: Role of cholecystokinin in the gastrocolonic response to a meal. Gastroenterology 85:17–21, 1983
92. Narducci F, Bassotti G, Granata MT, et al: Colonic motility and gastric emptying in patients with irritable bowel syndrome. Dig Dis Sci 31:241–246, 1986

93. Harvey RF, Read AE: Effect of cholecystokinin on colonic motility and symptoms in patients with the irritable bowel syndrome. Lancet i:1–3, 1973
94. Sullivan MA, Snape WJ Jr, Matarazzo SA, et al: Gastrointestinal myoelectrical activity in idiopathic intestinal pseudoobstruction. N Engl J Med 297:233–238, 1977
95. Snape WJ Jr, Sullivan MA, Cohen S: Abnormal gastrocolic response in patients with intestinal pseudoobstruction. Arch Intern Med 140:386–387, 1980
96. Battle WM, Snape WJ Jr, Wright S, et al: Abnormal colonic motility in progressive systemic sclerosis. Ann Intern Med 94:749–752, 1981
97. Taylor I, Duthie HL: Bran tablets and diverticular disease. Br Med J 1:988–990, 1976
98. Havia T, Manner R: The irritable colon syndrome. Acta Chir Scand 137:569–572, 1970
99. Suchowiecky M, Clarke PD, Bhasker M, et al: Effect of secoverine on colonic myoelectric activity in diverticular disease of the colon. Dig Dis Sci 32:833–840, 1987
100. Trotman IF, Misiewicz JJ: Sigmoid motility in diverticular disease and the irritable bowel syndrome. Gut 29:218–222, 1988
101. Ritchie JA, Truelove SC, Ardran GM, et al: Propulsion and retropulsion of normal colonic contents. Dig Dis Sci 16:697–704, 1971
102. Reynolds JC, Ouyang A, Lee CA, et al: Chronic severe constipation. Gastroenterology 92:414–420, 1987
103. Cook IJ, Van Eeden A, Collins SM: Patients with irritable bowel syndrome have greater pain tolerance than normal subjects. Gastroenterology 93:727–733, 1987
104. Bueno L, Fioramonti J, Frexino J, et al: Colonic myoelectrical activity in diarrhea and constipation. Hepato-Gastroenterology 27:381–389, 1980
105. Wangel AG, Deller D: Intestinal motility in man. III. Mechanisms of constipation and diarrhea with particular reference to the irritable colon syndrome. Gastroenterology 48:69–84, 1965
106. Narducci F, Bassotti G, Gaburri M, et al: Twenty-four hour manometric recording of colonic motor activity in healthy man. Gut 28:17–25, 1987
107. Thaysen EH, Pedersen L: Idiopathic bile acid catharsis. Gut 17:965–970, 1976.
108. Taylor I, Basu P, Hammond P, et al: Effect of bile acid perfusion on colonic motor function in patients with the irritable colon syndrome. Gut 21:843–847, 1980
109. Flynn M, Hammond P, Darby C, et al: Fecal bile acids and the irritable colon's syndrome. Digestion 22:144–149, 1981
110. Shiff SJ, Soloway RD, Snape WJ Jr: Mechanisms of deoxycholic acid stimulation of the rabbit colon. J Clin Invest 69:985–992, 1982
111. Almy TP: The irritable bowel syndrome. Back to square one? Dig Dis Sci 25:401–404, 1980
112. Burkitt DP, Walker ARP, Painter NS: Effect of dietary fibre on stools and transit-times, and its role in the causation of disease. Lancet ii:1408–1412, 1972
113. Painter NS: Pressure in the colon related to diverticular disease. Proc R Soc Med 63:144–145, 1970
114. Manning AP, Heaton KW, Harvey RF: Wheat fibre and irritable bowel syndrome. Lancet 2:417–418, 1977
115. Fox JET, Kostolanska F, Daniel EE, et al: Mechanisms of excitatory actions of neurotensin on canine small intestinal circular muscle in vivo and in vitro. Can J Pharmacol 65:2254–2259, 1987
116. Soltoft J, Krag B, Gudmand-Hoyer E, et al: A double-blind trial of the effect of wheat bran on symptoms of irritable bowel syndrome. Lancet 2:270–271, 1976
117. Ivey KJ: Are anticholinergics of use in the irritable colon syndrome? Gastroenterology 68:1300–1307, 1975
118. Ormas P, Bellobi C, Sagradi A, et al: Possible mechanism of action of caerulein on intestinal motility of sheep. Ann Res Vet 15:557–562, 1984
119. Chang RSL, Lotti VJ, Monaghan RL, et al: A potent nonpeptide cholecystokinin antagonist selective for peripheral tissues isolated from Aspergillus alliaceus. Science 230:177–179, 1985
120. Liddle RA, Kanayama S, Beccaria C, et al: The effect of a new cholecystokinin receptor antagonist, L-364,718 to inhibit gall bladder contraction in humans. Clin Res 36:398A, 1988
121. Jurna I, Zetler G: Antinociceptive effect of centrally administered caerulein and cholecystokinin octapeptide. Eur J Pharmacol 73:323–331, 1981
122. Kreek MJ, Schaefer RA, Hahn EF, et al: Naloxone, a specific opioid antagonist, reverses chronic idiopathic constipation. Lancet i:261–262, 1983
123. Karaki H, Weiss GB: Calcium channels in smooth muscle. Gastroenterology 87:960–970, 1984

124. Rasmussen H: The calcium messenger system. N Engl J Med 314:1164–1170, 1986
125. Bolton TB: Mechanisms of action of transmitters and other substances on smooth muscle. Physiol Rev 59:607–643, 1979
126. Bortolotti M, Labo G: Clinical and manometric effects of nifedipine in patients with esophageal achalasia. Gastroenterology 80:39–44, 1981
127. Hester KR, Weiss GB, Frey WJ: Differing actions of nitro-prusside and D-600 on tension and Ca fluxes in canine renal arteries. J Pharmacol Exp Ther 208:155–166, 1979
128. Lincoln TM, Fisher-Simpson V: A comparison of the effects of forskalin and nitro prusside on caplic nucleotides and relaxation in the rat aorta. Eur J Pharmacol 101:17–27, 1983
129. Mellow M: Effect of isosorbide and hydralazine in painful primary esophageal motility disorders. Gastroenterology 83:364–370, 1982
130. Swamy N: Esophageal spasm: Clinical and manometric response to nitroglycerine and long acting nitrate. Gastroenterology 72:23–27, 1977
131. Snape WJ Jr: Influence of papaverine on bethanechol or OP-CCK stimulation of feline colonic muscle. Gastroenterology 80:498–503, 1981
132. Shirley JA, Eykyn SJ, Pearson TC: Treating irritable bowel syndrome with peppermint oil. Br Med J iii:835–836, 1979
133. Dew MJ, Evans BK, Rhodes J: Peppermint oil for the irritable bowel syndrome: A multicentre trial. Br J Clin Pract 394–398, 1984
134. Nash P, Gould SR, Barnardo DE: Peppermint oil does not relieve the pain of irritable bowel syndrome. Br J Clin Pract 40:292–293, 1986
135. Ritchie JA, Truelove SC: Treatment of irritable bowel syndrome with lorazepam, hyoscine butylbromide, and ispaghula husk. Br Med J 1:376–378, 1979
136. Svedlund J, Ottosson JO, Sjodin I, et al: Controlled study of psychotherapy in irritable bowel syndrome. Lancet ii:589–591, 1983
137. Blanchard EB, Randnitz C, Schwarz SP: Psychological changes associated with self-regulatory treatments of irritable bowel syndrome. Biofeedback Self Regul 12:31–37, 1987
138. Marzuk PM: Biofeedback for gastrointestinal disorders: A review of the literature. Ann Intern Med 103:240–244, 1985
139. Preston DM, Lennard-Jones JE: Pelvic motility and response to intraluminal bisacodyl in slow-transit constipation. Dig Dis Sci 30:289–294, 1985
140. Hepner GW, Hofmann AF: Cholic acid therapy for constipation. Mayo Clin Proc 48:356–358, 1973
141. Lipton AB, Krauer CM: Pseudo-obstruction of the bowel—Therapeutic trial of metoclopramide. Dig Dis Sci 22:263–265, 1977
142. Fox S, Behar J: Pathogenesis of diabetic gastroparesis: A pharmacologic study. Gastroenterology 78:757–763, 1980
143. Malagaelada J, Rees WW, Mazzotta LJ, et al: Gastric motor abnormalities in diabetic and post vagotomy gastroparesis: Effect of metoclopramide and bethanechol. Gastroenterology 78:286–293, 1980
144. Schuurkes JJ, Akkerman L, Van Nueten J: Computer analysis of antroduodenal coordination: Comparison between cisapride and metoclopramide. Gastroenterology 90:1622, 1986
145. Van Nueten JM, Van Paele PGH, Reyntjens AJ, et al: Gastrointestinal motility stimulating properties of cisapride, a non-antidopaminergic non-cholinergic compound, in Roman C (ed): Proc. 9th Int. Symp. Gastrointestinal Motility. Lancaster, MTP Press, pp 513–520, 1986
146. Burleigh DE, Trout SJ: Evidence against an acetylcholine releasing action of cisapride in the human colon. Br J Clin Pharmacol 20:475–478, 1985
147. Moriartz KJ, Higgs NB, Woodford M, et al: Inhibition of the effect of serotonin on rat ileal transport by cisapride: Evidence in favour of the involvement of 5HT-2 receptors. Gut 28:844–848, 1987
148. Basilisco G, Camboni G, Bozzani A, et al: Oral naloxone antagonizes loperamide-induced delay of orocecal transit. Dig Dis Sci 32:829–832, 1987
149. Rattan S, Culver PJ: Influence of loperamide on the internal anal sphincter in the opossum. Gastroenterology 93:121–128, 1987
150. Coyne MJ, Bonorris GG, Chung A, et al: Propranolol inhibits bile acid and fatty acid stimulation of cyclic AMP in human colon. Gastroenterology 73:971–974, 1977

12

Association between Disturbances in Gastrointestinal Transit and Functional Bowel Disease

C. D. Lind and R. W. McCallum

Although irritable bowel syndrome (IBS) has classically been defined with regard to colonic symptoms,[1] mounting evidence points to a diffuse motility disturbance in many patients with IBS.[2] Further, as discussed elsewhere in this volume, specific functional disorders of esophageal, gastroduodenal, small intestinal, and colonic motility are being recognized as our ability to measure gastrointestinal electrophysiology, motility, and transit has improved. In this chapter, we will summarize the evidence for altered GI transit in IBS and delineate the relationship, if any, between altered transit of luminal contents and symptoms in IBS. Because of its relationship to IBS, we will also summarize the evidence for stress-related changes in normal GI transit. Finally, treatment regimens which may reverse these disturbances in GI transit, and their associated symptoms, will be discussed.

1. ESOPHAGEAL TRANSIT

A number of disorders of the esophagus including achalasia, diffuse esophageal spasm, nutcracker esophagus, and scleroderma esophagus are characterized by abnormal esophageal motor function. Generally, these disorders are identified using barium cine-esophagram or esophageal manometry, but neither of these assess esophageal transit with a high degree of accuracy. More recently, radionuclide techniques have been developed to quantitatively assess esophageal transit.[3,4] Although specific techniques vary, all utilize 10–15 ml of water labeled with 150–500 μCi of ^{99m}Tc-sulfur colloid as the radionuclide marker.[3–10] While supine, patients drink the technetium-labeled water in one[6,7] or more[3–

C. D. Lind and R. W. McCallum • Department of Internal Medicine, Division of Gastroenterology, University of Virginia Medical Center, Charlottesville, Virginia 22908.

[5,8,9] timed swallows and images are obtained at frequent intervals (5–15 sec) for up to 10 min. Using this technique, overall quantitative esophageal transit of a liquid bolus can be assessed[3] as well as patterns of abnormal transit when specific segments of the esophagus are differentiated.[4] When compared with conventional barium cineradiography, radionuclide transit studies were much more sensitive in identifying esophageal motility disorders (75 versus 30% sensitive) in one large study of 150 patients.[5]

A number of groups have compared esophageal radionuclide transit with routine esophageal manometry for the evaluation of functional motility disorders.[3–11] In general, transit studies are abnormal with a high sensitivity in patients with disorders of propagation involving loss of peristalsis (e.g., achalasia, scleroderma, diffuse esophageal spasm), whereas transit studies are generally normal in patients with abnormally high-amplitude contractions that are still peristaltic (e.g., nutcracker esophagus, nonspecific motor disorder). Disorders in which dysphagia is a prominent symptom, rather than chest pain, appear to be more likely to have abnormal transit studies, with a sensitivity as high as 93%.[6] In addition, the pattern of disordered transit may help to differentiate these motor disorders. Transit studies showing complete loss of the normal distinct propagating peaks of activity ("adynamic" scans) are suggestive of achalasia or scleroderma, whereas studies showing multiple simultaneous peaks of activity ("incoordination" scans) are suggestive of diffuse esophageal spasm.[4] In a careful comparison of simultaneous esophageal manometry and radionuclide transit, Richter et al.[9] showed that normal liquid bolus transit is dependent on the presence of a peristaltic wave front, as long as that wave has an amplitude of 30 mm Hg or greater. Above this threshold pressure, transit was not affected by abnormally high-amplitude or prolonged-amplitude contractions (i.e., nutcracker esophagus). [Conversely, prolonged transit was observed only with nonperistaltic contractions or peristaltic waves of very low (< 30 mm Hg) amplitude.] This study would support the finding of most other investigators that esophageal radionuclide transit studies are most useful in evaluating disorders of altered propagation, rather than disorders of altered wave form. Hence, transit studies would likely be most useful in the evaluation of dysphagia rather than in the evaluation of noncardiac chest pain. Sensitivity of the transit study will be highest in achalasia or scleroderma patients, intermediate in patients with diffuse esophageal spasm, and lowest in patients with nutcracker esophagus or nonspecific esophageal motor disorder. Unfortunately, this leaves little practical value for radionuclide transit testing of the esophagus at the clinical level. The diagnosis of achalasia or diffuse spasm is fairly obvious by radiology and/or esophageal motility. If the transit test is negative, motility must still be tested to exclude nutcracker esophagus as well as conditions such as "hypertensive lower esophageal sphincter." Therefore, as a screening test it has little or no role—esophageal motility testing is the choice.

It has been recognized that some patients with IBS have esophageal symptoms of dysphagia, chest pain, or heartburn.[12–14] This raises the question as to whether these symptoms are associated with abnormal esophageal motility and transit in these patients. Whorwell et al. reported that approximately 20% of 100 IBS patients had dysphagia and 20% were found to have heartburn.[13] This prevalence of heartburn was no different than in a control group, but the frequency of dysphagia was significantly increased. In addition, when evaluated with esophageal manometry, patients with IBS have been found to have significantly reduced lower esophageal sphincter pressure (13.8 versus 23.8 cm H_2O) and an increased incidence of spontaneous, repetitive, or simultaneous esophageal contractions as compared to controls.[15] Similarly, patients with known contraction abnormalities of the esophagus (nutcracker esophagus or diffuse esophageal spasm) have an increased incidence of lower GI symptoms compatible with IBS than do patients who have achalasia.[16] This would suggest an association of altered esophageal motility and IBS, supporting the concept of diffuse neuromuscular abnormalities in the GI tract in IBS. However, there are no studies which specifically evaluate esophageal transit in IBS, and it is unlikely that there will be a strong association between IBS and disordered esophageal transit. Peristaltic esophageal contraction abnormalities such as nutcracker esophagus or nonspecific esophageal motor disorders, which are the most commonly found in association with IBS, usually have a normal esophageal transit. In contrast, achalasia and scleroderma esophagus, which are not associated with IBS, are the disorders most likely to reflect abnormal transit. Despite these observations, the subset of IBS patients with associated dysphagia[13] may be expected to have altered esophageal transit.

There is a very high correlation between symptoms of dysphagia and altered esophageal transit. Patients with dysphagia in whom mechanical obstruction has been ruled out may still have altered radionuclide transit and the pattern of transit may be useful in helping to distinguish achalasia or scleroderma from diffuse esophageal spasm or nonspecific motor disorder. Patients with symptoms of chest pain may or may not have abnormal esophageal transit, depending upon the propagation of esophageal contractions. Chobanian et al.[17] found esophageal radionuclide transit studies useful in the evaluation of 73 patients with noncardiac chest pain, with an overall sensitivity of 79%. However, even in this study, the two most common diagnoses, nutcracker esophagus and nonspecific esophageal motility disorder, had the lowest frequency in abnormal transit studies. In contrast, all patients in this study with diffuse esophageal spasm or achalasia had abnormal radionuclide esophageal transit. Those with gastroesophageal reflux comprise another group of patients with noncardiac chest pain who may show abnormalities in esophageal transit studies. In these patients, radionuclide studies of the esophagus may show a "to-and-fro" movement of isotope in the distal esophagus despite completely normal esophageal manometry.[18] However, it is very difficult to interpret the position of the diaphragm and lower esophageal sphincter during a transit study. The diagnosis of gastroesophageal reflux will be made by other means (e.g., endoscopy, barium esophagus, acid perfusion test, pH monitoring) and radionuclide studies have been clearly demonstrated to be less sensitive and not recommended in evaluating gastroesophageal reflux disease.

2. GASTRODUODENAL TRANSIT

Because upper GI tract symptoms of nausea, bloating, dyspepsia, vomiting, early satiety, and abdominal pain have been recognized in some patients with IBS, a disorder of gastric emptying and/or gastroduodenal transit has been appreciated as a manifestation of IBS. A wide range of clinical settings may be associated with impaired gastroduodenal transit as shown in Table I.[19]

Once mechanical or inflammatory diseases are ruled out with upper GI x-rays or endoscopy, evaluation of suspected gastroparesis will need to focus on motor function of the stomach and duodenum. Current methods available to evaluate gastroduodenal motor

Table I. Delayed Gastric Emptying States

Mechanical factors
    Gastric carcinoma
    Duodenal, pyloric, or prepyloric ulcers
    Idiopathic hypertrophic pyloric stenosis
Acid-peptic diseases
    Gastroesophageal reflux
    Gastric ulcer disease
Gastritis
    Atrophic gastritis ± pernicious anemia
    Viral gastroenteritis (acute—? chronic)
Metabolic and endocrine
    Diabetic ketoacidosis (acute)
    Diabetic gastroparesis (chronic)
    Hypothyroidism
    Pregnancy?
    Uremia?
Collagen vascular diseases—scleroderma
Pseudoobstruction
    Idiopathic
    Secondary, e.g., amyloidosis, muscular dystrophies
Postgastric surgery
    Postvagotomy and/or postgastric resections
Medications
    Anticholinergics, narcotic analgesics, L-dopa
Hormones (pharmacologic studies)
    Gastrin, cholecystokinin, somatostatin
Anorexia nervosa—? bulimia
Idiopathic
    Gastric dysrhythmias—tachygastria
    Gastroduodenal dyssynchrony
    ? Role of central nervous system—e.g., depression

function include radiographic emptying tests, intubative emptying tests, radionuclide emptying studies, and gastroduodenal electrogastrography. Manometric studies and electrogastrography measure pressure activity and electrical activity of the stomach (and duodenum), respectively. However, these studies do not directly measure gastroduodenal transit. Barium radiography has been used for decades as a test to delineate gastric emptying[20–22]; however, its sensitivity and specificity for diagnosing gastroparesis is clearly very poor when compared to radionuclide techniques.[23] Intubative emptying tests, in which the instillation and subsequent aspiration of nonabsorbable markers directly from the stomach or duodenum is used to calculate emptying, have been useful as research tools. However, the invasiveness of these studies and the alteration of motility caused by intubation[24] have made this technique less useful in assessing gastroduodenal transit in the clinical setting.

    Currently, the most reliable technique for measuring gastric emptying of liquids and digestible solids appears to be the use of a radionuclide marker and scintillation camera.[25,26] Gastric emptying of liquids is largely determined by the gastroduodenal pressure gradient generated by fundic tone, whereas digestible solid emptying is determined by antral contractions which serve to triturate food into particles less than 1 mm in diameter. In both cases, gastroduodenal transit is further regulated by small intestinal feedback inhibition in response to stimulation of specific caloric, osmotic, pH, and nutrient receptors. Because of this distinction between liquid and solid emptying, dual isotope techniques which label the liquid and solid portions of a meal with different isotopes (indium and technetium)[25] have been the most useful in assessing specific disorders of transit related to fundic and/or antral dysfunction. When applied clinically,[27,28] these techniques appear to identify abnormalities of gastric emptying with a much greater degree of accuracy than older radiographic techniques.

One radiographic technique which remains helpful is the use of radioopaque markers to assess emptying of indigestible solids. Emptying of indigestible solids depends upon the antral contractions induced during late phase II and phase III of the migrating motor complex (MMC) which occur only during the fasted state. Feldman et al.[29] showed that delayed emptying of radioopaque markers (i.e., indigestible solids) may be a more sensitive test for diabetic gastroparesis than radionuclide methods. This technique appears useful for assessing gastroduodenal transit in the fasted state and can be modified to utilize radionuclide capsules, instead of radioopaque markers, in an effort to minimize radiation exposure from the test.[29a] Other techniques to more accurately assess gastric emptying are being developed, including ultrasound and three-dimensional computerized tomography, but these techniques remain investigative at present.

As stated earlier, techniques to directly assess gastroduodenal motility have been developed using flexible probes positioned to measure gastric and upper small bowel pressure via manometric (perfusion) catheters[30,31] or semiconductor transducers.[32] In addition, cutaneous and mucosal electrogastrography have been developed to assess gastric electrical activity. Neither technique directly measures gastroduodenal transit, but these approaches have been useful in identifying abnormal motility[33] or electrical patterns[34,35] in some upper GI functional bowel diseases. In addition, several studies compared abnormalities of motility with abnormalities of transit.[36-42] In a series of studies in which simultaneous measurements of gastroduodenal motility and gastric emptying were made during cold stress or labyrinthine stimulation, Malagelada and colleagues[36-38] identified delayed gastric emptying in association with an altered postprandial pattern of duodenal motility which resembled the fasting pattern in some individuals. In addition, these studies and others[30,39-42] have consistently shown a relationship between delayed gastric emptying of digestible solids and decreased antral motility in both the fed and fasted states. Settings in which reduced antral motility and delayed emptying are most consistently found include diabetic[30] and postvagotomy gastroparesis.[41] Patients with idiopathic gastroparesis[33,42] also may have altered antral contractility. Similarly, abnormal small intestinal motility manifested by prolonged burst of nonpropagated contractions has been associated with impaired gastric emptying in some clinical settings, including diabetes,[31] sympathetic autonomic neuropathy,[43] and idiopathic gastroparesis.[40] The association of abnormal gastroduodenal transit and altered gastric or duodenal electric patterns has been less well established. Gastric dysrhythmias, most notably tachygastria, have been identified in patients with delayed gastric emptying from various causes including idiopathic gastroparesis,[35] diabetes, anorexia nervosa, and drug-induced gastroparesis.[35] However, the observation that transient periods of gastric dysrhythmias occur in asymptomatic persons (normal subjects) raises the question of whether gastric dysrhythmias are reliably associated with altered transit. Certainly at this point we do not know which is primary, the gastric dysrhythmia or an underlying motor dysfunction. Also, the dysrhythmia could be a manifestation of the patient's nausea and epigastric discomfort.

As summarized above, many disorders have been associated with altered gastroduodenal transit, despite the absence of mechanical obstruction. Many of these disorders, including diabetes, Parkinson's disease, Shy–Drager syndrome, postvagotomy gastroparesis, and scleroderma, have identifiable neuropathic or myopathic changes when carefully evaluated. The next question is whether patients with classic IBS have similar abnormalities in gastroduodenal transit. Upper GI tract symptoms of nausea and vomiting have been identified in up to 50% of IBS patients, which is markedly higher than in a group of matched controls.[2] In addition, other symptoms of functional dyspepsia, including postprandial bloating, early satiety, and upper abdominal pain, have been frequently recognized in IBS patients.[33] A number of investigators have studied radionuclide gastric emptying in patients with IBS and compared findings in controls.[44–47] Each of these four studies, comprising over 100 IBS patients and 100 controls, failed to demonstrate any significant alteration of gastric emptying in IBS. Some studies did reveal alterations in small bowel transit or colonic motility (discussed below), but gastric emptying was not consistently altered in these patients. None of these studies specifically focused on that subset of IBS patients with dominant upper GI tract symptoms and, hence, a relationship between altered gastroduodenal transit and symptoms in these patients may have been missed. In review of these reports it may be concluded that the high prevalence of nausea, vomiting, and abdominal distension in IBS patients as a whole suggest that many of the upper gut symptoms seen in IBS are not related to gastric emptying. This does not imply that gastric motor function and gastroduodenal transit may not play a role in the generation of symptoms in IBS. Gastric function appears intimately related to the gastrocolonic response, where gastric distension and intestinal lipid delivery serve as potent stimuli for increased rectosigmoid motility seen postprandially.[48] As will be discussed, this postprandial gastrocolonic response may be altered in IBS and hence subtle alterations in gastroduodenal transit may theoretically influence the colonic symptoms seen in these patients.

The discordance between gastric emptying and upper GI tract symptoms in IBS also raises the question: how well does impaired gastric emptying correlate with symptoms of nausea, vomiting, bloating, or abdominal pain in other clinical settings? Pellegrini et al.[49] evaluated 48 patients with clinically suspected gastroparesis, mostly secondary to surgery or diabetes, using radionuclide emptying studies. They found that 50% of these patients had documented slow emptying, but the other 50% had normal or rapid gastric emptying. Similarly, Malagelada's group[33] studied 104 patients with functional upper gut symptoms using a manometric probe as described previously. They found that specific symptoms did not predict the presence or site of GI manometric abnormalities, although patients with known neurologic or metabolic diseases (e.g., Parkinson's, postvagotomy, hollow visceral myopathy, diabetes mellitus) usually had manometric abnormalities when upper gut symptoms were present. Similarly, some treatment trials in patients with significant diabetic gastroparesis have shown a poor correlation between improvement in gastric emptying and symptoms,[50,51] while other studies have shown a fairly good correlation,[52] particularly with symptoms of nausea and postprandial fullness. In cases of severe gastric stasis and bezoar formation, for example in postvagotomy states, upper tract symptoms parallel alterations in gastric emptying, particularly symptoms of postprandial fullness, nausea, and vomiting. Similarly, in cases of the dumping syndrome, which occurs most commonly after vagotomy and partial gastrectomy, symptoms of epigastric discomfort, nausea, diarrhea, palpitations, sweating, and weakness may correlate fairly well with rapid gastric emptying.[19] However, the overall difficulty in identifying a consistent relationship between alterations in gastric emptying and symptoms points to both the nonspecific nature of many upper GI symptoms and the recognized day-to-day variability of gastroduodenal transit seen in pathologic states. This realization makes the failure to show altered gastric emptying in IBS patients much more understandable.

Many patients with gastric stasis do not actually vomit. They have slow gastric emptying of solids but normal liquid emptying. Small quantities of liquid/soft foods can be tolerated, often with reasonably good maintenance of weight. Hence, waiting for patients to report vomiting before suspecting and investigating for gastric stasis is not necessary and vomiting is not a crucial criterion for pursuing a diagnosis of slow gastric emptying.

Summary. The authors are attempting to develop the concept that IBS may have diffuse manifestations throughout the GI tract, including the stomach. It would be useful for the reader to look at the full symptom complex of IBS as perhaps representing the total accumulation of symptoms arising from a number of areas in the GI tract, which one terms "irritable." The concept of "irritable" esophagus will be discussed in the context of the role of stress in the GI tract. There are patients being evaluated for chest pain who have essentially a normal manometric pattern but have painful responses to the acid infusion test (Bernstein test) and/or intravenous injection of ediophonium (Tensilon), suggesting an esophagus with a low pain threshold or increased sensitivity of mucosal receptors (in the case of the Bernstein test) or muscarinic receptors (in the case of the Tensilon injection). External stress can also be superimposed on this setting. It is also reasonable to accept the notion of the "irritable stomach." This is typically a setting of "idiopathic" gastric stasis, sometimes gastric stasis termed "nonulcer dyspepsia" or gastric stasis perhaps representing the motor sequelae of tachygastria or bradygastria. Also, disordered small bowel motility can contribute to slowing gastric emptying by changing duodenal small bowel impedance. Those patients may have more prominent abdominal pain due to motor abnormalities in the proximal small bowel. This abdominal pain can sometimes require significant pain medication to the point of concern about addiction potential.

Finally, the symptoms of nausea, bloating, fullness, and vomiting may represent an isolated small bowel motor disturbance and here the gastric emptying may or may not be abnormal. The finding of normal gastric emptying here may be confusing but highlights the nonspecificity of nausea, bloating, fullness, increased satiety, and vomiting and reminds us also to consider the small bowel as the origin of these symptoms. With this background the discussion will now move to small bowel motility abnormalities in IBS and the concept of "irritable small bowel."

3. SMALL BOWEL TRANSIT

Because IBS is often characterized by painful constipation or diarrhea (or both), much work has been done to evaluate the possible association of altered lower GI transit (small bowel or colonic) and the primary symptoms of IBS. Intuitively, slowed small bowel transit might be associated with symptoms of abdominal bloating and constipation, whereas rapid small bowel transit might be associated with diarrhea. In order to accurately evaluate small bowel transit, two major techniques have been developed: (1) breath hydrogen testing and (2) radionuclide scintigraphic techniques.

Breath hydrogen small bowel transit studies rely on colonic bacteria to metabolize carbohydrates, leading to a sustained rise in the concentration of hydrogen in expired air.[53,54] Typically, lactulose is ingested orally and the time from ingestion to the sustained rise in breath hydrogen concentration, measured every 10 min by a simple electrochemical detector and chromatographic system, is defined as the orocecal transit time. This technique gives an estimate of small bowel transit which may be influenced by altered gastric emptying, small bowel bacterial overgrowth, or the absence of hydrogen-producing bacteria, but has been validated with reasonable reproducibility in normals[53] and patients with chronic diarrhea.[54,55] Furthermore, it can be combined with radionuclide techniques for simultaneous assessment of gastric emptying and the breath hydrogen small bowel transit time.[55] The breath hydrogen test does not provide for assessing the contributions of gastric emptying or segments of the small bowel to the final results. McCallum and colleagues[55a] showed that technetium-labeled lactulose accurately measured small bowel transit when compared to breath hydrogen and had the added benefit of providing continuous scanning from mouth to cecum. Careful analysis of the breath hydrogen transit time using simultaneous radionuclide small bowel transit techniques has shown that the breath hydrogen transit time reflects the time when the "leading edge" of the unabsorbed carbohydrate reaches the cecum, and not necessarily when all of the carbohydrate has reached the colon.[56] This same study revealed that most subjects undergoing the lactulose breath hydrogen test in conjunction with a meal will have an early nonsustained rise in breath hydrogen concentration that represents emptying of the remnants of a previous meal from the ileum into the colon. The phenomenon of postprandial distal small bowel emptying may play a role in the symptoms of some patients with IBS.

The other major technique to measure small bowel transit has also utilized radioisotope markers and scintigraphy. Routine barium studies have been poor measures of small bowel transit because of the influence barium has on intrinsic intestinal motility. In addition, the lactulose used to measure small bowel transit by the breath hydrogen technique may itself influence the rate of transit and may not correlate well with transit time of a meal.[55] Consequently, radionuclide techniques have been developed in which various components of a meal, or indigestible solids, are labeled with a radioisotope and the passage of this marker is monitored using a scintillation camera. Indigestible solids used to assess small bowel transit have included ^{99m}Tc-labeled pellets[47] or capsules[57] and ^{131}I-labeled fiber.[58,59] Similarly, labeled technetium has been added to the digestible component of a meal by labeling the water used to prepare the meal[56,60] or by directly labeling bran cereal.[61] These techniques can then quantitatively determine the rate at which the radionuclide reaches the cecum allowing for the measurement of small bowel transit times for any proportion of a labeled meal. Interestingly, unlike the stomach where emptying of solids and liquid occurs at different rates, transit of the solid or liquid portion of a meal through the small bowel appears to occur at the same rate.[59] As noted above, however, the amount of nonabsorbed nutrient ingested, for example lactulose, can alter the overall small bowel transit time of a meal, depending on the osmotic concentration of the lactulose.[55]

One concern about using breath hydrogen or radionuclide techniques to assess small bowel transit arises from the fact that differences in gastric emptying may alter the orocecal transit and thereby make the interpretation of small bowel transit times difficult. A series of studies by Read and co-workers[45,62-64] addressed this problem using simultaneous radionuclide gastric emptying and small bowel transit studies, combined with breath hydrogen techniques. These studies suggest that changes in small bowel transit time can occur independently of changes in gastric emptying. Delaying gastric emptying by increasing fiber bulk or adding fat to a meal did not affect small bowel transit, as assessed by the breath hydrogen technique.[62,63] Similarly, no correlation could be found between gastric emptying times and time to 50% colonic filling (i.e., small bowel transit $T_{1/2}$) when both were measured by radionuclide techniques.[63,64] Hence, these techniques which specifically measure orocecal transit appear to be reasonable methods for estimating small bowel transit. As mentioned earlier, most investigators combine one of these small bowel transit techniques with a radionuclide gastric emptying technique, so the various components of the transit of a meal can be carefully distinguished. We prefer a dual isotope gastric emptying where the liquid phase is ^{111}In-labeled lactulose. During the 2 hr of assessing gastric emptying of the solid meal component (chicken liver labeled with ^{99m}Tc-sulfur colloid), gastric emptying of a liquid (lactulose) and its arrival time in the cecum can be simultaneously assessed.

The relationship of small bowel motility, as measured by intraluminal pressure activity, and small bowel transit has been less well investigated than gastric motility and transit. Again, Read et al.[64] have provided some insight into this question. In subjects given a radiolabeled solid meal, increased small intestinal pressure activity in the first 3 hr following meal ingestion did correlate with faster colonic filling times. In addition, colonic filling times were faster if a postprandial activity front (phase III of the MMC) migrated throughout the small bowel when the subject resumed the fasted (interdigestive) motility pattern. Hence, small bowel transit for a meal appears to be related to both the fasted and fed intraluminal pressure activity of the small intestine. How transit relates to abnormal patterns of small bowel motility still remains an area of active research.

As noted elsewhere in this chapter, abnormal small bowel motility has been suspected to be a component of IBS, particularly after Thompson et al.[65] described abnormal patterns of small bowel motility in a patient with irritable colon using radio-telemetric pressure pills. A number of subsequent studies investigated whether abnormal small bowel transit is a characteristic finding in patients with IBS, and whether alterations in transit can be associated with specific symptoms. Results of these studies have been inconsistent, but a relationship between symptoms in IBS and small bowel transit may exist. When IBS patients are divided into diarrhea-predominant, constipation-predominant, and pain/distension-predominant types, Read et al.[45,54,63] found that diarrhea-predominant patients had significantly faster small bowel transit (3.3 versus 4.2 hr) and constipation or pain/distension patients had significantly slower transit (5.4 versus 4.2 hr) than controls. McCallum et al. utilizing isotope-labeled lactulose also found this pattern. In addition, they found that patients with alternating constipation and diarrhea had essentially normal small bowel transit. Using a different technique, Nielsen et al.[47] found a similar slowing of small bowel transit in constipation patients (376 versus 202 min) but failed to show a difference between diarrhea patients and controls (205 versus 202 min). However, other groups using radionuclide techniques have shown rapid small bowel transit compared to controls in patients with functional diarrhea.[60] Although not all studies confirm this,[66] there does seem to be a general trend in IBS patients for those with diarrhea to have rapid small bowel transit and those with constipation to have slowed transit.

One other interesting aspect of small bowel transit in IBS is ileocecal transit in these patients. As noted earlier, breath hydrogen studies have shown an early, nonsustained rise in breath hydrogen following a meal. This hydrogen peak appears to reflect the emptying of remnants of a previous meal from ileum to cecum.[56] Trotman and Price[61] evaluated this phenomenon in IBS patients with postprandial bloating by administering ^{99m}Tc-labeled bran cereal to patients and then performing a dynamic scan of the cecum 3 hr later following a standard meal. In this study, IBS patients had slower ileal emptying and lower ileocecal clearance than controls. Read and colleagues also noted that in most patients with IBS and right iliac fossa pain, the pain was temporally associated with the arrival of a test meal in the cecum.[45] These studies suggest that one component of IBS may be altered ileocecal transit and this alteration may be partially related to abnormal cecal filling (or cecal compliance) in these patients.[67] Again, this is an area of ongoing active research.

One should realize that a consistent relationship between diarrhea or constipation and altered small bowel transit does not exist in all pathophysiologic states. In a group of diabetics with diarrhea, intestinal transit using the breath hydrogen technique did not differ from controls.[68] This most likely reflects the fact that diabetics with "diabetic diarrhea" may have either abnormally rapid small bowel transit leading to diarrhea or abnormally slow intestinal transit leading to bacterial overgrowth and associated diarrhea. Similarly, patients with inadequately treated celiac disease and associated steatorrhea were found to have delayed small bowel transit time as compared to controls or patients without steatorrhea.[69] This may reflect the "ileal brake" mechanism in which fat delivered to the ileum serves to decrease gastric and proximal small bowel motility and thereby slow transit. In addition, in normal subjects given increasing doses of lactulose with a meal, total stool weight for 48 hr after meal ingestion was related to whole gut transit time but not to small intestinal transit time.[55] This suggests that diarrhea in the setting of unabsorbed carbohydrate (i.e., osmotic diarrhea) may depend more on lack of colonic accommodation than the rate of small bowel transit. Clearly, the pathophysiology leading to diarrhea (or constipation) may influence whether small bowel transit abnormalities are seen in a group of patients.

4. COLONIC TRANSIT

Historically, IBS has been defined with regard to colonic symptoms. Those symptoms which most reliably identify IBS patients include abdominal distension, pain relief with a bowel movement, and more frequent or looser stools with the onset of pain.[1] In addition, chronic constipation, diarrhea, or alternating constipation and diarrhea, particularly when associated with pain, have been typical features of IBS. All of these findings in the past have been attributed to colonic dysfunction, although we have already reviewed how recent research suggests that gastric or small bowel abnormalities may contribute to these symptoms. Nevertheless a considerable focus to explain a major contribution to IBS symptoms rests on disorders of colonic motility and transit.

Unfortunately, colonic transit has been very difficult to specifically quantitate and data on colonic transit in IBS are surprisingly sparse. Major techniques to evaluate colonic transit have included stool analysis (stool weight, volume, and frequency), utilization of radioopaque markers, and radionuclide techniques. Stool weight and volume are often used to evaluate symptoms of diarrhea or constipation, but day-to-day variability of stool weights (up to tenfold differences) in normal individuals[70] makes stool analysis in IBS patients difficult to interpret. Similarly, when radioopaque markers are ingested and then recovered in stool collections (by x-raying the stool) to assess whole gut transit, which is an estimate of colonic transit, transit times may vary from 1 to 5 days in normal subjects.[70] This variability between and within normal subjects makes analysis of whole gut or whole colon transit times difficult to interpret in IBS patients.

Techniques to assess segmental colonic transit have been developed to better understand possible abnormalities in colonic transit. Using radioopaque markers, patients ingest a finite number of markers daily and abdominal x-rays are taken every 24 hr until all markers have passed.[71] By counting the total number of markers in each section of the colon (e.g., right colon, left colon, and rectosigmoid) on each day, segmental transit of the colon can be calculated. Similarly, by ingesting different-shaped markers on three successive days and taking a single film on day 4, segmental colonic transit can be calculated.[72] Using these techniques in normal adults, segmental transit times for right colon, left colon, and rectosigmoid have been 11–14, 11–14, and 11–12 hr, respectively. Colonic transit scintigraphy, using a radionuclide instilled directly into the cecum, has recently been described to more accurately quantitate segmental transit of the colon in normal humans.[73] Using this technique, the cecum and ascending colon were found to empty rapidly, with half-emptying time of 87.6 min, whereas the transverse colon was found to be the primary site for fecal storage. Overall, by 48 hr over 70% of ileal effluent had traversed the entire colon and been defecated.

Because colonic transit has been so difficult to quantitate, there are very few data which directly compare colonic motility, myoelectric activity, and transit. Although transit was not directly measured, Whitehead et al.[74] investigated rectosigmoid motor function in IBS patients with either diarrhea-predominant or constipation-predominant patterns of symptoms. In this study, fast colonic contractions having durations of less than 15 sec and occurring in runs at frequencies of 6–9 cycles/min were more frequent in diarrhea patients than in normals or IBS constipated patients. Severity of bowel symptoms also correlated with the overall motility index in these patients with diarrhea. Although this may suggest an association between colonic motor activity and transit, clearly things are more complex. In another group of patients with diarrhea, namely patients with ulcerative colitis, careful transit studies by Read's group[75] showed that patients with active colitis and diarrhea had proximal colonic stasis and rapid rectosigmoid transit. Hence, diarrhea in this group of patients was associated with rectosigmoid irritability rather than rapid colonic transit. Again, when comparing colonic transit and colonic motility, the pattern of motility and the segment of colonic transit being evaluated will be important to specify.

Despite these difficulties in evaluating normal colonic motility, altered colonic motility and myoelectric activity have been identified in patients with IBS,[76–78] as has been discussed elsewhere in this monograph. Whether changes in the colonic slow-wave frequency and basal motor activity are specific for IBS remains controversial,[78] but this implies that alterations in colonic transit may also be identified in these patients. Specifically, it has been thought that pain in IBS is caused by hypersegmentation in the colon, which also tends to delay transit.[79] The best evidence for an association between altered colonic transit and IBS comes from careful work by Marcus and Heaton[80] on 44 patients with chronic constipation, most of whom had documented slow intestinal transit. When questioned carefully about other symptoms of IBS, namely bloating, passage of mucus, rectal dissatisfaction, and pain relieved by defecation, all symptoms were more prevalent in the constipated patients than in a control group. Further, when 12 normal subjects were made constipated by loperamide administration, all developed one or more of these IBS symptoms. Notably, when effective laxative treatment was given to a group of these patients, the prevalence and severity of these IBS symptoms fell markedly. Their conclusion was that in some patients the slowing of whole gut transit (reflecting primarily colonic transit) is associated with IBS. This same group performed a 28-day longitudinal study of four patients with classic IBS in an attempt to identify a relationship between symptoms and transit.[81] In this study, a careful diary of symptoms and bowel movements was kept by each patient for 28 days. In addition, mean whole gut transit time was measured during the entire study, using a radioopaque marker technique, and every stool was collected and analyzed for weight, form, and consistency. Unfortunately, this study failed to show any temporal relationship between symptoms of IBS and the objective measurements of whole gut transit time, stool form or consistency. This study points out that the relationship between colonic motility, transit, and symptoms, particularly in patients with IBS, remains quite complex and poorly understood.

Altered large bowel function is almost certain to be involved in some of the symptoms of IBS, but whether this altered function results in disordered transit, either segmental or total colonic, remains unclear. In addition, the symptoms often attributed to colonic dysfunction, particularly abdominal pain and bloating, may be difficult to distinguish from symptoms that originate in the small intestine. The most reliable association between altered colonic transit and symptoms in IBS appears in those patients with clear delayed transit and constipation,[80] and this is most likely true in other functional disorders complicated by constipation (e.g., chronic idiopathic intestinal pseudoobstruction, Parkinson's disease, diabetes mellitus). An association between altered transit and symptoms in patients with diarrhea is less easily made. As noted in patients with diarrhea and ulcerative colitis,[75] proximal colonic transit may be slow while patients have symptomatic diarrhea. On the other hand, people with diarrhea due to carbohydrate malabsorption appear to have rapid colonic transit.[55] Again, the pathophysiology of the cause of diarrhea is critical in understanding the association of symptoms and disordered transit.

5. STRESS- AND MEAL-RELATED ALTERATIONS IN GI TRANSIT

Many symptoms in IBS are more prevalent during the postprandial period or during times of stress. Similarly, normal people often have irritable bowel-like symptoms during times of stress, which subsequently resolve after the stressful period abates. It has been well recognized that many people, perhaps 20–30% of the general population, have symptoms of classic IBS, but never seek medical care for these symptoms.[82–84] Consequently, a basic question in IBS has been whether these patients have a basic physiologic abnormality of the GI tract (the "epilepsy" model) or whether these patients simply have an enhanced, but qualitatively normal, physiologic response to stress, meals, or drugs (the "weeping" model).[85-87] This has led to a great deal of work, particularly in the past decade, in the evaluation of normal physiologic responses in the GI tract to meals or stress. Meal- or stress-related changes in transit are summarized here.

As mentioned earlier, Malagelada's group investigated the effects of labyrinthine stimulation and cold stress on gastroduodenal transit of a solid meal in a group of healthy volunteers.[36-38] Labyrinthine stimulation at subnauseant levels was induced by ear irrigation with ice water, and simultaneous measurements of gastroduodenal motility, gastric emptying, gastric acid secretion, and pancreatic trypsin output following a test meal were made.[36] Similarly, in a separate study, cold pain was induced by hand immersion in ice water and the same parameters were studied.[37] In both studies, the stressful stimulus led to a consistent, reproducible delay in gastric emptying in conjunction with a decreased antral pressure response to solids. When plasma levels of β-endorphin, catecholamines, and gut peptides were measured during these studies,[38] the delayed gastric emptying coincided with elevations in β-endorphin and norepinephrine. Hence, centrally acting external stressful stimuli of two types led to altered antral feeding activity and delayed gastroduodenal transit, perhaps mediated by β-endorphin and norepinephine. Using a different type of stress, Read and colleagues[88] investigated the effects of psychologic stress on the passage of a standard meal through the stomach and small intestine in normal volunteers. Gastric emptying, measured by radionuclide techniques, and mouth-to-cecum transit, measured by breath hydrogen techniques, were monitored in patients during times of psychologic stress induced by a dichotomous listening test. In this study, gastric emptying was not consistently affected by this stimulus but mouth-to-cecum transit times were significantly faster (276 versus 381 min) than during nonstressful control periods. In sum, studies on gastric emptying and stress suggest that certain types of stress may lead to delayed gastroduodenal transit whereas other types of stress have no effect.

The effects of stress on small intestinal transit have been less extensively studied than gastroduodenal transit. As just summarized, Read and associates[88] found that mouth-to-cecum transit of a standard meal was faster during times of psychologic stress. In contrast, the physical stress of immersion of a hand in cold water has been shown to decrease orocecal transit when measured by the same technique.[89] When upper small bowel motor activity has been measured during times of stress, there also appears to be an inhibition of motor activity.[90,91] In these studies, small bowel motor activity was monitored with radiotelemetric pills while the healthy volunteers were given mental stressors which included dichotomous listening, driving in traffic, delayed auditory feedback, and electronic video game or sleep interruption. All of these stressors significantly inhibited the incidence of fasting MMCs when compared to a control period. Of note, the small bowel effect of stress did not correlate with the cardiovascular response to stress and, hence, is likely not mediated by adrenergic mechanisms. Further, the small bowel effects of stress in this study occurred independent of the conscious perception of stress and did not produce specific symptoms. These studies did not correlate the stress-induced alterations in small bowel motility with transit because only the fasting state was evaluated. Importantly, however, when similar stressors were applied to a group of patients with IBS, significant additional motor abnormalities were seen in IBS patients, often associated with typical symptoms.[92] In this study, Kumar and Wingate reported the effects of three different stressors on small bowel motility in 22 patients with IBS, 10 healthy controls, and 5 patients with inflammatory bowel disease. Nineteen of twenty-two IBS patients versus one of ten controls showed additional motor abnormalities which included total abolition of MMCs under stress and abnormal irregular contractile activity which was either spontaneous or stress-induced. In 8 IBS patients, abnormal irregular contractile activity was associated with their typical abdominal discomfort. Again, transit was not assessed in these patients and only fasting motor patterns were evaluated. However, this does suggest that stress-induced alterations in small bowel motility occur normally, and that these alterations may be intermittently enhanced in IBS patients.

Besides stress, other factors including meal composition, drugs, or hormones clearly do influence small bowel transit. As discussed previously, the amount of unabsorbed carbohydrate in a meal will influence small bowel transit.[55,62] Similarly, hormonal alterations during a normal menstrual cycle will alter small bowel transit.[93] When measuring mouth-to-cecum times by the breath hydrogen technique, transit is significantly delayed during the luteal phase (when progesterone levels are increased) as compared to the follicular phase. Even significant diurnal variations in the fasting small bowel motor patterns have been well documented,[94,95] although diurnal alterations in transit have not been studied. These observations point out the multiplicity of normal, physiologic factors which may influence small bowel transit and emphasize the difficulty in identifying specific alterations in transit that may be seen in IBS patients.

Stress- and meal-related alterations in colonic myoelectric and motor function have been a major focus of investigation in IBS for decades.[96] An increase in rectosigmoid myoelectric and motor activity after a standard meal has been well recognized.[46,48,97,99] Both gastric mechanoreceptors, induced by gastric distension, and nutrient-specific intestinal chemoreceptors, induced by lipid delivery to the duodenum, participate in this gastrocolonic response and the response is partially mediated by cholinergic neural pathways.[48,98] Hormonal factors may also influence this response,[97] although it appears that cholecystokinin is not a physiologic mediator. Of note, patients with IBS have a prolonged postprandial colonic spike and motor response when compared to normals,[46,99] with some patients showing a continuous increase in colonic motor activity for over 180 min after eating. This suggests that IBS patients may have an enhanced gastrocolonic response to a meal, although there still remains the question of whether this is a physiologically different response (e.g., with altered basal electrical activity) or simply a quantitatively enhanced physiologically normal response.[100] Despite these studies on meal-related colonic myoelectric and motor function, virtually no human studies on meal-related alterations in colonic transit have been performed. Possible alterations in meal-related ileocecal transit between IBS patients and normals has already been discussed.

Stress-induced changes in colonic motility have been investigated by many techniques since the early studies of Almy and co-workers in the 1940s.[96] Recent studies[101,102] using various stressors, including ice-water immersion, stimulus differentiation testing, ball sorting, and anger, confirm that rectosigmoid myoelectric and motor activity increase significantly during times of stress. Further, these studies suggest that the stress-induced increase in colonic activity is significantly greater in IBS patients than in healthy controls. Again, correlations between the stress-induced motility changes and altered colonic transit have not been carefully studied in humans. However, cold-restraint stress in rats has been shown to increase fecal pellet output and colonic transit[103] and diarrhea is a common symptom of acute stress in humans. Consequently, there is some evidence that the increased colonic motor activity seen during stress may be reflected in increased colonic transit and diarrhea. However, this model more closely approximates the acute setting of a "fear and fright" reflex we all have with resultant diarrhea rather than the intermittent exacerbations of chronic IBS.

Exciting recent research into stress-induced alterations in GI transit and IBS has focused on a possible animal model for IBS. Williams et al.[104] developed a technique of mild restraint (wrap restraint) in rats and have shown that this model leads to analgesia and typical plasma elevations of β-endorphin and adrenocorticotropic hormone (ACTH) seen in stress. Further, this model did not induce GI ulcers. Using this model to evaluate GI transit changes induced by stress, gastric emptying was not affected, small intestinal transit was inhibited, and large intestinal transit was stimulated, leading to an increase in fecal excretion. As already summarized, these stress-induced changes in transit parallel the stress-induced changes in humans. A circadian influence to these stress-induced changes in intestinal motility was also noted, correlating with the timing of ACTH release. However, neither exogenous ACTH nor β-endorphin had any similar effect on transit, and neither adrenalectomy nor hypophysectomy prevented this stress-induced effect on the intestine. Further work by these same investigators has shown that exogenous corticotropin-releasing factor (CRF) will induce similar changes in GI transit in the rat[105]: delayed gastric emptying, inhibited small intestinal transit, stimulated colonic transit, and increased fecal excretion. The effects of CRF on gastric emptying have been confirmed by others in a dog model.[106] More importantly, administration of a CRF antagonist prevented the stress-induced changes in transit seen in the mild restraint rat model. The actions of CRF on stimulating ACTH, β-endorphin, and catecholamine secretion have been described,[107,108] and the central role of CRF in response to stress has been emphasized.[108] The work by Williams et al.,[104,105] taken in sum, suggests that stress-induced changes in GI transit may be mediated by CRF, independent of its effects on ACTH, β-endorphin, or catecholamine secretion. Hence, blunting of an enhanced GI response to stress (i.e., IBS?) may require blunting of the secretion or peripheral action of CRF. Clearly, this exciting area requires further extensive research.

6. EFFECTS OF TREATMENT ON ALTERED GI TRANSIT

Most treatment regimens in IBS have focused on amelioration of symptoms or normalization of motor activity seen in patients with IBS. Few treatment regimens have focused specifically on the normalization of altered intestinal transit. As summarized in this chapter, the difficulties in addressing altered GI transit in IBS have been difficulties in measuring intestinal transit in these patients and then clearly correlating any abnormalities in transit to specific symptoms. Despite these drawbacks, a few comments on how treatment changes intestinal transit can be made.

Disorders in esophageal transit are not clearly associated with IBS, but altered esophageal transit is associated with other functional esophageal diseases, notably achalasia, scleroderma, and sometimes, diffuse esophageal spasm. In patients with achalasia and delayed esophageal transit, both isosorbide dinitrate and nifedipine have been shown to accelerate transit when assessed by radionuclide methods.[11] Isosorbide dinitrate improved transit with greater efficacy than nifedipine in this study, and symptom improvement correlated closely with faster transit. Improved transit in vigorous achalasia using nifedipine has been confirmed by others.[109] Similarly, successful pneumatic dilation or surgical myotomy has been shown to improve esophageal emptying when assessed by radiographic or radionuclide techniques, and improved emptying generally correlates with improved symptoms in these patients. Specific treatment of altered esophageal emptying in scleroderma or diffuse esophageal spasm has been less well studied than in achalasia. Esophageal spasm patients with significant dysphagia sometimes improve with nitrate, calcium channel blocker, or dilation therapy, although much less reliably than achalasia patients. Presumably, these treatment responders would show improvements in transit if studied.

Functional disorders in gastroduodenal transit have been more extensively evaluated with regard to treatment than disorders in esophageal transit. As discussed previously, many causes of disordered gastroduodenal transit have been identified.[19] When delayed gastric emptying is due primarily to decreased antral contractility (e.g., postvagotomy or diabetic gastroparesis), dietary manipulation to avoid digestible solids may alone improve gastric emptying and symptoms of gastric stasis. Similarly, surgical antrectomy may be expected to improve gastroduodenal transit in these patients, although results are quite inconsistent. Most attention to the treatment of delayed gastroduodenal transit has focused on pharmacologic therapy designed to increase antral contractility and emptying. Although many agents have been evaluated, the best studied "prokinetic" agents for gastroduodenal transit have included metoclopramide,[50,52,110] domperidone,[52] and cisapride.[110,111] With each of these agents, patients with diabetic gastroparesis showed short-term improvement in emptying of solids (digestible or indigestible) on the prokinetic agent, and this correlated with improved symptoms in some of the studies.[52,111] Both esophageal and gastric emptying were improved with cisapride in insulin-dependent diabetics in the most recent of these studies.[111] Although correlation between improved gastric emptying and improved upper GI tract symptoms is far from perfect, these studies do suggest that delayed transit can be improved in certain gastroparetic states and this treatment may lead to improved symptoms. Of note, while cholinergic agonists (e.g., bethanechol) have been shown to increase antral contractility in gastroparetic states,[30] they do not qualify for the term "prokinetic" agent, since they do not coordinate contractions in the antrum, pylorus, and duodenum to result in a net acceleration in gastric emptying.

Treatment of altered small intestinal transit in IBS has not been carefully studied, with difficulties in showing a specific disorder in small bowel transit in these patients. However, agents known to alter small bowel motility and transit are commonly used to symptomatically treat patients with various functional disorders. As mentioned, unabsorbed carbohydrate (e.g., lactulose) will enhance small bowel transit[62] and is often used in settings of constipation to decrease whole gut transit time. Indigestible fiber, on the other hand, does not appear to alter small bowel transit,[59] but may affect whole gut transit time by its action in the colon (see below). Metoclopramide has been shown to block the stress-induced inhibition of small bowel motility while domperidone did not inhibit these stress-induced changes.[91] Cisapride has been shown to enhance propagated contractions in the small bowel in the fasting state.[112] Whether these drug effects on motility enhance small bowel transit in pathologic states has not been well studied. Many more agents are known to inhibit small intestinal motility and transit including opioids, anticholinergic agents, phenothiazines, dopamine agonists, and adrenergic agonists. Of these, opioids and anticholinergics are commonly used to treat functional diarrheal disorders [e.g., diphenoxylate with atropine (Lomotil), loperamide (Imodium)], often with success.[113] In addition, elimination of any of these agents in a patient with constipation and suspected pseudoobstruction may enhance transit and improve symptoms. Obviously, the effects of these agents on small bowel or colonic transit cannot always be clinically separated.

Most studies on normalization of transit in the treatment of IBS have focused on whole gut transit or colonic transit. Acceleration of whole gut transit has been shown to occur in patients with constipation when treated with dietary fiber or bran.[114,115] Further, patients with rapid transit and diarrhea were shown to have a prolongation in whole gut transit time with dietary fiber in one of these studies,[114] although this has not been confirmed by others.[115] Another form of fiber supplement, ispaghula husk, has been thought to be efficacious in IBS,[116–118] although it did not alter whole gut transit time when specifically measured.[116] When compared with placebo, dietary fiber in the form of bran[115,119] or psyllium[120] did not significantly improve symptoms in IBS, despite acceleration of whole gut transit.[115] Ispaghula husk, on the other hand, did improve symptoms of IBS[116,118] without changing whole gut transit.[116] Despite these inconsistencies, a general correlation between increased dietary fiber, accelerated whole gut transit, and symptom improvement in patients with constipation can be gleaned from these studies.

Other agents commonly used for IBS besides fiber include anticholinergic agents, opioid agonists, antidepressants, and minor tranquilizers (e.g., benzodiazepines). Few of these agents have been evaluated with respect to alterations in intestinal transit. As mentioned, opioids have been used with success in settings of diarrhea to slow small bowel and colonic transit. The effects of anticholinergic agents (including antidepressants) on transit are more complex. Anticholinergics decrease small intestinal motor activity and, presumably, transit. In the colon, anticholinergics will decrease the abnormal postprandial motor response seen in IBS patients,[46,99] theoretically leading to improvement in postprandial symptoms in these patients. However, the effects of these anticholinergics on colonic transit remain unclear because they may inhibit both propagating contractions and segmental (nonpropagating) colonic contractions. Most of the effects of antidepressants on intestinal transit are likely due to their anticholinergic properties, and in general, they are agents which lead to constipation. However, antidepressants may also modify the CNS response to stress in IBS patients and influence transit by this mechanism. Similarly, benzodiazepines have been shown to blunt the stress-induced increase in colonic motility seen in IBS patients,[101] presumably acting both in the CNS and as a peripheral smooth muscle relaxant. Again, these effects on colonic motility by benzodiazepines and antidepressants have not been directly correlated with alterations in transit.

Because many symptoms in IBS are meal- or stress-related, one final approach to normalizing abnormal intestinal motility and transit in these patients has focused on behavior modification. Postprandial propulsive activity has been shown to occur in the colon of physically active subjects, whereas it may be absent in sedentary individuals.[121] Hence, patients with postprandial abdominal pain and constipation may benefit simply from increased physical activity.[122] Similarly, behavior modification using relaxation techniques and operant conditioning[123] may help to modify the exaggerated colonic motility response to stressful stimuli. The influence of these techniques on colonic transit still awaits evaluation.

7. SUMMARY

IBS and other functional bowel diseases have been associated with disordered intestinal motility, often resulting in altered transit. We have attempted to develop a concept of diffuse smooth muscle effects in IBS, a condition that in the past had specific connotations for the colon. We suggest that the stomach, esophagus, small bowel, and colon can be regarded, either collectively or independently, as being "irritable," and have described the symptoms and clinical settings of these states. Classic IBS still implies that certain well-agreed-upon symptoms are present and in this sense this traditional entity reflects "irritable colon." The term *irritable bowel* by current understanding therefore means an irritable colon with the possibility of contributions of variable severity from the small bowel, stomach, and/or esophagus. This emphasizes the heterogeneous makeup of any irritable bowel patient population. We have summarized the techniques most frequently used to measure transit in each segment of the GI tract. With specific attention to IBS, the evidence for altered transit in functional bowel disorders has been delineated and various treatments for disordered transit summarized. As pointed out, the relationships between altered transit and symptoms in IBS are not completely understood. Specific disorders of esophageal, gastroduodenal, small intestinal, and colonic transit are being recognized with increasing frequency. As our ability to investigate the alterations in GI function improve, a better understanding of the relationships between altered transit and symptoms will surely follow. The interrelationship and sometimes symbiotic setting of personal stress and IBS symptoms was explored and finally a review of treatment approaches and their effects on transit and symptoms was included.

REFERENCES

1. Manning AP, Thompson WG, Heaton KW, et al: Towards positive diagnosis of the irritable bowel. Br Med J 2:653–654, 1978
2. Whorwell PJ, McCallum M, Creed FH, et al: Non-colonic features of irritable bowel syndrome. Gut 27:37–40, 1986
3. Tolin RD, Malnud LS, Reilley J, et al: Esophageal scintigraphy to quantitate esophageal transit (quantitation of esophageal transit). Gastroenterology 76:1402–1408, 1979
4. Russel COH, Hill LD, Holmes ER, et al: Radionuclide transit: A sensitive screening test for esophageal dysfunction. Gastroenterology 80:887–892, 1981
5. DeCaestecker JS, Blackwell JN, Adam RD, et al: Clinical value of radionuclide oesophageal transit measurement. Gut 27:659–666, 1986
6. Llamas-Elvira JM, Martinez-Paredes M, Sopena-Monforte R, et al: Value of radionuclide oesophageal transit in studies of functional dysphagia. Br J Radiol 59:1073–1078, 1986
7. Mughal MM, Marples M, Bacewicz J: Scintigraphic assessment of oesophageal motility: What does it show and how reliable is it? Gut 27:946–953, 1986
8. Blackwell JN, Hannan WJ, Adam RD, et al: Radionuclide transit studies in the detection of oesophageal dysmotility. Gut 24:421–426, 1983

9. Richter JE, Blacwell JN, Wu WC, et al: Relationship of radionuclide liquid bolus transport and oesophageal manometry. J Lab Clin Med 109:217–224, 1987

10. Davidson A, Russel C, Littlejohn GO: Assessment of esophageal abnormalities in progressive systemic sclerosis using radionuclide transit. J Rheumatol 12:472–477, 1985

11. Gelfond M, Rozen P, Gilat T: Isosorbide dinitrate and nifedipine treatment of achalasia: A clinical, manometric and radionuclide evaluation. Gastroenterology 83:963–969, 1982

12. Watson WC, Sullivan SN, Corke M, et al: Incidence of oesophageal symptoms in patients with irritable bowel syndromes. Gut 17:827, 1976

13. Whorwell PJ, McCallum M, Creed FH, et al: Non-colonic features of irritable bowel syndrome. Gut 27:37–40, 1986

14. Thompson WG, Heaton, KW: Functional bowel disorders in apparently healthy people. Gastroenterology 79:283–288, 1980

15. Whorwell PJ, Clouter C, Smith CL: Oesophageal motility in the irritable bowel syndrome. Br Med J 282:1101–1102, 1981

16. Clouse RE, Eckert TC: Gastrointestinal symptoms of patients with esophageal contraction abnormalities. Dig Dis Sci 31:236–240, 1986

17. Chobanian SJ, Benjamin SB, Curtins DJ, et al: Systematic esophageal evaluation of patients with non-cardiac chest pain. Arch Intern Med 146:1505–1508, 1986

18. de Caestecker JS, Brown J, Blackwell JN, et al: The oesophagus as a cause of recurrent chest pain: Which patients should be investigated and which tests should be used? Lancet 2:1143–1146, 1985

19. Minami H, McCallum RW: The physiology and pathophysiology of gastric emptying in humans. Gastroenterology 86:1592–1610, 1984

20. Kassander P: Asymptomatic gastric retention in diabetics (gastroparesis diabeticorum). Ann Intern Med 48:797–812, 1958

21. Zitomer BR, Gramm HF, Zozak GP: Gastric neuropathy in diabetes mellitus: Clinical and radiologic observations. Metabolism 17:199–211, 1968

22. Pelot D, Dana ER, Berk JE: Comparative assessment of gastric emptying by the ''barium-burger'' and saline load tests. Am J Gastroenterol 58:411–416, 1971

23. McCallum RW: Diagnosing motility disorders of the upper gastrointestinal tract. South Med J 77:947–955, 1984

24. Read NW, Al-Janabi MN, Bates TE, et al: Effect of gastrointestinal intubation on the passage of a solid meal through the stomach and small intestine in humans. Gastroenterology 84:1568–1572, 1983

25. Collins PJ, Horowitz M, Cook DJ, et al: Gastric emptying in normal subjects—A reproducible technique using a single scintillation camera and computer system. Gut 24:117–125, 1983

26. Meyer JH, MacGregor IL, Gheller R, et al: ^{99m}Tc-tagged chicken liver as a marker of solid food in the human stomach. Dig Dis Sci 21:296–303, 1976

27. Scarpello JHB, Barber DC, Hogue RV, et al: Gastric emptying of solid meals in diabetics. Br Med J 2:671–673, 1976

28. Campbell IW, Heading RC, Tothill P, et al: Gastric emptying in diabetic autonomic neuropathy. Gut 18:462–467, 1977

29. Feldman M, Smith HJ, Simon TR: Gastric emptying of solid radioopaque markers: Studies in healthy subjects and diabetic patients. Gastroenterology 87:895–902, 1984

29a. Valenzuela G, Stubbs J, Plankey M, et al: Radionuclide to quantitate gastric emptying of indigestible solids. Am J Gastroenterol 83, 1988 (abstr)

30. Fox S, Behar J: Pathogenesis of diabetic gastroparesis: A pharmacologic study. Gastroenterology 78:757–763, 1980

31. Camillery M, Malagelada JR: Abnormal intestinal motility in diabetics with gastroparesis syndrome. Eur J Clin Invest 14:420–427, 1984

32. Mathias JR, Sninsky CA, Millar HD, et al: Development of an improved multi-pressure-sensor probe for recording muscle contraction in human intestine. Dig Dis Sci 30:119–123, 1985

33. Malagelada JR, Stanghellini V: Manometric evaluation of functional upper gut symptoms. Gastroenterology 88:1223–1231, 1985

34. Telander RL, Morgan KG, Kreulen DL, et al: Human gastric atony with tachygastria and gastric retention. Gastroenterology 75:497–501, 1978

35. Kim CH, Malagelada JR: Electrical activity of the stomach: Clinical implications. Mayo Clin Proc 61:205–210, 1986
36. Thompson DG, Richelson E, Malagelada JR: Perturbation of gastric emptying and duodenal motility through the central nervous system. Gastroenterology 83:1200–1206, 1982
37. Thompson DG, Richelson E, Malagelada JR: Perturbation of upper gastrointestinal function by cold stress. Gut 24:277–283, 1983
38. Stanghellini V, Malagelada JR, Zinsmeister AR, et al: Stress-induced gastroduodenal motor disturbances in humans: Possible humoral mechanisms. Gastroenterology 85:83–91, 1983
39. Rees WDW, Miller LJ, Malagelada JR: Dyspepsia, antral motor dysfunction, and gastric stasis of solids. Gastroenterology 78:360–365, 1980
40. Camilleri M, Brown ML, Malagelada JR: Relationship between impaired gastric emptying and abnormal gastrointestinal motility. Gastroenterology 91:94–99, 1986
41. Malagelada JR, Rees WDW, Mazzotta LJ, et al: Gastric motor abnormalities in diabetic and postvagotomy gastroparesis: Effect of metoclopramide and bethanechol. Gastroenterology 78:286–293, 1980
42. Labo G, Bortolotti M, Vezzadini P, et al: Interdigestive gastroduodenal motility and serum motilin levels in patients with idiopathic delay in gastric emptying. Gastroenterology 90:20–26, 1986
43. Camillery M, Malagelada JR, Stanghellini V, et al: Gastrointestinal motility disturbances in patients with orthostatic hypotension. Gastroenterology 88:1852–1859, 1985
44. Acharya, U, White N, Howlett P, et al: Failure to demonstrate altered gastric emptying in irritable bowel syndrome. Dig Dis Sci 28:889–892, 1983
45. Cann PA, Read NW, Brown C, et al: Irritable bowel syndrome: Relationship of disorders in the transit of a single solid meal to symptom patterns. Gut 24:405–411, 1983
46. Narducci F, Bassotti G, Granata MT, et al: Colonic motility and gastric emptying in patients with irritable bowel syndrome. Effect of pretreatment with octylonium bromide. Dig Dis Sci 31:241–246, 1986
47. Nielsen OH, Gjorup T, Christensen FN: Gastric emptying rate and small bowel transit time in patients with irritable bowel syndrome determined with ^{99m}Tc-labeled pellets and scintigraphy. Dig Dis Sci 31:1287–1291, 1986
48. Wiley J, Tatum D, Keinath R, et al: Participation of gastric mechanoreceptors and intestinal chemoreceptors in the gastrocolonic response. Gastroenterology 94:1144–1149, 1988
49. Pellegrini CA, Broderick WC, Dyke DV, et al: Diagnosis and treatment of gastric emptying disorders. Clinical usefulness of radionuclide measurements of gastric emptying. Am J Surg 145:143–150, 1983
50. Snape WJ, Battle WM, Schwartz SS, et al: Metoclopramide to treat gastroparesis due to diabetes mellitus. A double-blind, controlled trial. Ann Intern Med 96:444–446, 1982
51. Horowitz M, Harding PE, Chatterton BE, et al: Acute and chronic effects of domperidone on gastric emptying in diabetic autonomic neuropathy. Dig Dis Sci 30:1–9, 1985
52. McCallum RW, Ricci DA, Rakatansky H, et al: A multicenter placebo-controlled clinical trial of oral metoclopramide in diabetic gastroparesis. Diabetes Care 6:463–467, 1983
53. Bond JH, Levitt MD: Investigation of small bowel transit time in man utilising pulmonary hydrogen (H_2) measurements. J Lab Clin Med 85:546–555, 1975
54. Corbett CL, Thomas S, Read NW, et al: Electrochemical detector for breath hydrogen determination: Measurement of small bowel transit time in normal subjects and patients with the irritable bowel syndrome. Gut 22:836–840, 1981
55. Read NW, Miles CA, Fisher D, et al: Transit of a meal through the stomach, small intestine and colon in normal subjects and its role in the pathogenesis of diarrhea. Gastroenterology 79:1276–1282, 1980
55a. Caride VJ, Propop EK, McCallum RW, et al: Scintigraphic determination of small intestinal transit time: Comparison with hydrogen breath technique. Gastroenterology 86:714–720, 1984
56. Read NW, Al-Janabi MN, Bates TE, et al: Interpretation of the breath hydrogen profile obtained after ingesting a solid meal containing unabsorbable carbohydrate. Gut 26:834–842, 1985
57. Kaus LC, Fell JT, Sharma H, et al: On the intestinal transit of a single non-disintegrating object. Int J Pharm 20:315–323, 1984
58. Carryer PW, Brown ML, Malagelada JR, et al: Quantification of the fate of dietary fiber in humans by a newly developed radiolabeled fiber marker. Gastroenterology 82:1389–1394, 1982
59. Malagelada JR, Robertson JS, Brown ML, et al: Intestinal transit of solid and liquid components of a meal in health. Gastroenterology 87:1255–1263, 1984

60. Jian R, Najean Y, Bernier JJ: Measurement of intestinal progression of a meal and its residues in normal subjects and patients with functional diarrhoea by a dual isotope technique. Gut 25:728–731, 1984

61. Trotman IF, Price CC: Bloated irritable bowel syndrome defined by dynamic ^{99m}Tc bran scan. Lancet 2:364–366, 1986

62. Read NW, Cammack J, Edwards C, et al: Is the transit time of a meal through the small intestine related to the rate at which it leaves the stomach? Gut 23:824–828, 1982

63. Read NW, Al-Janabi MN, Holgate AM, et al: Simultaneous measurement of gastric emptying, small bowel residence and colonic filling of a solid meal by the use of the gamma camera. Gut 27:300–308, 1986

64. Read NW, Al-Janabi MN, Edwards CA, et al: Relationship between postprandial motor activity in the human small intestine and the gastrointestinal transit of food. Gastroenterology 86:721–727, 1984

65. Thompson DG, Laidlaw JM, Wingate DL: Abnormal small bowel motility demonstrated by radiotelemetry in a patient with irritable colon. Lancet 2:1321–1323, 1979

66. Lami F, Callegari C, Bozzola M: Small bowel transit time (letter). Gut 27:468–469, 1986

67. Heaton KW: Irritable bowel syndrome: Still in search of its identity. Br Med J 287:852–853, 1983

68. Keshavarzian A, Iber FL: Intestinal transit in insulin-requiring diabetics. Am J Gastroenterol 81:257–260, 1986

69. Spiller RC, Lee YC, Edge C, et al: Delayed mouth–caecum transit of a lactulose labelled liquid test meal in patients with steatorrhea caused by partially treated coeliac disease. Gut 28:1275–1282, 1987

70. Wyman JB, Heaton KW, Manning AP, et al: Variability of colonic function in healthy subjects. Gut 19:146–150, 1978

71. Arhan P, Devroede G, Jehannin B, et al: Segmental colonic transit time. Dis Colon Rectum 24:625–629, 1981

72. Metcalf AM, Phillips SF, Zinsmeister AR, et al: Simplified assessment of segmental colonic transit. Gastroenterology 92:40–47, 1987

73. Krevsky B, Malmud LS, D'ercole F, et al: Colonic transit scintigraphy. A physiologic approach to the quantitative measurement of colonic transit in humans. Gastroenterology 91:1102–1112, 1986

74. Whitehead WE, Engel BT, Schuster MM: Irritable bowel syndrome. Physiological and psychological differences between diarrhea-predominant and constipation-predominant patients. Dig Dis Sci 25:404–413, 1980

75. Rao SSC, Read NW, Brown C, et al: Studies on the mechanism of bowel disturbance in ulcerative colitis. Gastroenterology 93:934–940, 1987

76. Snape WJ, Carlson GM, Cohen S: Colonic myoelectric activity in the irritable bowel syndrome. Gastroenterology 70:326–330, 1976

77. Snape WJ, Carlson GM, Matarazzo SA, et al: Evidence that abnormal myoelectrical activity produces colonic motor dysfunction in the irritable bowel syndrome. Gastroenterology 72:383–387, 1977

78. Latimer P, Sarna S, Campbell D, et al: Colonic motor and myoelectrical activity: A comparative study of normal subjects, psychoneurotic patients, and patients with irritable bowel syndrome. Gastroenterology 80:893–901, 1981

79. Connell AM, Avery-Jones F, Rowlands EN: Motility of the pelvic colon. IV. Abdominal pain associated with colonic hypermotility after meals. Gut 6:105–112, 1965

80. Marcus SN, Heaton KW: Irritable bowel-type symptoms in spontaneous and induced constipation. Gut 28:156–159, 1987

81. Oettle GJ, Heaton KW: Is there a relationship between symptoms of the irritable bowel syndrome and objective measurements of large bowel function? A longitudinal study. Gut 28:146–149, 1987

82. Thompson WG, Heaton KW: Functional bowel disorders in apparently healthy people. Gastroenterology 79:283–288, 1980

83. Drossman DA, Sandler RS, McKee DC, et al: Bowel patterns among subjects not seeking health care. Use of a questionnaire to identify a population with bowel dysfunction. Gastroenterology 83:529–534, 1982

84. Whitehead WE, Winget C, Fedoravicius AS, et al: Learned illness behavior in patients with irritable bowel syndrome and peptic ulcer. Dig Dis Sci 27:202–208, 1982

85. Almy TP: The irritable bowel syndrome. Back to square one? Dig Dis Sci 25:401–403, 1980

86. Drossman DA: Diagnosis of the irritable bowel syndrome. Ann Intern Med 90:431–432, 1979

87. Thompson WG: The irritable bowel. Gut 25:305–320, 1984

88. Cann PA, Read NW, Cammack J, et al: Psychological stress and the passage of a standard meal through the stomach and small intestine in man. Gut 24:236–240, 1983

89. O'Brien JD, Thompson GD, Holly J, et al: Stress disturbs human gastrointestinal transit via a beta-adrenoreceptor-mediated pathway. Gastroenterology 88:1520, 1985 (abstr)

90. McRae S, Younger K, Thompson DC, et al: Sustained mental stress alters human jejunal motor activity. Gut 23:404–409, 1982

91. Valori RM, Kumar D, Wingate DL: Effects of different types of stress and of "prokinetic" drugs on the control of the fasting motor complex in humans. Gastroenterology 90:1890–1900, 1986

92. Kumar D, Wingate DL: The irritable bowel syndrome: A paroxysmal motor disorder. Lancet 2:973–977, 1985

93. Wald A, Van Thiel DH, Hoechstetter L, et al: Gastrointestinal transit: The effect of the menstrual cycle. 80:1497–1500, 1981

94. Kellow JE, Borody TJ, Phillips SF, et al: Human interdigestive motility: Variations in patterns from esophagus to colon. Gastroenterology 91:386–395, 1986

95. Kumar D, Wingate D, Ruckebusch Y: Circadian variation in the propagation velocity of the migrating motor complex. Gastroenterology 91:926–930, 1986

96. Almy TP, Tulin M: Alteration in colonic function in man under stress: Experimental production of changes simulating the "irritable colon." Gastroenterology 8:616–626, 1947

97. Snape WJ, Matarazzo SA, Cohen S: Effect of eating and gastrointestinal hormones on human colonic myoelectrical and motor activity. Gastroenterology 75:373–378, 1978

98. Snape WJ, Wright, SH, Battle WM, et al: The gastrocolic response: Evidence for a neural mechanism. Gastroenterology 77:1235–1240, 1979

99. Sullivan MA, Cohen S, Snape WJ: Colonic myoelectrical activity in irritable-bowel syndrome. Effect of eating and anticholinergics. N Engl J Med 298:878–883, 1978

100. Sarna S, Latimer P, Campbell D, et al: Effect of stress, meal and neostigmine on rectosigmoid electrical control activity (ECA) in normals and in irritable bowel syndrome patients. Dig Dis Sci 27:582–591, 1982

101. Narducci F, Snape WJ, Battle WM, et al: Increased colonic motility during exposure to a stressful situation. Dig Dis Sci 30:40–44, 1985

102. Welgan P, Meshkinpour H, Bceler M: Effect of anger on colon motor and myoelectric activity in irritable bowel syndrome. Gastroenterology 94:1150–1156, 1988

103. Borone FC, Deegan JF, Fowler PJ, et al: A model of stress-induced increased fecal output and colonic transit. Gastroenterology 90:1337, 1986

104. Williams CL, Villar RG, Peterson JM, et al: Stress-induced changes in intestinal transit in the rat: A model for irritable bowel syndrome. Gastroenterology 94:611–621, 1988

105. Williams CL, Peterson JM, Villar RG, et al: Corticotropin-releasing factor directly mediates colonic response to stress. Am J Physiol 253:G582–G586, 1987

106. Pappas T, Debas H, Taché Y: Corticotropin-releasing factor inhibits gastric emptying in dogs. Regul Peptides 11:193–199, 1985

107. Rivier CL, Plotsky PM: Mediation by corticotropin releasing factor (CRF) of adenohypophyseal hormone secretion. Annu Rev Physiol 48:475–494, 1986

108. Lenz HJ, Raedker A, Greten H, et al: CRF initiates biological actions within the brain that are observed in response to stress. Am J Physiol 252:R34–R39, 1987

109. Berger K, McCallum RW: Nifedipine in the treatment of achalasia. Ann Intern Med 96:61–62, 1982

110. Feldman M, Smith HJ: Effect of cisapride on gastric emptying of indigestible solids in patients with gastroparesis diabeticorum. A comparison with metoclopramide and placebo. Gastroenterology 92:171–174, 1987

111. Horowitz M, Maddox A, Harding PE, et al: Effect of cisapride on gastric emptying and esophageal emptying in insulin-dependent diabetes mellitus. Gastroenterology 92:1899–1907, 1987

112. Stacher G, Gaupmann G, Mittelbach G, et al: Effects of oral cisapride on interdigestive jejunal motor activity, psychomotor function, and side-effect profile in healthy man. Dig Dis Sci 32:1223–1230, 1987

113. Cann PA, Read NW, Holdsworth CD, et al: Role of loperamide and placebo in management of irritable bowel syndrome (IBS). Dig Dis Sci 29:239–247, 1984

114. Harvey RF, Pomare EW, Heaton KW: Effects of increased dietary fibre on intestinal transit. Lancet 1:1278–1280, 1973

115. Cann PA, Read NW, Holdsworth CD: What is the benefit of coarse wheat bran in patients with irritable bowel syndrome? Gut 25:168–173, 1984

116. Kumar A, Kumar N, Vij JC, et al: Optimum dosage of ispaghula husk in patients with irritable bowel syndrome: Correlation of symptom relief with whole gut transit time and stool weight. Gut 28:150–155, 1987

117. Ritchie JA, Truelove SC: Comparison of various treatments for irritable bowel syndrome. Br Med J 281:1317–1319, 1980

118. Ritchie JA, Truelove SC: Treatment of irritable bowel syndrome with lorazepam, hyoscine butylbromide, and ispaghula husk. Br Med J 1:376–378, 1979

119. Lucey MR, Clark ML, Lowndes JO, et al: Is bran efficacious in irritable bowel syndrome? A double blind placebo controlled crossover study. Gut 28:221–225, 1987

120. Longstreth GF, Fox DD, Youkeles L, et al: Psyllium therapy in the irritable bowel syndrome. A double-blind trial. Ann Intern Med 95:53–56, 1981

121. Holdstock DJ, Misiewics JJ, Smith T, et al: Propulsion (mass movements) in the human colon and its relationship to meals and somatic activity. Gut 11:91–99, 1970

122. Connell AM: Intestinal motility and the irritable bowel. Postgrad Med J 60:791–796, 1984

123. Bueno-Miranda F, Cerulli M, Schuster MM: Operant conditioning of colonic motility in irritable bowel syndrome (IBS). Gastroenterology 70:867, 1976

13

Abdominal Pain and Biliary Tract Dysmotility

Walter J. Hogan, Wylie J. Dodds, and Joseph E. Geenen

1. INTRODUCTION

Motor dysfunction of the gastrointestinal tract without discernible structural alteration is suspected frequently in patients with episodic or chronic abdominal pain. The biliary tract [gallbladder/sphincter of Oddi (SO)] assumes a "leadership" role in this clinical arena when the patient with "biliary-type" pain fails conventional diagnostic testing. A convincing relationship between dysmotility and pain is often difficult or impossible to establish. A motility disorder may simply be an epiphenomenon without meaningful clinical correlation or relevance to the patient's symptoms. On the other hand, a valid relationship may exist between smooth muscle dysfunction in the biliary tract and the patient's "biliary-like" pain complaints. Theoretically, functional disorders of bile flow may arise from a disturbance in motor function anywhere within the biliary tract. Similar speculation has persisted since the late 19th century, in fact.[1] To help deal with this dilemma and to focus on the more meaningful clinical issues, a brief review of biliary flow dynamics, the mechanisms of biliary-type pain, and the spectrum of functional biliary tract disorders is useful.

2. BILE FLOW WITHIN THE BILIARY TRACT

Delivery of bile into the duodenum involves a series of complex interrelationships between hepatic secretion of bile and pressure differentials generated within the gallbladder, cystic duct, and SO (Fig. 1). Bile flow occurs in a low-pressure, low-flow system that

Walter J. Hogan • Department of Medicine, Medical College of Wisconsin, Milwaukee, Wisconsin 53226.
Wylie J. Dodds • Department of Radiology, Medical College of Wisconsin, Milwaukee, Wisconsin 53226.
Joseph E. Geenen • Department of Medicine, St. Luke's Hospital, Racine, Wisconsin 53403.

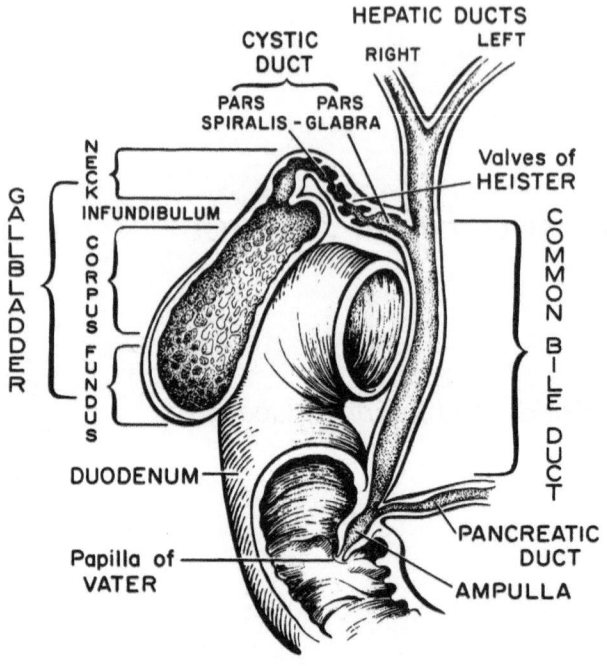

Figure 1. Delivery of bile into the duodenum involves complex physiologic interrelationships within the biliary system. The sphincter of Oddi conducts this orchestration in a low-pressure, low-flow environment.

involves hepatic secretion and gallbladder contraction. Partition of bile into the common bile duct (CBD) and gallbladder is influenced by the relative resistances of the cystic duct and SO. These resistances have both active and passive components.

Approximately 75% of hepatic bile enters the gallbladder during periods of fasting.[2] The gallbladder contracts periodically in orchestration with the migratory myoelectrical activity that periodically sweeps through the small intestine.[3] Following a meal, the gallbladder empties 50% or more of its contents within a half hour during sustained contraction.[4] During this time, resistance within the zone of the SO decreases. Gallbladder emptying, however, occurs at a slow, sustained rate of 2% per minute ensuring small pressure gradients within the ductal system and across the SO segment.

Gallbladder filling occurs when a small negative pressure gradient develops across the cystic duct area during simultaneous relaxation of the gallbladder and increased resistance to bile flow at the SO.[5]

Tonic and rhythmic contractions have been described within the SO zone.[6] Periodic fluctuation of a sustained basal SO pressure appears to modulate the flow of bile into the duodenum a majority of the time, while rhythmic SO contractions may aid in monitoring bile flow during peak secretion or in clearing the high-pressure zone of residual secretory debris. Although these contractions are myogenic, they appear to be modulated by neurohormonal stimuli. Basal SO pressure activity may vary in parts of the sphincter zone or transiently disappear during continuous pressure monitoring. Phasic SO contractions, which are superimposed on basal pressure, appear to originate in the proximal sphincter margin and propagate antegrade fashion toward the duodenum.[7] Some phasic SO contractions propagate retrograde fashion toward the gallbladder, while some contractions occur simultaneously over the length of the sphincter. These latter types of sphincteric contractions, obviously, do not enhance bile flow into the duodenum. Sphincter contractions of any variety transiently disrupt passive flow of bile from the common duct into the duodenum. The sphincter segment appears to fill during the intervals between contractions when basal SO pressure does not rise above resting common duct pressure.[8] The rate of phasic SO contractions alters synchronously with the migrating motor complex (MMC) which cycles repetitively through the gastrointestinal tract. The highest rates of phasic SO contractions occur in phases II and III of MMC activity cycle.[9]

Bile flow from the CBD can be enhanced by: SO decrease in basal pressure, increase in rate of peristaltic contractions, increase in proportion of antegrade contractions, and increase in stroke volume of the contractions. On the other hand, bile flow from the CBD can be retarded by: SO increase in basal pressure, decrease in proportion of antegrade peristalsis, and decrease in stroke volume of contractions. The primary physiologic role of the SO is regulation of pressure within the biliary tract.[10] Irrespective of the bile flow rate, the SO maintains pressure within a low range that enables hepatic secretion to proceed against negligible hydrostatic pressure.

3. BILIARY-TYPE PAIN—REFERRED VERSUS REAL

How accurately can abdominal pain be identified as originating from a specific focus such as the biliary tract? Does biliary tract pain possess unique qualities such as an exclusive right upper quadrant location or pure colicky nature? Unfortunately, the answer to both of these important clinical questions is in the negative. For instance, motor dysfunction in the biliary tract may cause pain in a variety of anatomic locations, e.g., upper abdomen, back, or chest areas. The difficulty in distinguishing true hepatobiliary pain from that arising from other organs of the body such as the coronary arteries or esophagus is legend. Studies as far back as 1949, for example, demonstrated that patients were unable to distinguish pain originating from the CBD and the gullet following balloon distension of either organ.[11]

The relationship between pain originating in the coronary arteries and biliary tract was demonstrated almost 50 years ago.[12] Balloon distension of the gallbladder and CBD in animals decreased coronary blood flow; rapid balloon distension of the CBD adversely affected circulatory dynamics. Subsequent animal studies demonstrated that bilateral cervical vagotomy prevented alteration in pulse rate and blood pressure caused by balloon distension of the CBD.[13] Biliary disease as a cause of chest pain in humans was first demonstrated in 1942[14] and later confirmed by other investigators. In patients with underlying coronary artery disease, balloon distension of the CBD produced angina-like pain; the chest pain disappeared upon balloon deflation.[15] These studies demonstrate the unique overlap in afferent sensory innervation between the esophagus, heart, and gallbladder, which often confounds the clinician who deals with this possibility in day-to-day practice.

Biliary tract pain is described classically as intermittent colicky pain which lasts from one to several hours and is usually related to food intake. In early studies, patterns of pain response were observed during gallbladder distension in 6 patients who were "awakened" during cholecystectomy operation.[16] All 6 patients experienced severe, penetrating pain in the epigastrium. Additionally, distension of the CBD caused intense epigastric pain. In another study, electrical stimulation of the CBD during operation caused right upper quadrant pain and/or epigastric pain in 5 of 8 patients but, interestingly, produced periumbilical pain in 3 of the patients. Radiation of pain to the intrascapular area was experienced in 4 of these patients.[17] Similar pain patterns were found during infusion of saline under pressure, through a T-tube, into the CBD of 30 postcholecystectomy patients.[18] Twenty-nine of the thirty patients experienced epigastric or right upper quadrant pain, while 11 patients noted radiating pain to the interscapular or right subscapular region. Balloon distension of the CBD through an indwelling T-tube caused similar distress in 45 of 56 patients who were recuperating from a cholecystectomy.[19] The majority of the 45 patients complained of a painful sensation in the lower substernum and epigastrium, while the minority perceived the pain to be in the right upper quadrant, intrascapular zone, and low back. Eleven patients, however, did not experience pain, despite distension of the CBD. Lastly, in the majority of clinical studies, the distress experienced by balloon distension, electrical stimulation, or manipulation of the biliary tract is not colicky, but rather a steady, penetrating-type pain.

True biliary pain, therefore, is neither predictable during distension of the CBD nor predictable in relationship to anatomic referral point(s). Why is it that the majority of clinicians focus exclusively on the biliary tract when they encounter the patient with "right upper quadrant" pain? There seems to be a unique clinical tradition surrounding "right upper quadrant" pain that mesmerizes the physician's attention to the biliary tract long after a litany of negative diagnostic studies exclude this organ system from further etiologic consideration. Despite our knowledge to the contrary, the location of bodily pain is often assumed to be organ specific.

In a recent enlightening report, balloon distension of the esophagus, stomach, intestine, and colon was performed in 22 patients with undiagnosed chronic right upper quadrant pain of many years' duration.[20] The right upper quadrant pain was reproduced in 21 of the patients during balloon distension of the small or large intestine in at least one site. In 12 of the 22 patients, however, more than one "trigger site" was demonstrated at locations as far removed as the jejunum and cecum. This is ample demonstration why some, perhaps the majority of, patients with chronic right upper quadrant pain do not have demonstrable biliary tract disease despite repetitive and exhaustive diagnostic pursuits directed toward that organ system.

A last word about abdominal pain. Abdominal pain is a major determinant to clinical decision-making by the physician or surgeon. Abdominal pain is also the apparent keystone to the majority of suspected functional disorders of the biliary tract. Patients with suspected functional gastrointestinal tract disorders often seem to have an overresponsiveness or hypersensitivity to hollow visceral distension. Routine visceral stimulation, for instance, sometimes appears magnified beyond acceptable boundaries of sensation for these patients, e.g., severe biliary-type pain can occur during initial injection of a few cubic centimeters of contrast during diagnostic ERCP study without apparent distension of the duct.

Shortly after his classic description of the distal choledochal sphincter which ultimately came to bear his name, Oddi[1] suggested that functional "spasm" of the sphincter could cause pain and jaundice. Within the next 30 years, Meltzer demonstrated that SO dysfunction could produce both biliary colic and jaundice.[21] Since that time, the pursuit of this phenomenon as a clinical explanation for "idiopathic" right upper quadrant pain has been relentless.

4. BILIARY TRACT DISORDERS OF FUNCTIONAL NATURE

4.1. Gallbladder

Motor dysfunction of the gallbladder could involve either an excessive contractility state (hyperkinesia) or a depressed contractility state hypokinesia. There is virtually no direct information to confirm the clinical existence of either possibility, however. Despite this lack of "hard evidence," a hyperkinetic gallbladder has been proposed to explain the biliary-type pain in patients who demonstrate exaggerated gallbladder contraction in response to injection of cholecystokinin octapeptide (CCK-OP).[22] The test is sequenced as follows: The gallbladder is initially opacified by oral cholecystography and subsequently CCK-OP is administered. A positive test results when the gallbladder demonstrates an exaggerated contractile response after CCK-OP associated with reproduction of the patient's symptoms. Complete evacuation of gallbladder dye within 5 to 10 min is considered an abnormal response. Distension of the CBD during rapid gallbladder evacuation could also be a major or contributing mechanism to pain symptoms. Post-CCK-OP radiographic configuration of the gallbladder, on the other hand, suggests abnormal contractility to some investigators. For instance, a globular configuration of the gallbladder image after CCK-OP injection with impaired emptying of contrast suggests to some observers obstruction to flow caused by hypercontractility of the gallbladder neck or cystic duct. The entity of gallbladder hyperkinesia has received little clinical confirmation, however. Cholecystectomy performed on suspected hyperkinesia patients who have had a positive CCK-OP cholecystography exam has shown histologically normal gallbladders—or only the presence of adenomyomatosis. The latter finding, unfortunately, only compounds the controversy.

In some patients, decreased muscle contraction of the gallbladder could be a contributing factor to formation of gallstones. This possibility has been considered in the past but, recently, the introduction of diisopropyl iminodiacetic acid (DISIDA) scintigraphy has been used to study this question during CCK-OP-stimulated emptying of the gallbladder. In one report, a group of "symptomatic" patients with normal oral cholecystography and gallbladder sonography exams was evaluated by this technique.[23] Mean gallbladder ejection fraction was significantly smaller in those patients with cholesterol crystals in their bile compared to those patients without bile crystals. Subsequent cholecystectomy disclosed histologic changes of chronic cholecystitis in the patients with "crystals" in their bile. In some patients with overt gallstones, cholescintigraphy has also demonstrated abnormalities of gallbladder contractions in response to meals or CCK-OP injection. Impaired contraction conceivably could be caused by decreased postprandial CCK release, wereas increased gallbladder contractility possibly indicates a hypersensitivity to CCK-OP.

Quantitative hepatobiliary scintigraphy has been performed recently in 100 nonjaundiced, cholecystectomized patients with unexplained upper abdominal pain and suspected partial CBD obstruction.[24] The patient group consisted of 80 women and 20 men aged 52 ± 15 (S.D) years. DISIDA was administered intravenously and the time of peak isotope activity and isotope clearance curves were derived from a region over the hepatic hilum. Values from patients were compared with those from 22 asymptomatic cholecystec-tomized controls. The "validity" of the test for each patient was derived from the results of an ERCP exam, accompanied by SO manometry in those patients with possible cryptic obstructive dysfunction of the SO. Of the 100 patients, 31 were judged true-positive and 69 true-negative. The positive patients included 17 with common duct stones, 10 with SO dysfunction, and 4 with benign stricture, tumor, or choledochocoele. The SO dysfunction patients had either sphincter stenosis or dyskinesia. Overall sensitivity was 78%, includ-ing 76% for common duct stones and 80% for SO dysfunction. False-positive findings occurred in 14% of the true-negatives for a specificity of 86%.

In the prairie dog model of cholelithiasis, gallstones are prevented by sphincter-otomy. Gallbladder filling is diminished and stasis is reduced following ablation of the SO zone.[25]

Gallbladder motility could be adversely affected by abnormal hormonal or neural influences. Pregnancy, vagotomy, and diabetes are well-known clinical conditions that have been associated with defective emptying, possible stasis, and increased incidence of gallbladder calculi. High circulating levels of progesterone associated with pregnancy may cause depression of gallbladder contractility,[26] while diabetes and vagotomy may impair emptying by interfering with innervation of the gallbladder.

4.2. Sphincter of Oddi

A condition prompting partial obstruction at the SO zone can cause intermittent or persistent upper abdominal pain (classically, aggravated by food intake), deranged liver function tests, and distension or delayed emptying of contrast from the CBD after ERCP injection. An overabundance of eponyms has been associated with clinical conditions suspected to be the result of partial obstruction of the distal choledochus. This not only has confused the issue, but has failed to separate structural (stenosis) from functional (dys-kinesia) disorders of the SO segment.

SO stenosis is a structural alteration of the sphincteric segment which may result in inflammatory stricture or scarring of the sphincteric zone, thereby increasing resistance to bile flow.

SO dyskinesia, on the other hand, is a functional disturbance of the sphincteric mechanism which may cause hypertonicity, altered motility and impedance to bile flow. Subsequent increase in intraductal pressure may cause distension of the ductal system, stimulate sensory fibers, and produce pain. A primary motor abnormality of the SO may be difficult to distinguish from a structural "stenosis," however. Dyskinesia can fre-quently be distinguished from stenosis by the use of SO manometry and concordant administration of intravenous drugs and hormones which relax smooth muscle.

5. SPHINCTER OF ODDI MANOMETRY

Following the development of diagnostic ERCP, direct pressure recording of the human SO motor function became a reality. Similar to diagnostic ERCP cannulation, a

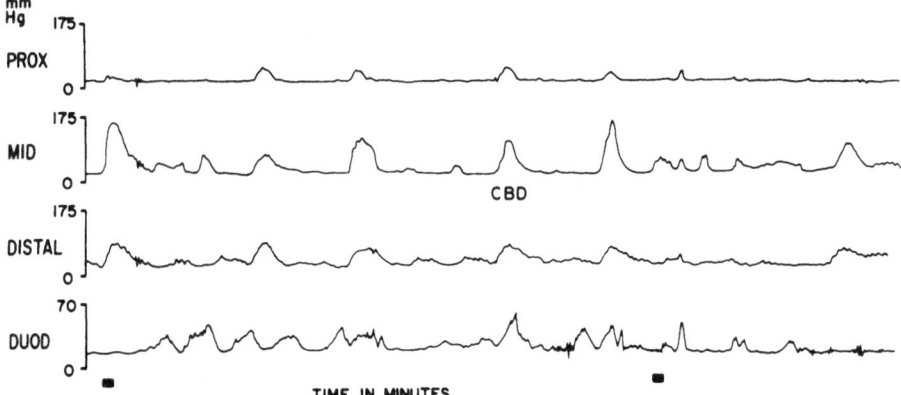

Figure 2. Manometric pressure measurement obtained within the zone of the sphincter of Oddi. A triple-lumen catheter records both basal and phasic sphincter activity over a 4-mm segment (proximal to distal). Discordant duodenal luminal pressure activity is noted at the bottom of the trace.

triple-lumen manometric catheter is passed through the biopsy channel of the duodenoscope and inserted into the papillary orifice. Unlike diagnostic cannulation, however, the manometric device must pass through the zone of the SO so that it lies "free" with the CBD or pancreatic duct. Accurate recording of sphincteric pressure transients requires a noncompliant catheter infusion pump system.[27] Manometric pressure recording is obtained from within the SO zone during incremental withdrawal of the catheter into the duodenum or by stationing two or more recording orifices within the sphincter segment for 5- to 10-min periods. A separate catheter is attached to the shaft of the endoscope to monitor concurrent intraduodenal pressure.[6] During station pull-through of the catheter orifice across the SO zone, a typical pressure profile is obtained. A pressure gradient of approximately 15 to 20 mm Hg exists between the duct and the duodenum within the SO segment. A basal pressure of 19 ± 7 (S.D.) mm Hg exists above the CBD or pancreatic duct pressure. Basal SO pressure may occasionally be isobaric with the ductal pressure or may appear and disappear from one or two orifices for prolonged intervals during extended recording periods.

Prominent phasic contractions are recorded along the 6- to 8-mm length of the SO. The phasic wave activity is superimposed on the SO basal pressure (Fig. 2). Phasic contractions occur at a mean frequency of 4 per min, for a mean duration of 4 to 5 sec and a mean peak amplitude of 150 mm Hg. Phasic SO contractions may be propagated in antegrade sequence toward the duodenum, in retrograde sequence toward the gallbladder, or they may occur in simultaneous sequence throughout the sphincter zone (Fig. 3). In patients without ductal abnormalities[7] compared to control subjects,[28] the frequency of antegrade phasic waves has been reported to vary from 60 to 22%. Discrete high-pressure zones have not been identified within the SO to correspond to the anatomic sphincters (choledochal, ampullary, and pancreatic) described by Boyden[29] (Fig. 4). Instead, we have found a continuum of pressure over the SO zone, and we routinely record pressure from a pancreatic duct portion of the sphincter which was not predicated from his human SO dissections. Indeed, we have determined that basal and phasic wave contractions are

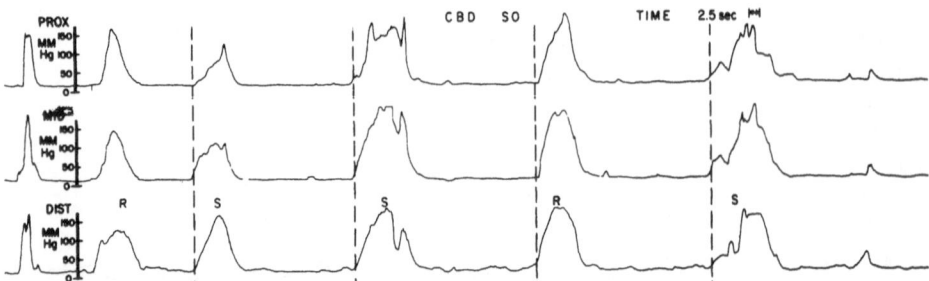

Figure 3. An example of phasic sphincter of Oddi contractile activity. In this sequence, scored from onset of the major upstroke, three of the wave sequences appear simultaneous, and two sequences appear retrograde, i.e., distal to proximal.

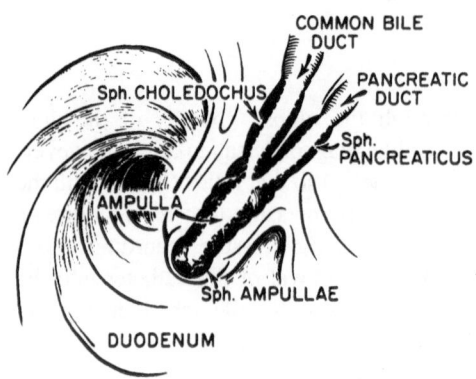

Figure 4. Schema of the sphincter of Oddi segment demonstrating a series of "minisphincters" suggested by the anatomic dissections of Boyden.[29] During manometric study, however, a continuum of pressure is recorded over this 6- to 8-mm-long segment whether the catheter is directed into the common duct or the pancreatic duct.

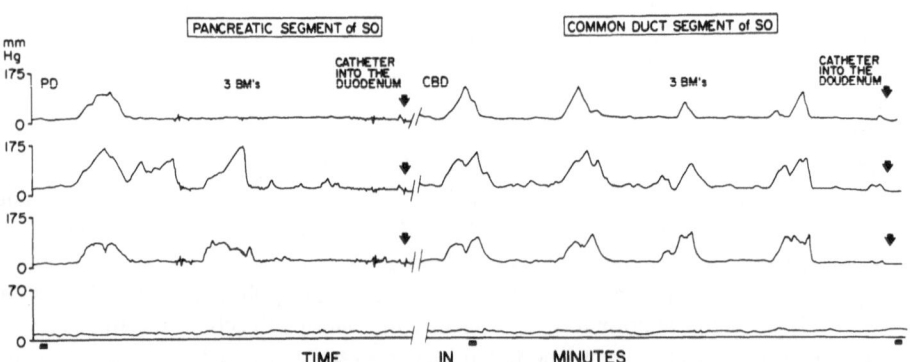

Figure 5. Sphincter of Oddi manometric study showing pressure recordings from the pancreatic duct segment and the common duct segment in the same patient. Basal pressure and phasic wave contraction amplitude are equivalent in either limb of the sphincter of Oddi. [3 BM's refers to the insertion depth of the pressure recording catheter as determined by the serial concentric marks (0.5 mm apart) seen by the endoscopist.]

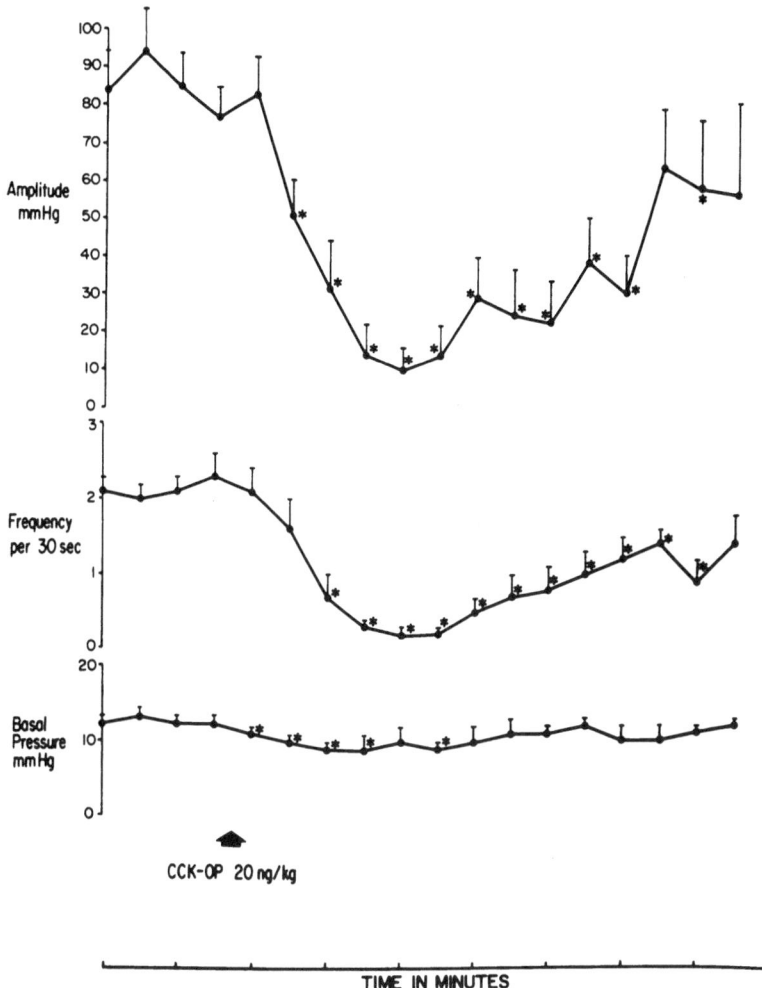

Figure 6. The effect of cholecystokinin octapeptide (CCK-OP) (20 µg/kg i.v.) on sphincter of Oddi phasic contraction amplitude (top), frequency (middle), and basal pressure (bottom) in 20 patients with normal biliary tract anatomy during sphincter of Oddi manometry. Following CCK-OP injection, there is a rapid and significant decrease in all sphincter of Oddi motor activity within 3 min.

uniform along the SO zone whether the recording catheter is directed into the CBD or pancreatic duct[30] (Fig. 5).

Intravenous CCK-OP (Fig. 6), glucagon, and amyl nitrite (Fig. 7) relax both tonic and phasic SO contractions.[31] (The reduction in basal sphincter pressure suggests that there is active sustained contraction of the sphincteric muscle.) Morphine has a powerful excitatory action on the SO. Small doses of morphine increase the frequency of SO phasic contractions and cause minimal effect on basal SO pressure; larger doses increase basal pressure and cause generalized ''spasm'' of the SO.[32]

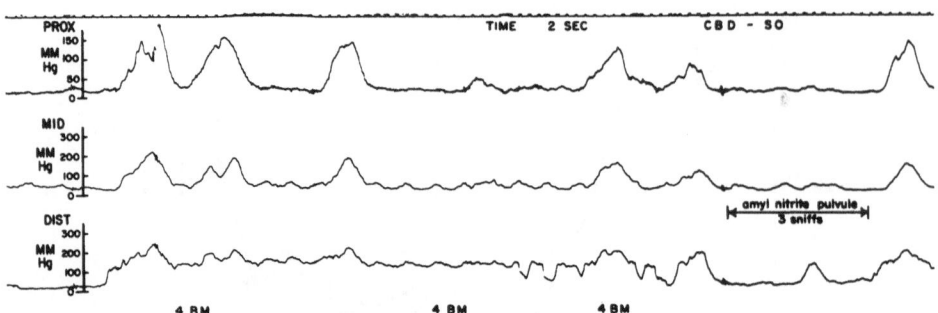

Figure 7. The effect of amyl nitrite vapors inhaled by the patient on basal sphincter of Oddi pressure is demonstrated in all three recording tips in this segment of tracing.

6. CLINICAL CLASSIFICATION OF PATIENTS WITH SUSPECTED SPHINCTER OF ODDI DYSFUNCTION

SO dyskinesia may cause a hypotonic, or more commonly a hypertonic, sphincter which impedes bile passage into the duodenum. Papillary stenosis, on the other hand, results from inflammation and scarring of the papilla of Vater. It is sometimes difficult, if not impossible, to differentiate patients with primary SO dyskinesia from those patients with papillary stenosis. To deal with the dilemma caused by overlapping etiology, we have developed the following clinical classification of patient groups with suspected SO dysfunction.

6.1. Biliary Type I

6.1.1. Definition

Type I patients have biliary-like pain, abnormal liver function tests [primarily aspartate transaminase (AST) and alkaline phosphatase] confirmed on two or more occasions, delayed CBD drainage of ERCP contrast beyond 45 min, and a dilated CBD greater than 12 mm in diameter measured at ERCP examination.

6.1.2. Example

A 62-year-old housewife was hospitalized for recurrent epigastric pain with radiation to the right subscapular zone and transient elevation of liver function test. The patient had a cholecystectomy 20 years earlier because of symptomatic multiple gallstones. Serum AST and alkaline phosphatase values were elevated three to four times normal upon admission. Abnormal liver function tests had been noted 2 weeks earlier during an office visit prompted by colicky abdominal pain. Diagnostic ERCP study disclosed a 15-mm CBD diameter with a smoothly tapered, narrowed distal choledochal segment. Drainage time of ERCP contrast, despite the absence of preendoscopic narcotic medication, was incomplete at the 60-min fluoroscopic inspection of the CBD. Ductal calculi, or structural irregularities, were not appreciated on radiographs; the sphincteric segment was noted to be "tight" during catheter insertion, which initially presented problems for the endoscopist.

6.1.3. Discussion

This patient's biliary tract problem is most likely caused by a structural alteration, i.e., stenosis, rather than a primary functional disorder of the SO. Although the specific pathological abnormality is frequently not completely elucidated, there is little controversy about the need for improving biliary drainage in this patient by operative or endoscopic sphincterotomy. Although SO manometric pressure measurement may be useful in this patient, it is an optional diagnostic modality.

6.2. Biliary Type II

6.2.1. Definition

Type II patients have biliary-like pain but only one or two of the previously noted criteria, i.e., abnormal liver function tests documented on at least two occasions, delayed drainage, or dilated CBD.

6.2.2. Example

A 40-year-old female realtor was hospitalized for the fifth time in the last 2 years for severe right upper quadrant pain. The pain is nonradiating and "steady" in quality. Originally, the distress was episodic, but has been persistent and periodically "incapacitating" for the last 6 weeks. The pain is more intense after meals, although this is not an exclusive event. A cholecystectomy had been performed 2 years earlier at the onset of her difficulty, but no stones were found. Serum AST levels have been elevated on two other occasions during emergency room visits and, on this admission, AST and alkaline phosphatase are both twice normal values. A DISIDA scan, abdominal computed tomography (CT) scan, and serum amylase studies all have been unremarkable.

At ERCP examination, pancreaticobiliary structures were normal-appearing and contrast drainage time from both ducts was normal. SO manometric study disclosed an elevated basal pressure of 55 mm Hg above resting duodenal pressure. Basal SO pressure and phasic contractile activity were transiently, but dramatically, ablated following i.v. injection of CCK-OP (20 μg/kg). Subsequently, an endoscopic sphincterotomy was done and the patient has had no further pain episodes during a 5-year follow-up.

6.2.3. Discussion

In Biliary Type II patients, a definitive explanation for apparent partial biliary obstruction is unlikely. The response to CCK-OP, however, in this patient strongly suggests a primary dyskinesia rather than a stenosis as the cause of this problem.

We have recently reported the results of a 1-year randomized study of a group of postcholecystectomy Biliary Type II patients to determine the efficacy of endoscopic sphincterotomy as a treatment modality.[33] Forty-seven patients were involved in this prospective study; they were randomized to endoscopic sphincterotomy or sham procedure treatment. SO manometry was performed on all patients, but it was not used as a criterion to determine study entry or randomization. The clinical results of endoscopic sphincterotomy versus sham procedure were evaluated in relationship to several modalities, i.e., CBD diameter and contrast drainage time; liver function test abnormalities; results of the morphine/prostigmin (Nardi) test and SO manometry. The only significant predictor of clinical outcome was SO manometry. Patients who had an elevated basal SO pressure > 40 mm Hg and underwent endoscopic sphincterotomy demonstrated significant improvement in objective clinical findings, and symptoms at 1 year compared to the other high basal pressure group who had the sham procedure—or the remaining two groups with normal SO pressures. At the end of the 1-year follow-up, 7 of the sham patients with elevated basal SO pressure elected to have endoscopic sphincterotomy. After 4 years of following these patients, 17 of 18 patients (94%) with elevated basal SO pressure who had endoscopic sphincterotomy have remained improved. SO manometry is a very useful modality in predicting outcome of endoscopic sphincterotomy in this patient group.

6.3. Biliary Type III

6.3.1. Definition

Type III patients have biliary-like pain exclusively; there are no other objective clinical abnormalities.

6.3.2. Example

A 50-year-old unmarried practical nurse was referred for postprandial lower substernal and epigastric distress first noticed approximately 6 years earlier. It had recently become "unmanageable." A cholecystectomy had been performed 5 years ago at the onset of her symptoms, and the pathology report indicated "acalculous cholecystitis." The pain returned 2 months following the operation, however. The abdominal pain was variably described as "toothache-like, burning or pressure." It was associated with bloating and diarrhea with the onset of distress. The patient was being seen in the emergency room weekly and was taking pain medication chronically. Liver function tests, abdominal CT scan, and serum amylase tests all had been normal. However, an ERCP study performed by the referring physician suggested "distal narrowing of the common bile duct" and the patient was referred for SO manometry.

Repeat diagnostic ERCP showed a normal distal CBD and contrast drainage time. SO manometric pressures were normal. Basal sphincter pressure average of 24 mm Hg and phasic contractions were normal in amplitude, frequency, and duration. Interestingly, immediately upon injection of the first few cubic centimeters of contrast into the CBD, the patient experienced abdominal pain reproducing her symptoms. The pain dissipated within 5 min during drainage of contrast from the CBD. Incidentally, an ultrasound study with fatty-meal performed the day prior to ERCP showed no change in the CBD diameter 45 min after ingestion of lipomul (1.5 ml^3/kg). This is a normal response.

Further history was obtained about the patient. She was currently "very stressed" about her relationship with a fiancé of 10 years. The patient's mother was an invalid in a nursing home after a recent stroke, and a nursing shortage had increased our patient's overtime work considerably. She had failed psychological counseling on at least two occasions during the last 4 years. The patient was placed on calcium-channel blocker therapy, nonnarcotic analgesics, and was referred for psychiatric counseling. The influence of stress on the gastrointestinal tract is well described[34] and, undoubtedly, affects SO or distal CBD afferent responses.

6.3.3. Discussion

Although considerable numbers of patients attempt to qualify for inclusion into the Biliary Type III category of primary functional SO disorder, few gain admission to this relatively exclusive group. Primary SO dyskinesia is quite rare and still difficult to prove conclusively. SO manometry studies are mandatory in Biliary Type III patients.

7. PRIMARY SPHINCTER OF ODDI MOTOR DYSFUNCTION

It has been speculated that a variety of primary motor disorders could affect SO function and cause the clinical picture of pain and/or partial biliary tract obstruction. These speculations are based on the following clinical observations.

Hypertonicity of the SO (or spasm) impairs bile duct emptying by preventing passive flow of bile or decreasing filling of the sphincteric segment between phasic contractions. Patients with elevated basal SO pressure may have superimposed normal or hypertonic phasic contractions or may have no phasic wave activity whatsoever (Fig. 8). Spuriously "high" basal pressure can result from an impacted or acutely angulated manometry catheter wedged within the proximal ductal system. To avoid this pitfall, the manometry catheter must be freely inserted into the duct without obstruction. In many patients, an

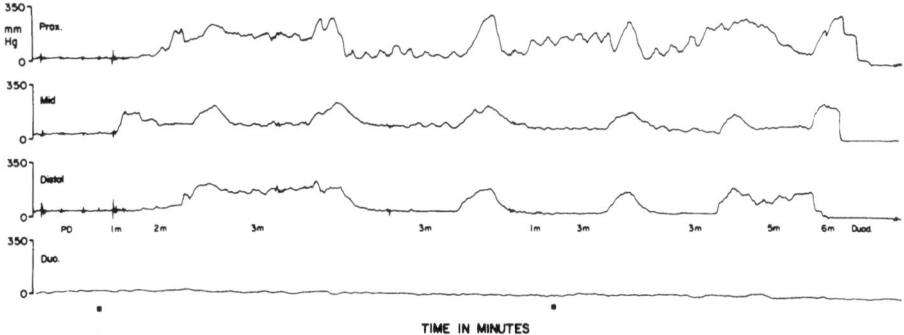

Figure 8. Elevated basal sphincter of Oddi pressure, with superimposed phasic contractions, demonstrated in all three recording tips during catheter pull-through from the pancreatic duct (PD) into the duodenum.

elevated basal SO pressure is dramatically reduced by a smooth muscle pharmacologic relaxant, indicating "muscular contraction" rather than "structural narrowing." In our experience to date, an elevated basal SO pressure is the most unique and significant finding on ERCP manometry.

Paradoxical contraction, rather than relaxation, of the SO following injection of CCK-OP suggests dyskinesia. This response to CCK was initially reported in 5 of 38 patients with elevated prestimulatory basal SO pressure[35] and subsequently described in 10 patients with suspected dysfunction. Basal SO pressure increased from a mean value of 31 to 82 mm Hg, and most patients noted a reproduction of their pain during the paradoxical response to CCK-OP.[36] Most recently, another group of 10 patients with suspected dyskinesia were reported to have a paradoxical SO response to CCK-OP. Prestimulatory basal SO pressure was elevated in 5 of the patients, and all experienced mild to moderate biliary-type symptoms following CCK-OP administration. Eight patients were treated by papillotomy and have experienced symptomatic relief during a 1-year follow-up.[37]

CCK-OP normally inhibits SO tonic and phasic contractions. In the cat model, the CCK effect is mediated by stimulating inhibitory nerves that override a direct effect of the hormone on SO muscle.[38] It is possible that an impaired inhibitory innervation "unmasks" this direct effect of CCK on the muscle prompting a "paradoxical" contraction of the SO.

Abnormal sequencing of SO phasic contractions has been described in patients with retained CBD stones.[7] Normally, the majority of phasic contractions propagate in an antegrade direction; in the patients with ductal stones, the majority of phasic contractions were noted to be retrograde in sequence. Abnormality in propagation direction of phasic contractions was also reported during manometric study in 12 patients with suspected SO dysfunction.[36] The frequency of retrograde wave propagation was 50% or higher in these patients. A predominance of retrograde phasic contractions could enhance bile stasis and retention of stones. In a recent study involving volunteer subjects, however, propagation of SO phasic contractions was noted to be simultaneous in 46%, retrograde in 32%, and antegrade in only 22%.[28]

Rapid SO contractile activity (tachyoddia) could retard or obstruct the flow of bile into the duodenum (Fig. 9). Low-dose, intravenous morphine has been shown to cause a dramatic increase in rate of SO phasic contractions in humans.[32] High-frequency phasic contractions were reported in 11 patients with suspected SO dysfunction ranging from 7 to 12/min (normal: 4/min).[36] In some of these patients, high-frequency phasic contractions occurred for 20 to 30 sec and were followed by quiescent periods of 30 to 60 secs. During these periods of rapid SO phasic contractions, the patients often experienced their primary abdominal distress.

On the other hand, long-term manometric recording from the SO in patients with indwelling T-tubes has shown that the frequency of phasic contractions varies cyclically in close relationship with the duodenal MMC.[9] This relationship had been demonstrated earlier in the opossum SO.[39] Whether or not prolonged "tachyoddia" occurs or accounts for clinical symptoms remains to be proven. We have recorded a continuous 8-min episode of tachyoddia in one patient with suspected biliary dyskinesia. Subsequent endoscopic sphincterotomy was associated with abrupt disappearance of symptoms which have not recurred over a 5-year follow-up period.

The exact role of SO dysfunction in causing clinical problems continues to be

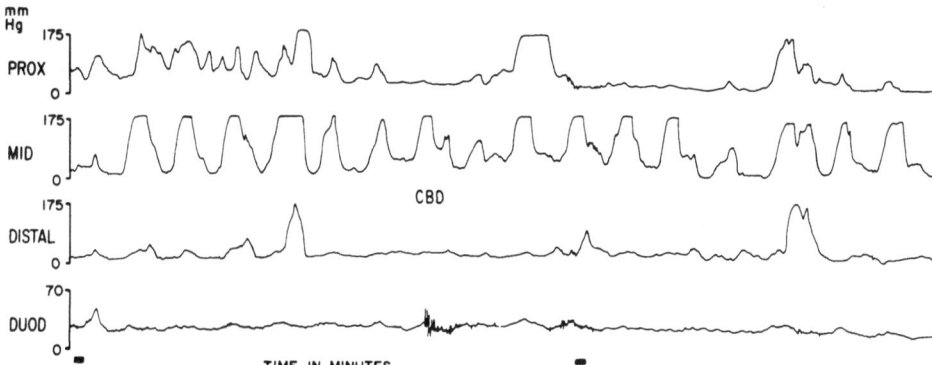

Figure 9. Rapid sphincter of Oddi contraction rate (tachyoddia) confined to the middle tip of the three-lumen manometric pressure recording catheter. Note that duodenal contractile activity is quiescent during this period.

defined. We have classified patients with suspected SO dysfunction into three groups. The prevalence of SO dysfunction is much higher in Group I than in Group III. SO manometry is especially useful and necessary to diagnose certain varieties of SO motor disorders (Types II and III). Although there is increasing evidence to support the existence of primary SO dyskinesia in humans, conclusive proof of this entity is still lacking.

REFERENCES

1. Oddi R: D'une disposition a'sphincter speciale de l'ouverture due canal choledogue. Arch Ital Biol 8:317–322, 1887
2. Krishnamurthy GT, Bobba VR, Kingston E: Radionuclide ejection fraction: A technique for quantitative analysis of motor function of the human gallbladder. Gastroenterology 80:482–490, 1981
3. Itoh Z, Takahashi I: Periodic contractions of the canine gallbladder during the interdigestive state. Am Physiol 240:6183–6189, 1981
4. Everson GT, Braverman DZ, Johnson ML, et al: A critical evaluation of real-time ultrasonography for the study of gallbladder volume and contraction. Gastroenterology 79:40–46, 1980
5. Ryan JP: Motility of the gallbladder and biliary tree, in Johnson LR (ed): Physiology of the Gastrointestinal Tract. New York, Raven Press, 1981, pp 473–494
6. Geenen JE, Hogan WJ, Dodds WJ, et al: Intraluminal pressure recording from the human sphincter of Oddi. Gastroenterology 78:317–324, 1980
7. Toouli J, Geenen JE, Hogan WJ, et al: Sphincter of Oddi motor activity: A comparison between patients with common bile duct stones and controls. Gastroenterology 82:111–117, 1982
8. Toouli J, Dodds WJ, Honda R, et al: Motor function of the opossum sphincter of Oddi. J Clin Invest 71:208–220, 1983
9. Torsoli A, Corazziari E, Habib FI, et al: Frequencies and cyclic pattern of the human sphincter of Oddi phasic activity. Gut 27:363–369, 1986
10. Hogan WJ, Dodds WJ, Geenen JE: The biliary tract, in Christensen J, Wingate D (eds): A Guide to Gastrointestinal Motility. London, Wright & Sons, 1983, pp 157–197
11. Chapman WP, et al: Comparison of pain produced experimentally in lower esophagus, common bile duct and upper intestine with pain experienced by patients with diseases of the biliary tract and pancreas. Surg Gynecol Obstet 89:573–582, 1949
12. Gilbert NC: Influence of extrinsic factors on the coronary flow and clinical course of heart disease. Bull NY Acad Med 18:83, 1942

13. Cullen M, Reese H: Myocardial circulatory changes measured by clearance of Na[24]; effect of common duct distention on myocardial circulation. J Appl Physiol 5:281, 1953

14. Ravdin IS, et al: Reflexes originating in the common duct giving rise to pain simulating angina pectoris. Ann Surg 115:1055, 1942

15. Ravdin IS, et al: Relation of gallstone disease to angina pectoris. Arch Surg 70:333, 1955

16. Zolinger R: Observations following distention of the gallbladder and common duct in man. Proc Soc Exp Biol Med 30:1260–1261, 1933

17. Zolinger R, Walter CW: Localization of pain following foradic stimulation of the common bile duct. Proc Soc Exp Biol Med 35:267–268, 1936

18. Layne JA, Bergh GS: An experimental study of pain in the human biliary tract induced by spasm of the sphincter of Oddi. Am J Physiol 128:18–24, 1940

19. Doran F: Sites of pain referred from the common bile duct. Br J Surg 54:599, 1967

20. Kingham JGC, Dawson AM: Origin of chronic right upper quadrant pain. Gut 26:783–788, 1985

21. Meltzer SJ: Disturbance of law of contrary innervation as a pathogenic factor in the diseases of the bile ducts and gallbladder. Am J Med Sci 153:469–482, 1917

22. Goldberg HI: Cholecystokinin cholecystography. Semin Roentgenol 11:175–179, 1976

23. Brugge WR, Brand DL, Atkins HL, et al: Gallbladder dyskinesia in chronic acalculous cholecystitis. Dig Dis Sci 31:461–467, 1986

24. Collins JSA, Dodds WJ, Geenen JE, et al: Efficacy of quantitative hepatobiliary scintigraphy (QHS) for evaluating a large series of patients with suspected partial common duct obstruction. Gut 29:A1458, 1988

25. Hutton SW, Siebert CEJ, Vennes JA, et al: The effect of sphincterotomy on gallstone formation in the prairie dog. Gastroenterology 81:663–667, 1981

26. Everson GT, McKinley C, Lawson M, et al: Gallbladder function in the human female: Effect of the ovulatory cycle, pregnancy and contraceptive steroids. Gastroenterology 82:711–719, 1982

27. Arndorfer RC, Steff JJ, Dodds WJ, et al: Improved infusion system for intraluminal esophageal manometry. Gastroenterology 73:23–27, 1977

28. Guelrud M, Mendoza S, Rossiter G, et al: Effect of nifedipine on sphincter of Oddi motor activity: Studies in healthy volunteers and patients with biliary dyskinesia. Gastroenterology 95:1050–1055, 1988

29. Boyden EA: The anatomy of the choledochoduodenal junction in man. Surg Gynecol Obstet 104:641–652, 1957

30. Raddawi H, Geenen JE, Hogan WJ, et al: Pressure measurement from the biliary and pancreatic segments of the sphincter of Oddi: Comparison between patients with functional, biliary or pancreatic disease. Gastroenterology 94:A363, 1988

31. Toouli J, Hogan WJ, Geenen JE, et al: Action of cholecystokinin-octapeptide on sphincter of Oddi basal pressure and phasic wave activity in humans. Surgery 92:497–503, 1980

32. Helm JF, Venu RP, Geenen JE, et al: Effects of morphine on the human sphincter of Oddi. Gut 29:1402–1407, 1988

33. Geenen JE, Hogan WJ, Dodds WJ, et al: The efficacy of endoscopic sphincterotomy in post-cholecystectomy patients with sphincter-of-Oddi dysfunction. N Engl J Med 320(2):82–87, 1989

34. Latimer R, Sarna S, Campbell D, et al: Colonic motor and myoelectrical activity: A comparative study of normal subjects, psychoneurotic patients and patients with irritable bowel syndrome. Gastroenterology 80:893–901, 1981

35. Hogan WJ, Geenen JE, Dodds WJ, et al: Paradoxical motor response to cholecystokinin-octapeptide (CCK-OP) in patients with suspected sphincter of Oddi dysfunction. Gastroenterology 82:1085, 1982

36. Toouli J, Roberts-Thomson IC, Dent J, et al: Manometric disorders in patients with suspected sphincter of Oddi dysfunction. Gastroenterology 88:1243–1250, 1985

37. Rolny P, Arleback A, Funch-Jensen P, et al: Paradoxical response of sphincter of Oddi to intravenous injection of cholecystokinin or ceruletide. Manometric findings and results of treatment in biliary dyskinesia. Gut 27:1507–1511, 1986

38. Behar J, Biancani P: Effect of cholecystokinin and the octapeptide of cholecystokinin on the feline sphincter of Oddi and gallbladder. Mechanisms of action. J Clin Invest 66:1231–1239, 1980

39. Honda R, Toouli J, Dodds WJ, et al: Relationship of sphincter of Oddi spike bursts to gastrointestinal myoelectric activity in the conscious opossum. J Clin Invest 69:770–778, 1982

14

Disorders of the Anal Sphincters

N. W. Read and Wei Ming Sun

1. ANATOMY

The anal sphincter is really two sphincters in one. It consists of an inner ring of smooth muscle, which is contiguous with the smooth muscle of the rectum, and an outer striated muscle ring, which is linked functionally to the puborectalis fibers of the levator ani complex (Fig. 1). The internal sphincter (IAS) is not under conscious control, but like all other smooth muscle sphincters, relaxes when the bowel immediately proximal to it contracts or is distended. The external sphincter (EAS) and puborectalis are under conscious control and tend to contract together, increasing the sphincter resistance and accentuating the anorectal angulation.

Nerve Supply

The IAS is connected by intrinsic nerve plexuses to the rectum. The extrinsic nerve supply comes from the pelvic parasympathetic nerves and from the lumbar sympathetic outflow via the hypogastric plexus. Stimulation of the sympathetic nerves increases the IAS tone via α receptors,[1,2] though β adrenoreceptor agonists reduce IAS tone.[3] In contrast, stimulation of the pelvic parasympathetic nerves can tend to relax the IAS via nonadrenergic, noncholinergic fibers.[3−5] The transmitter is probably vasoactive intestinal polypeptide.

The EAS receives its nerve supply from the pudendal nerve (S 2, 3, 4), which enters the perineum by winding around the ischial spine. The nerve supply of the puborectalis and levator ani complex is from direct branches of S2 and S3.

Sensation from the sphincter lining is conveyed by the pudendal nerve.

N. W. Read and Wei Ming Sun • Department of Human Gastrointestinal Physiology and Nutrition, Royal Hallamshire Hospital, Sheffield S10 2TN, England.

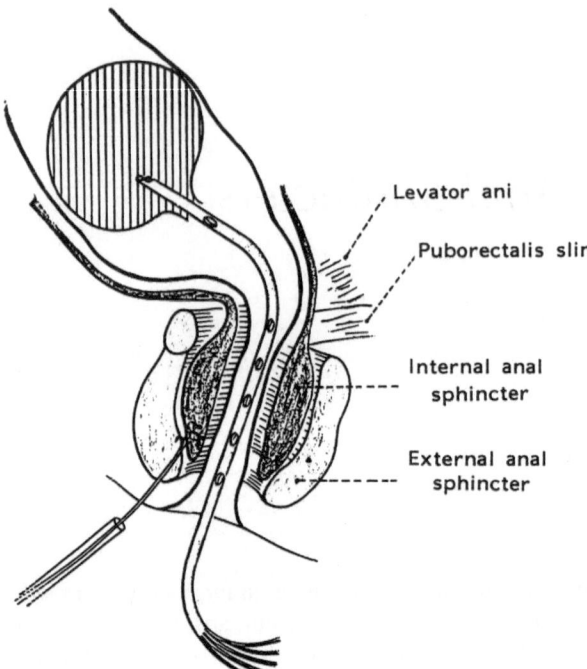

Levator ani

Puborectalis sling

Internal anal
sphincter

External anal
sphincter

Figure 1. Diagram of the anal canal,
showing the different muscle components and the probes used to measure
pressure in multiple sites in the anal
canal and the electrical activity of the
IAS and EAS.

2. THE INCOMPETENT SPHINCTER

2.1. Maintenance of Continence

Under resting conditions, continence to rectal mucus and small volumes of feces is
thought to be maintained by the tonic contraction of the IAS. The circular fibers of the
IAS, however, are unable to shorten sufficiently to seal off the anal canal unless they are
contracting around an anal lining that is sufficiently bulky to plug the orifice. The bulk of
the anal lining is enhanced by infolding when the sphincter is contracted, and also by the
presence of expansile vascular cushions, which act to seal the sphincter, at the same time
stretching the muscle so that the fibers can contract at a greater mechanical advantage.[6,7]
A radical hemorrhoidectomy is associated with a high incidence of anal seepage.[8] Tonic
contraction of the EAS can augment the resting tone of the IAS, but this muscle is almost
completely relaxed when the subject is asleep.[9]

The tonic contraction of the sphincter is unable to maintain continence when this is
threatened by rectal contraction, rectal distension, and increases in intraabdominal pressure. This is because rectal distension and contraction cause a reflex relaxation of the IAS,
mediated by intrinsic nerves; while increases in intraabdominal pressure are usually of
sufficient magnitude to overwhelm the resting sphincter pressure and may also induce
sphincter relaxation. Continence can only be maintained under these conditions by a
compensatory contraction of the EAS. Contraction of the EAS during relaxation of the

IAS increases the resistance of the sphincter, particularly in its outermost aspect, while allowing the composition of the rectal contents to be sampled by the sensitive anal lining.[10] The sampling of the rectal contents by the anal sensors has been proposed as the mechanism whereby people can discriminate between solid stool, liquid feces, and flatus. It is possible, however, that solid and fluid (gas or liquid) rectal contents may be discriminated by their ability to stimulate rapidly adapting rectal stretch receptors in the rectal wall, while feces (solid or liquid) and gas could be discriminated by stretch receptors in the pelvic floor,[11] providing the subject is in an upright position. More work is needed to elucidate the mechanism of discrimination of rectal contents.

Simultaneous contraction of the puborectalis assists the EAS in maintaining continence by making the anorectal angle more acute. It is easy to see how a more acute anorectal angle will impede the entry of a solid cylindrical stool into the anal canal, but it would be unlikely to aid continence to liquids, unless the upper anal canal was being compressed against a relatively fixed object, such as the cervix uteri or the prostate gland.

The relationship between contraction of the EAS and the IAS is poorly understood, because of the difficulty in recording the function of both muscles simultaneously in human subjects. Although both muscles relax during defecation, they contract in a reciprocal manner during attempts to maintain continence. For example, rectal distension and contraction relax the IAS, but contract the EAS, while micturition is associated with relaxation of the EAS and contraction of the IAS.[12] This reciprocal activity may explain why patients who have weakness of both the IAS and the EAS tend to be more incontinent than patients who have EAS weakness alone.

2.2. Investigation of Patients with Fecal Incontinence

The function of the IAS and EAS in patients with fecal incontinence can be discriminated by manometric and electrophysiological techniques.

The identification of abnormalities of internal or external sphincter function by manometric techniques is only possible if pressures are recorded at multiple closely spaced sites within the anal sphincter. This is because the two muscles often exhibit reciprocal activity; hence, the EAS contraction, which occurs, for example, during rectal distension, can mask IAS relaxation in the outermost anal channels, but not in the inner channels. Interpretation of the manometric profiles is greatly facilitated by simultaneous recording of the electrical activities of the EAS and IAS, allowing changes in pressure caused by the activity of those muscles to be identified.

In the technique employed in our laboratory (Fig. 1), pressures at multiple sites in the rectum and anal canal are measured with a narrow polyvinyl seven-lumen tube bearing a terminal inflatable balloon. The electrical activity of the sphincter is recorded at the same time by means of a bipolar electrode, consisting of two insulated wires (diameter 0.025 mm) with their ends bared, hooked, and offset to avoid electrical contact.[13] The wires are introduced into the superficial EAS or into the groove between the superficial EAS and the IAS inside a fine-gauge hypodermic needle, which is subsequently withdrawn. The activity of the IAS is represented on the raw EMG record as regular oscillations, which occur at a frequency of between 6 and 20 per minute and increase in amplitude as the activity of the muscle increases[14] (Fig. 2). The activity of the EAS appears on the raw

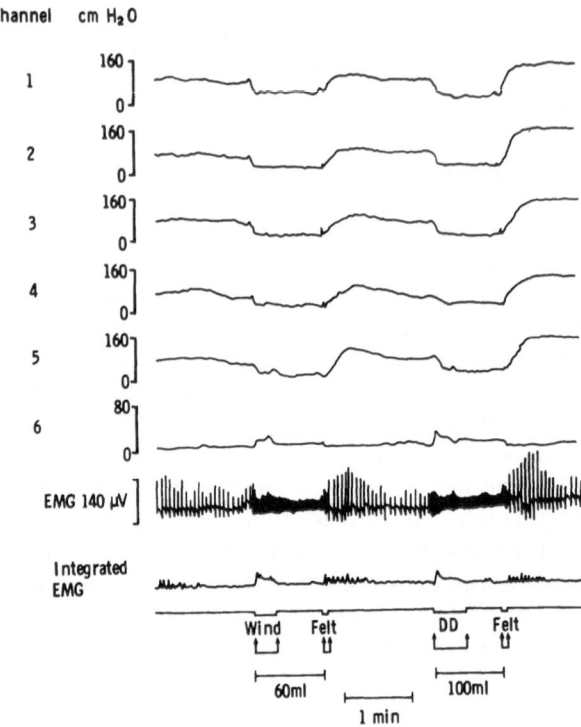

Figure 2. Recordings of anorectal pressure and the electrical activity of the EAS and IAS in the typical normal female subject before, during, and after inflation of rectal balloon with 60 and 100 ml of air. Channels 1–6 represent ports situated 0.5, 1.0, 1.5, 2.0, 2.5, and 4.5 cm from the anal verge. Note that rectal distension induces relaxation in sphincter pressure associated with abolition of the electrical oscillations, produced by IAS activity, and an increase in the electrical activity of the EAS, whereas deflation produces a rebound increase in pressure which is associated with marked increase in the slow-wave oscillations. The bar (⌣) indicates when subject experienced rectal sensations. DD, desire to defecate.

EMG record as successive spikes that increase in both amplitude and frequency as the activity of that muscle increases.

With this technique, anorectal motor activity and anal electrical activity were recorded at rest, and during maximum sphincter contraction, rectal distension and rises in intraabdominal pressure in over 200 patients, referred for investigation of fecal incontinence. This systematic procedure allowed us to study the response of the sphincter under basal conditions and during maneuvers that threatened continence. Rectal sensations were recorded during rectal distension, and leakage of perfusion fluid during any of the maneuvers was noted on the chart.

2.3. Normal Records

Inflation of the rectal balloon in the normal volunteers always caused reductions in pressure in all of the anal ports (Fig. 2). These anal relaxations increased in amplitude and duration as the distending volume increased, and were associated with increases in both rectal pressure and the electrical activity of the EAS (Fig. 2). The increased EAS activity became more prolonged as the distending volume and duration of sphincter relaxation increased and caused the pressure in the anal canal in normal volunteers to remain above the rectal pressure during rectal distension; so that leakage did not take place. Upon deflating the balloon, there was often a rebound increase in anal pressure to values that exceeded the preinflation pressure (Fig. 2). This postinflation rebound was associated with an increase in the amplitude of the IAS electrical slow waves (Fig. 2) and may be related to reflex activation of the sympathetic nerves supplying the IAS.

When normal subjects increased the intraabdominal pressure through a Valsalva maneuver, by blowing up a party balloon, the electrical activity in the EAS also increased and the pressures in the distal anal canal rose to levels that were consistently above rectal pressure, thus preserving continence.

2.4. Disturbances in Sphincter Function in Patients with Fecal Incontinence

There is no single mechanism responsible for fecal incontinence. In theory, fecal incontinence can be caused either by weakness of the IAS and/or the EAS/puborectalis complex or by disruption of any component of the nervous reflexes that control these muscles. In practice, the disturbances in sphincter function responsible for fecal incontinence can be grouped into several clinical entities (Table I), which can be characterized and discriminated by manometric and electrophysiological studies. The identification of the mechanism underlying fecal incontinence provides a useful basis for selection of an appropriate treatment option.

Table I. Disturbances in Sphincter Function Responsible
for Fecal Incontinence

Cause	Features	Treatment
Pudendal neuropathy	Perineal descent; weak EAS contraction; normal electrical response	Post-anal repair
Obstetric trauma	Circumferential electrical gap	Sphincter repair
Impaired rectal sensation	(1) IAS relaxes at volumes that fail to induce sensation and EAS response; (2) delayed EAS response	Training
Low spinal lesion	Absent EAS responses to rectal distension and increases in intraabdominal pressure	Training
High spinal lesion	Little conscious control of EAS; enhanced reflex control	Training
Irritable bowel syndrome	Enhanced rectal sensitivity; reduced rectal compliance; increased rectal contractility and anal relaxation in response to rectal distension	Drugs Diet Psychotherapy
Transient IAS relaxation	Inappropriate IAS relaxation under resting conditions and after squeeze and strain	? Drugs
Impaired IAS function	Very low pressures; no IAS relaxation on rectal distension	? Drugs

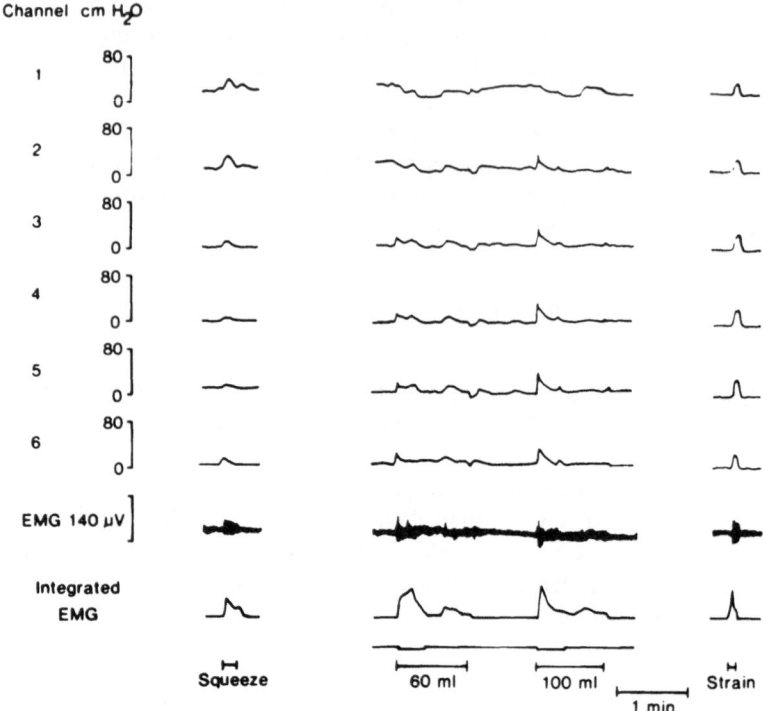

Figure 3. Recordings of anorectal pressure and the electrical activity of the EAS in a female patient with perineal descent, during conscious contraction of the EAS, during rectal balloon distension with 60 and 100 ml of air, and during straining. Channels 1–6 represent ports situated at 0.5, 1.0, 1.5, 2.0, 2.5, and 4.5 cm from the anal verge. Note that the electrical activity of the EAS is appropriate, but the mechanical effort is weak.

2.4.1. Pudendal Neuropathy

These patients have an abnormal degree of perineal descent, especially when they strain,[15] and weak conscious and reflex contraction of the EAS. The sphincter pressure often fails to increase above the rectal pressure during rectal distension and increases in intraabdominal pressure.[16] This often results in leakage of perfusion fluid from the anus. The EAS shows appropriate electrical responses to conscious contraction, rectal distension, and increases in intraabdominal pressure, but the mechanical effort is weak (Fig. 3). Neurophysiological measurements show increased fiber density and prolonged motor unit potential duration and increased pudendal nerve terminal motor latency,[15,17–19] features that are typical of neuropathy. The evidence suggests that the weakness of the EAS occurs because the distal segment of the pudendal nerve becomes stretched and compressed against the ischial spine. This situation is thought to arise as a consequence of weakness of the pelvic floor, caused either during childbirth or as a result of prolonged straining.[15,19] Moreover, there is a marked increase in terminal motor latency after childbirth in some women.[19] The mechanism of the apparent weakness of the pelvic floor is uncertain. Studies need to be carried out to determine whether this is related to disruption of the connective tissue fascia, to traumatic or neuropathic weakness of the levators, or to paradoxical relaxation of the levators during straining.

2.4.2. Impaired IAS

Most studies of fecal incontinence have emphasized the role of the puborectalis and EAS.[18,20–23] In contrast, the role of the IAS has been largely ignored, though it has been suggested that the low resting anal pressure in incontinent diabetics is caused by weakness of the IAS.[24] Twenty-five percent of the patients, referred to us for investigation of fecal incontinence, had abnormally weak sphincters that exhibited very low resting pressures and no relaxation when the rectum was distended, suggesting impaired function of the IAS.[25] The abnormally low pressures in this group would rule out Hirschsprung's disease.[26–28] Most of these patients showed no anal relaxation during rectal distension with any volume, and exhibited increases in anal pressure instead (Fig. 4). A few patients, however, showed no relaxation at low distending volumes, but because of the postinflation rebound in IAS tone, relaxations were observed at higher distending volumes (Fig. 5). The absent or delayed IAS relaxation in these patients was not associated with an

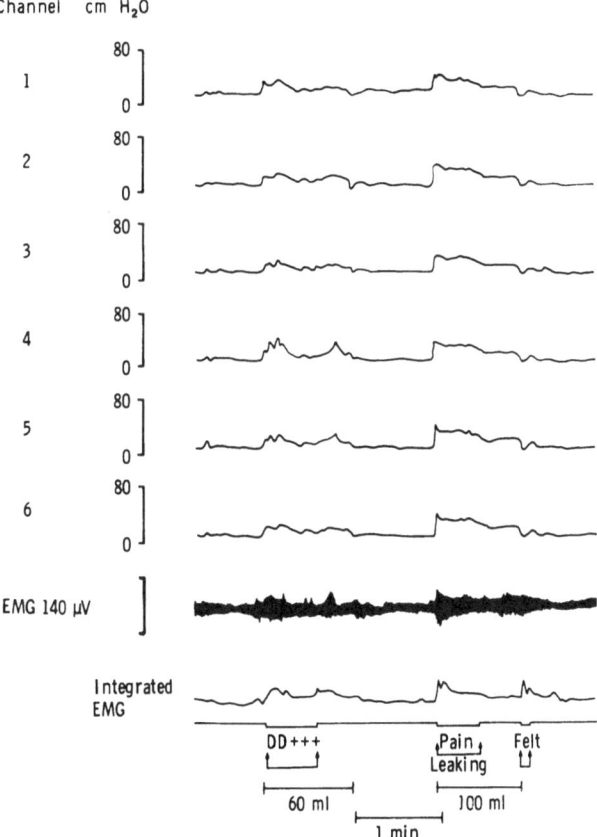

Figure 4. Recordings of anorectal pressure and the electrical activity of the sphincter in a female patient with impaired IAS function before, during, and after inflation of a rectal balloon with 60 and 100 ml of air. Channels 1–6 represent ports situated 0.5, 1.0, 1.5, 2.0, 2.5, and 4.5 cm from the anal verge. Note the absence of IAS electrical activity and the abnormally low basal anal pressures, and the absence of anal relaxation during rectal distension. This increase is associated with an increase in the electrical activity of the EAS. No rebound pressures were observed upon deflating the rectal balloon. The bars (⊔) indicate when the subject experienced rectal sensation. DD, desire to defecate; +++ indicates the severity of the sensation.

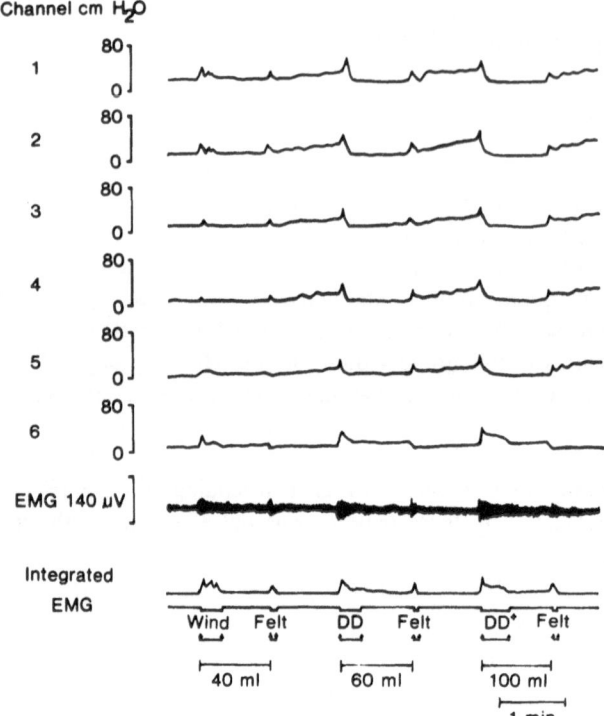

Figure 5. Recordings of anorectal pressure and the electrical activity of the sphincter in a female patient with impaired IAS function before, during, and after inflation of a rectal balloon with 60 and 100 ml of air. Channels 1–6 represent ports situated 0.5, 1.0, 1.5, 2.0, 2.5, and 4.5 cm from the anal verge. Note that rectal distension with volumes of 40, 60, and 100 ml evoked rebound increases in anal pressure upon deflation that persisted until the subsequent inflation, so that distension with 60 and 100 ml caused anal relaxation.

insensitive and hypercompliant rectum,[29,30] but was related instead to impaired IAS contractility and electrical activity. Further measurements showed that the maximum squeeze pressures and the EAS pressure responses to rectal distension and to increases in intraabdominal pressure were also abnormally low in patients who had impaired internal sphincters. Although these features were shared by many of the incontinent patients we have studied, EAS function was more severely impaired in the patients who had evidence of IAS dysfunction. Patients with combined weakness of the IAS and EAS were more severely incontinent than patients who had weakness of only the EAS.

The weakness of the IAS was not related to impairment in smooth muscle function in other parts of the gut or extraintestinal evidence of autonomic neuropathy. All of the patients had weakness of the EAS and 92% had abnormal pelvic floor descent. Perhaps the extremely weak striated muscle exposes the IAS to traction by the tissues of the pelvic floor. Alternatively, the abnormal descent of the pelvic floor may damage the delicate sympathetic nerves, which are thought to enhance the tone of the IAS. In a previous study, inhibition of the sympathetic outflow by high spinal anesthesia reduced the resting sphincter pressure by about 44%.[31]

Impaired IAS function is not confined to patients who present with fecal incontinence. In our experience, all patients with full thickness rectal prolapse exhibit the same phenomenon; presumably the rectal wall herniates through the defect caused by the weak sphincters. Loss of IAS tone is also seen in many constipated patients; is this related to a generalized reduction in gastrointestinal smooth muscle tone in these patients or is it

associated with perineal descent, caused by excessive straining? The reason that constipated patients with absent IAS tone do not usually complain of incontinence must be
because their stools are large and hard, though it is notable that many of these patients
have little control over their bowels after they have taken laxatives.

2.4.3. Inappropriate Transient Anal Relaxation

Inappropriate transient relaxation of the lower esophageal sphincter is regarded as a
major mechanism for reflux of acid from the stomach to the esophagus.[32,33] Approximately 20% of patients referred for investigation of fecal incontinence showed episodes
of spontaneous anal relaxation at rest.[34] These lasted at least 15 sec and reduced the
pressure in the outermost anal channels by at least 20 cm H_2O (Fig. 6). The same
phenomenon was observed in a similar percentage of normal controls. Spontaneous
reductions in sphincter pressure were always associated with attenuation or abolition of
the electrical oscillations of the IAS (Fig. 6), but no decrease in activity of the EAS. In
fact, 83% of episodes of transient relaxation recorded in normal subjects were associated
with compensatory increases in the electrical activity of the EAS (Fig. 6). IAS relaxations
are normally evoked by rectal distension, such as might be caused by the entry of feces
into the rectum, or by rectal contraction.[14,35,36] However, less than 50% of the episodes
of spontaneous sphincter relaxation, recorded in this study, were associated with corresponding increases in rectal pressure. Thus, the majority of the episodes appeared to be

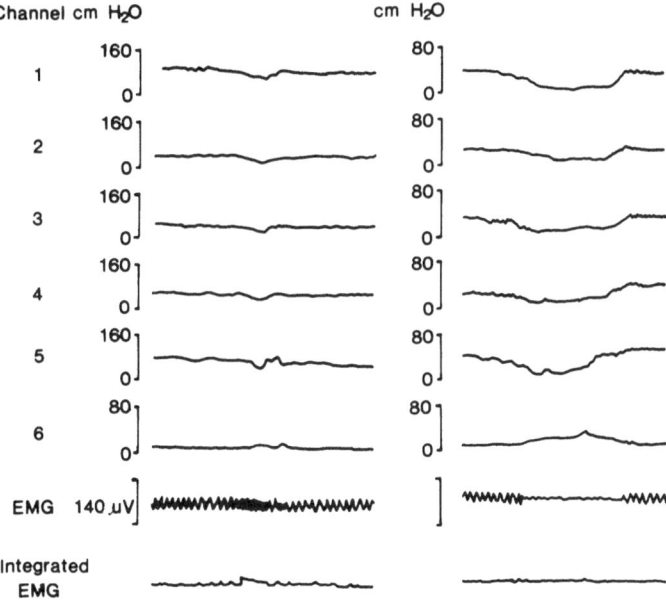

Figure 6. Multiport recordings of anal pressure and the electrical activity of the EAS and IAS during and after
an episode of spontaneous anal relaxation in a normal subject (left) and an incontinent patient (right). Channels
1–6 represent ports situated 0.5, 1.0, 1.5, 2.0, 2.5, and 4.5 cm from the anal verge. The relaxation lasted longer
in the patient and was not associated with a compensatory increase in EAS activity.

due either to autonomous losses of IAS tone or to reductions in tone, provoked by events that did not increase pressure in the rectum.[37] Naudy et al.[38] have shown that relaxation of the sphincter can be induced by distension of more proximal regions of the colon; so perhaps the "spontaneous relaxations" are related to contractile activity and movements of the contents in the more proximal colon.

Spontaneous relaxation of the IAS is probably of little or no significance in normal subjects, because simultaneous contraction of the EAS maintains the anal pressure barrier and guards against incontinence. It poses a much more serious threat to continence in patients who have impaired EAS function. Only 23% of the incontinent study group showed compensatory increases in EAS activity, and in the remainder the EAS response was weak.[34] Some patients, particularly those with diabetes mellitus and other causes of autonomic neuropathy, only have incontinent episodes at night while they are asleep. Since the EAS is unable to compensate for a relaxation of the IAS while the subject is asleep,[9] the possibility that transient relaxations of the sphincter are responsible for the episodes of nocturnal incontinence in these patients needs to be investigated.

Incontinent patients who exhibited spontaneous relaxations were more sensitive to rectal distension than the remainder of the incontinent patients.[34] The rectal volumes required to elicit anal relaxation, to induce sustained relaxation, to elicit a sensation of "wind," and to cause a desire to defecate were all much lower in the incontinent patients who showed spontaneous relaxations than in the remainder of the incontinent patients or in normal subjects. Rectal distension also induced more prolonged sphincter relaxation in response to lower volumes of rectal distension, and gave rise to higher rectal pressures in the incontinent study group compared with the incontinent control group. Fifty percent of the incontinent patients who showed spontaneous relaxation also showed postsqueeze or poststrain relaxations (Fig. 7), which were also associated with attenuation of the electrical activity of the IAS. These phenomena were rare in the remainder of the incontinent patients and in normal controls. All of these results indicate that patients with spontaneous IAS relaxations have an unusually sensitive rectum and a rather unstable sphincter that relaxes to the slightest provocation. A similar sensitivity of the rectum is found in patients with the irritable bowel syndrome or ulcerative colitis,[39-41] though transient IAS relaxations are not, in our experience, a common feature in such patients.

The resting tone of the IAS can be modulated by activity in the autonomic nervous system.[42] No patients, however, had evidence of a generalized visceral neuropathy affecting the sphincter, although two had diabetes mellitus, and another four had undergone hysterectomy, which could possibly have damaged the nerve supply to the sphincter.[43,44]

2.4.4. Impaired Rectal Sensation

The ability of the patients to perceive the distension of the rectum, caused by, for example, the arrival of feces, appears to be necessary for the prompt and appropriate contractile response of the EAS.[13] Conscious perception of rectal distension is not necessary for relaxation of the IAS. Thus, patients with impaired rectal sensation may fail to contract the EAS to compensate for a relaxation of the IAS, induced by rectal distension or contraction. Two abnormalities can be seen during manometric and electrophysiological tests. In the first, the rectal volume that induces IAS relaxation is lower than that which induces rectal sensation and an increase in EAS activity.[45] This abnormality is

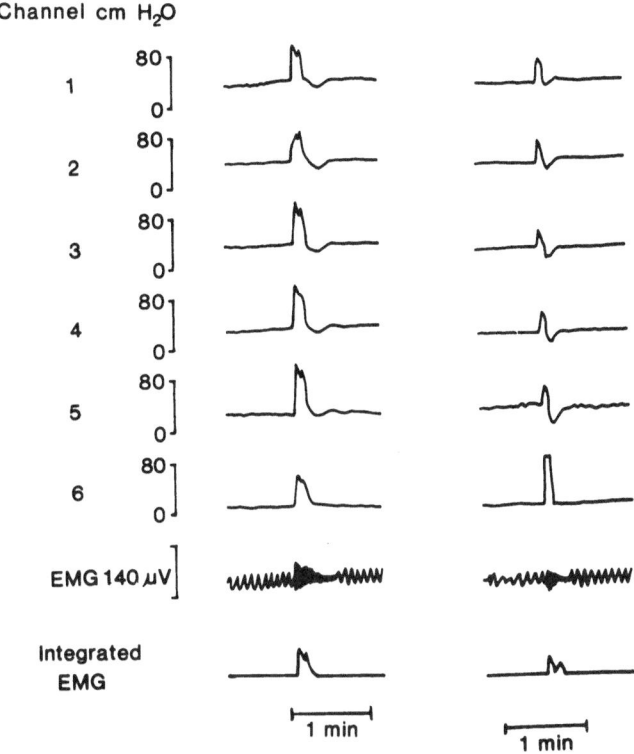

Figure 7. Recordings of anorectal pressure and the electrical activity of the sphincter during maximum conscious contraction of the EAS (left) and during straining (right) in a patient who exhibited spontaneous relaxation. Channels 1–6 represent ports situated 0.5, 1.0, 1.5, 2.0, 2.5, and 4.5 cm from the anal verge. Note postsqueeze and poststrain relaxations that are associated with suppression of the IAS slow wave, but no decrease in the electrical activity of the EAS below baseline values.

often found in patients with megarectum and fecal impaction. In the second, the EAS response is present, but delayed (Fig. 8).[46] Surgery and drugs are ineffective in such patients, but success can be achieved by biofeedback techniques of sensory and coordination training.

2.4.5. Spinal Lesions

About 10% of patients referred for fecal incontinence exhibited manometric and electrophysiological features which resemble those of patients with lesions in the spinal cord. Most of these patients also have difficulty in initiating defecation. In an analogous system, disturbances in micturition may be the presenting feature of neurological disease and the last to recover after spinal injury.[47] In both situations, conventional neurological examination and investigation fail to reveal a lesion. Neurology does not help. Therefore occult spinal disease may well be an important cause of disturbances in defecation as well as micturition.

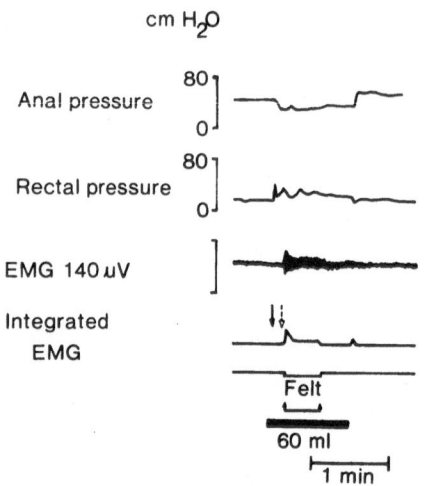

Figure 8. Recording of anorectal pressure and the electrical activity of the sphincter complex in a patient during rectal balloon distension with 60 ml of air. The IAS relaxes upon rectal distension, but rectal sensation and the EAS response are delayed. Solid arrow and dashed arrow represent the onset of rectal distension and rectal sensation, respectively.

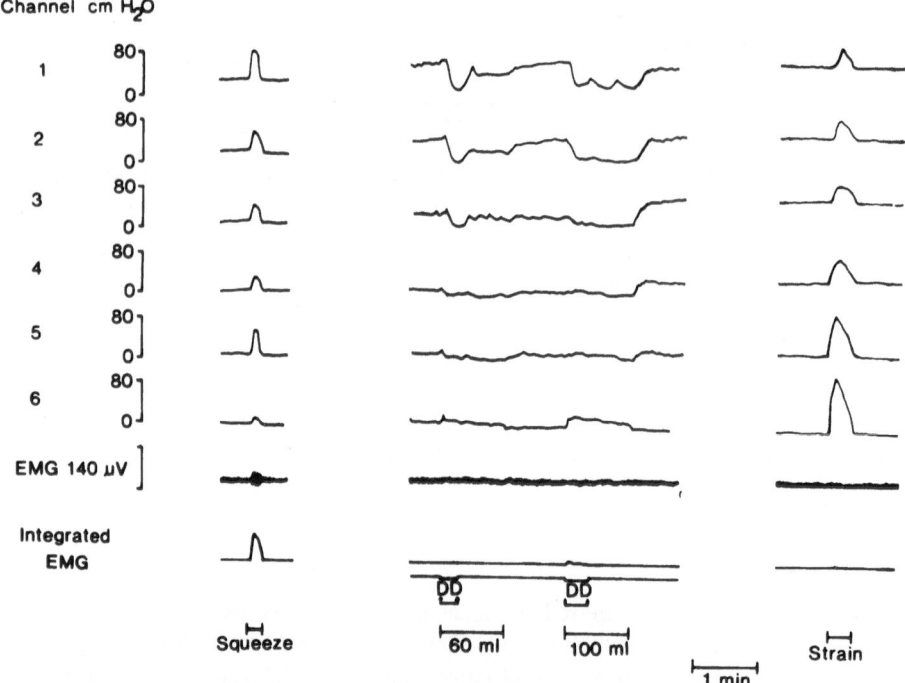

Figure 9. Multiport recordings of anal pressure and the electrical activity of the EAS during maximum conscious contraction of the EAS, during rectal distension, and during straining (as if to defecate) in a typical patient with low spinal lesion. Channels 1–6 represent ports situated 0.5, 1.0, 1.5, 2.0, 2.5, and 4.5 cm from the anal verge. Note that there is appropriate conscious contraction of the sphincter but no increase in activity generated by rectal distension and increase in intraabdominal pressure.

Tests in our laboratory showed that patients with established low spinal lesions had low basal pressures and squeeze pressures. In fact, 67% of these patients had no increase in pressure or in EAS electrical activity during conscious attempts to contract the sphincter. Rectal sensation was blunted, and EAS responses to either rectal distension or increases in intraabdominal pressure or both were absent or markedly attenuated or delayed (Fig. 9). Most of these patients leaked during the test. Such results have been observed by other groups.[48–50]

Patients with lesions in the cauda equina often have markedly impaired rectal sensation, increased rectal compliance, and weak or absent conscious and reflex contraction of the EAS.[51]

Patients with high spinal lesions also have low sphincter pressures, but none of the patients that we have tested were able to increase the activity in the sphincter consciously. Unlike the patients with low spinal lesions, reflex activity of the sphincter was often exaggerated. The EAS contracted vigorously when the patient moved and during increases in intraabdominal pressure and rectal distension (Fig. 10). Thus, the residual pressures during rectal distension were significantly higher in patients with high spinal

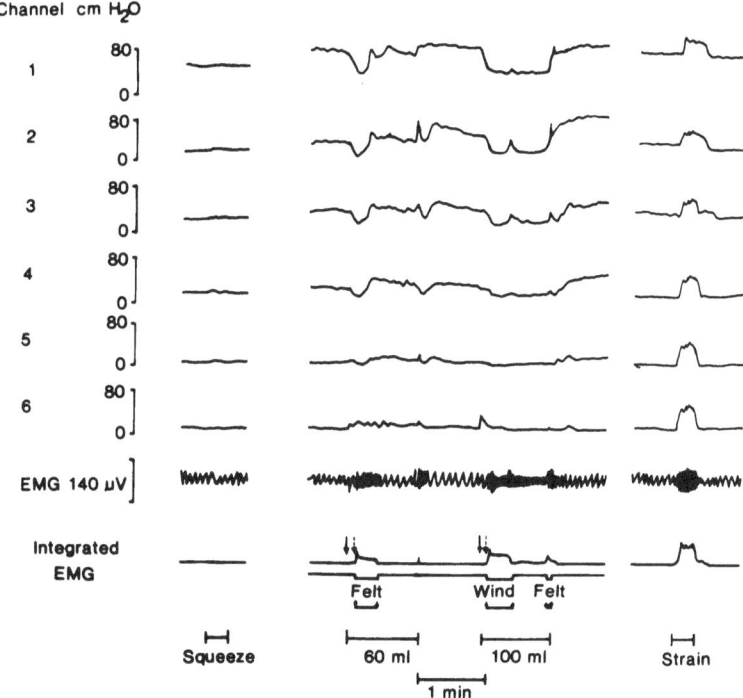

Figure 10. Recording of anorectal pressure at ports situated 0.5, 1.0, 1.5, 2.0, 2.5, and 4.5 cm from the anal margin (channels 1–6) and the electrical activity of the sphincter complex in a patient with a high spinal lesion during rectal balloon distension with 60 and 100 ml of air. There is no conscious contraction of the sphincter but reflex response to rectal distension and increase in intraabdominal pressure are much increased. Solid arrow and dashed arrow represent the onset of rectal distension and rectal sensation, respectively.

lesions compared with those with low spinal lesions, and a lower percentage of these patients leaked during the test.

3. THE OBSTRUCTED SPHINCTER

3.1. Normal Defecation

Defecation is a stereotyped sequence of actions, usually initiated by a conscious mechanism and involving a number of pelvic reflexes that are controlled and coordinated by a center in the brain stem.

Stool is propelled into the rectum by propagated colonic contractions. If the stool is large enough, the rectal distension and probably also the weight of the stool on the pelvic floor induce a desire to defecate. This sensation is usually associated with a rectal contraction and a relaxation of the IAS, both of which serve to tamp the stool down into the proximal anal canal (the firing position for defecation). This increases the defecatory urge, which can only be suppressed by a vigorous contraction of the EAS and puborectalis, closing the anal sphincter and propelling the stool back into the rectum.[52] When conditions are appropriate for defecation, the subject sits or squats, contracts the diaphragm, the abdominal muscles, and the levators, while relaxing the EAS and possibly also the puborectalis.[52,53] Contraction of the levators is thought by some to be necessary to lift the posterior pelvic wall, and together with relaxation of the puborectalis, opens up the anorectal angle so that the stool has a direct passage to the exterior.[54] Whether the puborectalis relaxes during defecation has not been established; it is possible that the angle opens up because the contraction of the fibers of the levators pulls the puborectalis posteriorly.[54,55] Once defecation has commenced, it can continue with no conscious effort, suggesting that the passage of stool through the anus may stimulate a strong colonic contraction resulting in effortless expulsion of a large volume of stool. Certainly, pediatricians and veterinarians can attest to the fact that examination of the rectum of very young children, paraplegic patients, and horses can induce a mass evacuation of the distal colon.

3.2. Causes of Impaired Defecation

Defecation may be impaired by failure of the IAS to relax, inappropriate contraction of the EAS and puborectalis, failure of the levators to lift the pelvic floor and open the anorectal angle, and luminal obstruction by hemorrhoids and partial rectal prolapse (see Table II).

3.2.1. Anismus

Many young women with severe constipation are unable to expel a simulated stool, inserted into the rectum and pulled down into the rectal ampulla,[56,57] even when they are allowed to do this in privacy.[57] Most normal subjects, tested under the same conditions, can expel the same objects without difficulty. The difficulty in expulsion is not usually caused by insufficient intraabdominal force,[56,58] but appears to be related to an inability of the patients to relax the puborectalis and EAS during attempts at defecation.[56,57,59] In

Table II. Causes of Obstructed Defecation, Identified by Combined Anorectal Manometry, Electromyography, and Sensory Testing

Cause	Features	Treatment
Anismus	Paradoxical EAS contraction during defecation	? Training
Short segment Hirschsprung's	High anal pressures; failure of IAS to relax on rectal distension	Sphincterotomy
Megarectum	Increased rectal compliance and capacity; reduced rectal sensation	Retraining
Low spinal lesion	Absent EAS responses to rectal distension and increases in intraabdominal pressure	Training
Irritable bowel syndrome	Enhanced rectal sensitivity; reduced rectal compliance; increased rectal contractility and anal relaxation in response to rectal distension	Drugs Diet Psychotherapy
Nonprolapsing hemorrhoids	Ultraslow waves	Banding
	High resting pressures	Electrocoagulation
	Failure of outermost anal canal to relax on rectal distension	Hemorrhoidectomy
Partial rectal prolapse	Very low resting pressures	Banding
	Failure of anal pressure to increase above rectal pressure during increases in intraabdominal pressure	? Post-anal repair

most cases, these muscles contract when the patient strains to defecate (Fig. 11). Some patients even have difficulty in expelling barium or saline from the rectum. This would explain why laxatives and even ileorectal anastomosis may be ineffective in some women with severe constipation.[60,61]

These observations suggest that some constipated patients are unable to inhibit the normal continence reaction whereby the activity of the EAS and puborectalis increases as the intraabdominal pressure rises. This difficulty may be related to impairment of rectal sensation. We found that the perception of a desire to defecate was blunted in young women with severe constipation,[57] whereas the perception of distension and pain during inflation of a balloon in the rectum was unaffected.

A failure of expulsion is not the only abnormality these patients exhibit; if it were, then feces would probably collect in the rectum as impacted masses. The rectum of these patients is usually empty, suggesting impaired colonic propulsion. Studies by Preston and Lennard-Jones[62] have shown that some of these patients have impaired propagated colonic pressure waves in response to laxatives.

3.2.2. Short Segment Hirschsprung's: Does It Exist?

The anus and variable lengths of the colon in children with Hirschsprung's disease are tonically contracted because the intrinsic innervation, which exhibits a predominantly inhibitory influence, has failed to develop.[63] If the condition only involves the anus, it

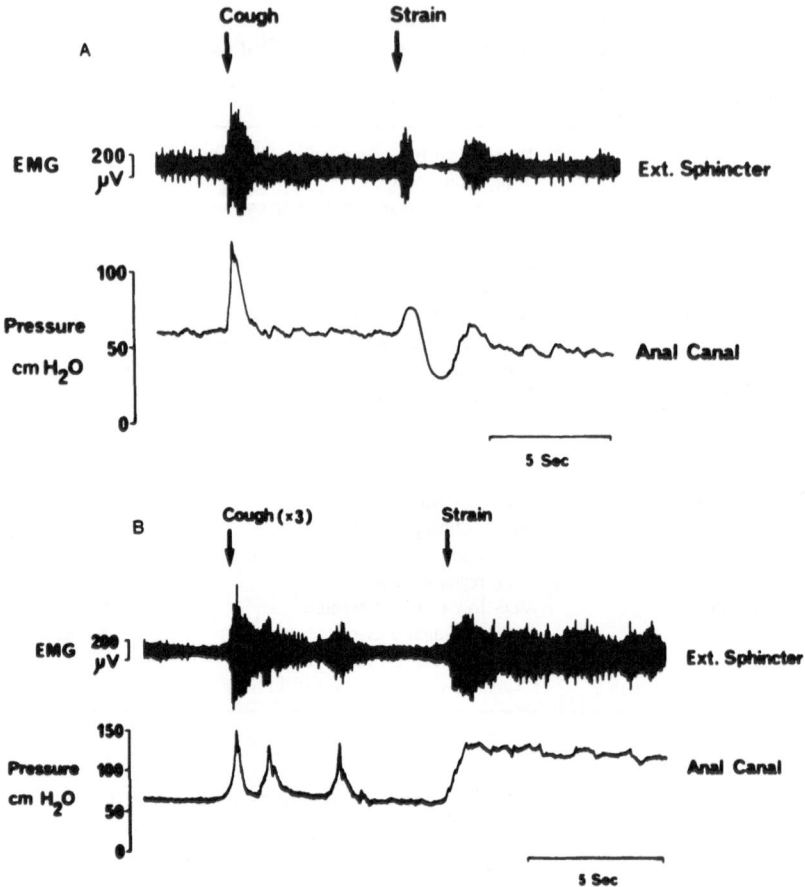

Figure 11. Recordings of anal pressure and the electrical activity of the EAS in a normal subject (A) and a constipated patient (B) during attempted defecation. Note that the pressure in the anal canal increases during straining in the constipated patient. From Preston and Lennard-Jones, Dig Dis Sci 30:413–418, 1985.

may not be diagnosed until adulthood. Thus, short segment and ultrashort segment Hirschsprung's disease are thought by some to be a significant cause of constipation in the adult.

Although the manometric characteristics of a high anal tone, which fails to relax upon rectal distension, are clear-cut, it can be very difficult to diagnose this condition with standard anal pull-through techniques or stationary sensors, positioned at the site of maximum anal pressure. One reason for this is that the relaxation of the IAS can be masked by a compensatory contraction of the EAS. When anal pressures are measured using multiple sensors spaced throughout the anal canal, it is usually possible to observe a reduction in pressure in the inner anal channels during rectal distension. In fact, we have not diagnosed a single case of short segment Hirschsprung's disease in manometric tests, carried out in 300 constipated adults. We have, however, observed failure of the sphincter

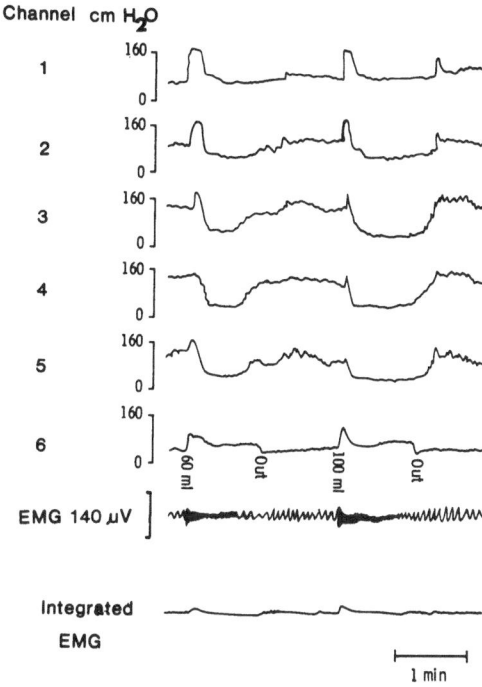

Figure 12. Recordings of anorectal pressure and the electrical activity of the EAS and IAS in patients with nonprolapsing hemorrhoids during rectal balloon distension with 60 and 100 ml of air. Channels 1–6 represent ports situated 0.5, 1.0, 1.5, 2.0, 2.5, and 4.5 cm from the anal verge. Note that there are no anal relaxations in the outermost channels, although the inner channels show normal relaxation and the IAS electrical activity is abolished.

to relax upon rectal distension, but there are other reasons for this. Patients with non-prolapsing hemorrhoids may fail to relax the outermost part of the sphincter because the high pressure in the vascular tissue buffers the decline in anal tone (Fig. 12). Patients with absent anal tone (see above) show no anal relaxation, but the pressures in these patients are much lower than those reported in Hirschsprung's disease. Finally, some patients with megarectum may require abnormally large distending volumes to stimulate the rectal tension receptors that mediate anal relaxation.

3.2.3. Fecal Impaction

Fecal impaction is common in the elderly patient and is often regarded as a conse-quence of mental and physical decline.[64] Confusion and depression may cause old people to ignore the sensation of stool in the rectum[65] until the fecal mass becomes too large to be passed. Additional factors such as immobility, weakness, and inadequate toilet facilities[65] may contribute to the situation while an increased use of laxatives may exacerbate the problem by damaging the myenteric plexus.[60]

Anal pressures are lower in elderly patients who suffer from fecal impaction than in an age- and sex-matched control group, and the sphincter relaxes normally during rectal distension with a balloon.[66] These observations indicate that the fecal impaction is not caused by outlet obstruction. Instead, the major physiological abnormality in this group appears to be a profound reduction in anal and rectal sensitivity.[67] The dulling of rectal sensitivity is almost certainly related to increases in rectal capacity and compliance,[67] so that much larger volumes are required to stimulate rectal tension receptors and induce a desire to defecate. After disimpaction, elderly patients are quite able to pass simulated stools from the rectum, once they have been told that something is there.[66] Thus, the data suggest that elderly patients become fecally impacted because they are unable to detect the presence of a fecal mass in the rectum until it is too large to be expelled.

One important and unanswered question concerns whether the insensitivity of the rectum is the initial problem that leads to retention or whether feces are retained because of immobility, confusion, and depression, and the chronic retention of feces desensitizes the rectum. It is certainly possible to train some children with fecal impaction to defecate and to acquire normal rectal sensitivity if the rectum is evacuated regularly. Can elderly patients be treated in the same manner? Perhaps the concomitant blunting of anal and perianal sensation is more in favor of a primary defect in nervous control. In fact, the combination of a weak EAS, poor anal sensation, and a hypercompliant insensitive rectum resembles the features of patients with low spinal or cauda equina lesions.[49–51,67]

3.2.4. Levator Syndrome

Some patients with severe constipation have severe perineal descent and cannot straighten out the anorectal angle. Defecography reveals that they are attempting to pass their rectal contents directly through a bulging perineum (Fig. 13). It is usually assumed

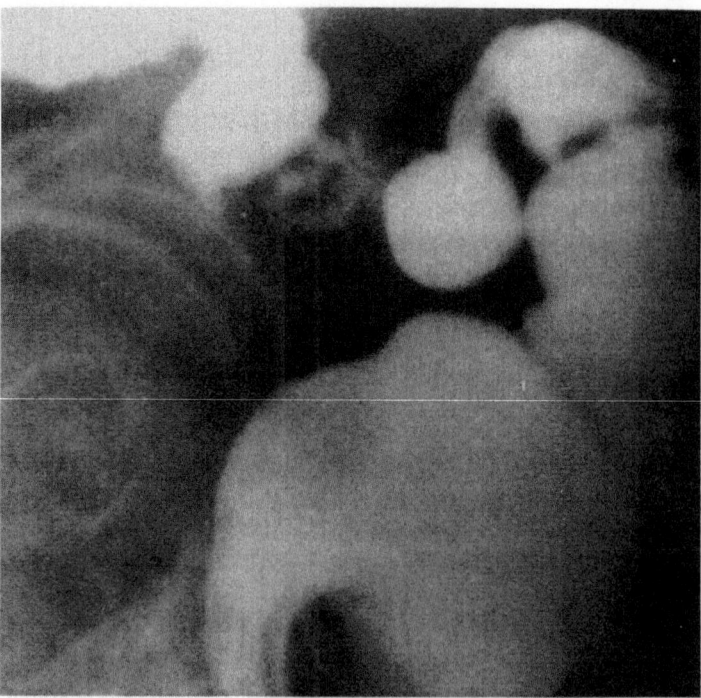

Figure 13. Perineal bulging during straining. The anal canal remains closed when the center of the levator muscle descends distally to the line drawn between the anorectal angle and the tip of the coccyx. From Kuijpers, Int. J. Colorec Dis 3:77, 1988.

that the apparently weak and abnormally descended pelvic floor is the result of prolonged straining at stool.[15] This may be a misconception; it is equally possible that the weakness of the levators may be the cause of the constipation.[54,55] During defecation, the levators contract to lift the pelvic floor while the puborectalis sling opens, the net effect being a less acute anorectal angle.[54,55] The stretching and bulging of a weak pelvic floor during attempts at defecation is associated with a contracted puborectalis and an accentuated anorectal angle. There are two possible reasons for this: first, the increased stretching of the pelvic floor may stimulate stretch receptors in the levators or in the pelvic fascia that cause a reflex contraction of the EAS and puborectalis. Second, if the puborectalis and the levators actually contract together, then if the bulk of the levators is damaged and weak, it would fail to oppose the action of the puborectalis in pulling the anorectum forwards. The crucial question is: can the levators and puborectalis function independently?

3.2.5. Hemorrhoids

Hemorrhoids are common in young women, particularly during pregnancy, but the pathogenesis of "anal piles" is not established. Contrary to popular belief, constipation does not appear to give rise to hemorrhoids. In a recent study, we found that hemorrhoids were no commoner in patients with severe slow transit constipation than they were in normal subjects, and manometric features associated with hemorrhoids were not seen in constipated patients.[68] Nevertheless, patients with nonprolapsing or first-degree hemorrhoids commonly complain of obstructed defecation.[69] Their stools are often small, require much effort to expel, and appear to stick in the anal canal behind the ballooning anal cushions. Straining exacerbates the obstruction by causing the "piles" to swell. Eventually the patient may strain so much that the hypertrophied anal cushions prolapse.[70] Although prolapse relieves the obstruction, it induces mucous discharge and pruritus ani.

Manometric studies in patients with nonprolapsing piles show abnormally high pressures.[69,71] When the rectum is distended with a balloon, the pressures in outer aspect of the anal canal remain elevated even when the IAS is relaxed and the activity of the EAS is not increased (Fig. 12).[71] This high residual pressure is probably caused by the high pressure within the vascular spaces, a distinct possibility in view of the histological resemblance of the anal cushions to erectile tissue.[70] This hypothesis is supported by direct measurements of pressures within the anal cushions; these are abnormally high in patients with hemorrhoids and show very large increases when the patient strains. Moreover, unlike normal subjects, the pressure fails to come down to normal levels for about 18–30 sec after straining (Fig. 14).

3.2.6. Partial Rectal Prolapse (Solitary Rectal Ulcer Syndrome)

Patients with partial prolapse of the anterior rectal wall into the anal canal complain of a frequent urge to defecate but an inability to expel any stool despite long periods of straining. Passage of stool does not usually abolish the urge to defecate, so that they often continue to strain. Some patients find that deflection of the anterior rectal wall with a finger in the anus may allow them to defecate. Prolonged straining may cause the rectal wall to emerge as a red berry at the anus; and it has been suggested that the very high

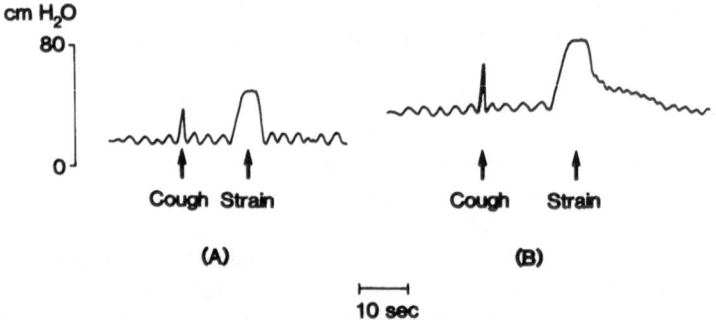

Figure 14. Pressure measurement within the anal cushions in a normal subject (A) and a patient with nonprolapsing hemorrhoids (B). Note that the patient had a higher basal pressure than the normal subject, and the pressures rose to higher levels during straining.

transmural pressures across the prolapsing rectal wall induce bleeding and mucosal disruption, resulting in a solitary rectal ulcer.[72]

Rectal prolapse, anterior mucosal prolapse, and solitary rectal ulcer are usually found in patients who have perineal descent and very low anal pressures.[73] Many of these patients complainof incontinence, and absent IAS tone is a common feature of patients with prolapse. The weak sphincters allow the rectal wall to enter the anal canal during increases in intraabdominal pressure.[73] In normal subjects, increases in intraabdominal pressure cause reflex contraction of the EAS so that the anal pressure always exceeds the rectal pressure. In patients with prolapse, the intraabdominal pressure often exceeds the anal pressure and causes the rectal wall to enter the anal canal (Fig. 15). Studies in patients with solitary rectal ulcer showed prolonged increases in activity of the puborectalis and EAS during attempts at defecation.[72] The presence of a mass in the anal canal causes an intense desire to defecate, encouraging further straining and prolapse of the rectum. Such intense straining may exacerebate the perineal descent that many of these patients have, causing further damage to the pudendal nerve and EAS weakness.

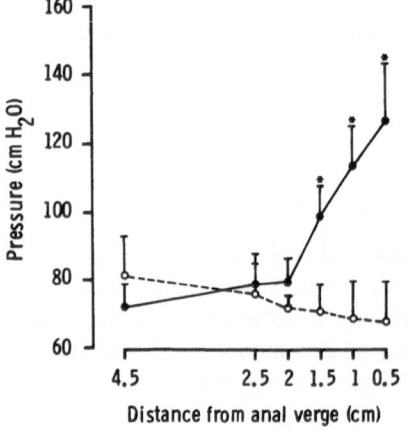

Figure 15. The highest pressures in the rectum (4.5 cm from the anal verge) and the anal canal when normal subjects (●) and patients with prolapse (○) increased their intraabdominal pressure by straining. Results are expressed as mean ± S.E.M. Note the pressure in the rectum was higher than anal pressures in patients with prolapse, while there was a pressure gradient with the highest pressure toward the outermost anal ports in normal subjects.

Partial rectal prolapse and solitary rectal ulcer are more common in women than men; this is probably because the sphincter is weaker in women than men[13,73] and can be further weakened by obstetric trauma and pudendal neuropathy following childbirth.[19,74]

3.2.7. Rectocoele

Defecography has revealed that some women appear to attempt to force the rectal contents through the posterior wall of the vagina.[75] The only way that some of these women say they can defecate is to insert their fingers into the vagina and press backwards as they strain. Unfortunately, there is no real evidence that surgical repair of the posterior vaginal wall facilitates defecation. Proctography showed that many of these patients also appear to contract the puborectalis, but fail to contract the bulk of the levators during attempts at defecation.

4. THE IRRITABLE ANORECTUM

A frequent desire to defecate, urgency, pain relieved by defecation, and a feeling of incomplete evacuation after defecation are common symptoms experienced by a large number of young women who are referred to gastroenterologists.[76] These sensations suggest a hypersensitive and irritable rectum. Some patients are able to expel small amounts of stool frequently and complain of diarrhea. Other patients, despite a frequent desire to defecate, are frustrated by their inability to expel the stool that they sense in the rectal ampulla and may complain of constipation. Their evacuation difficulties may be related to the caliber of their stools, since we found that normal subjects took longer and generated higher intraabdominal pressures to pass small solid objects than larger objects,[77] and irritable bowel syndrome patients (IBS) characteristically pass small fecal pellets.

Balloon distension of the rectum in patients who have the symptoms of IBS shows that the rectum is hypersensitive. Patients with IBS feel a desire to defecate, an urgent desire to defecate, and pain at much lower rectal volumes than normal subjects.[39] This enhanced sensitivity may be responsible for symptoms of urgency and frequent desire to defecate. Anorectal manometry reveals that a sustained relaxation of the IAS and repetitive rectal contractions are induced at lower rectal volumes in patients with IBS compared with normal subjects (Fig. 16).[39,41] Thus, the smooth muscle of the anorectum in patients with IBS readily adopts an activity that is appropriate for clearance of its contents. The rectum is not only hyperreactive to mechanical stimuli; it also reacts excessively to ingestion of a fatty meal,[78] injection of cholecystokinin,[79] and infusion of bile acids.[80]

Although these symptomatic and physiological features are typical of IBS, they can also be found in other conditions which sensitize the rectum. These include inflammatory conditions such as ulcerative colitis[40] and the solitary rectal ulcer syndrome[73] and also bile acid malabsorption. Eastwood and colleagues have shown that 14% of patients with "functional diarrhea" have impaired absorption of bile acids on the SeHCat test.[81] Bile acids are not absorbed in the colon, but are converted to secondary bile acids, which stimulate colonic motility and secretion, and sensitize the bowel. We have recently found

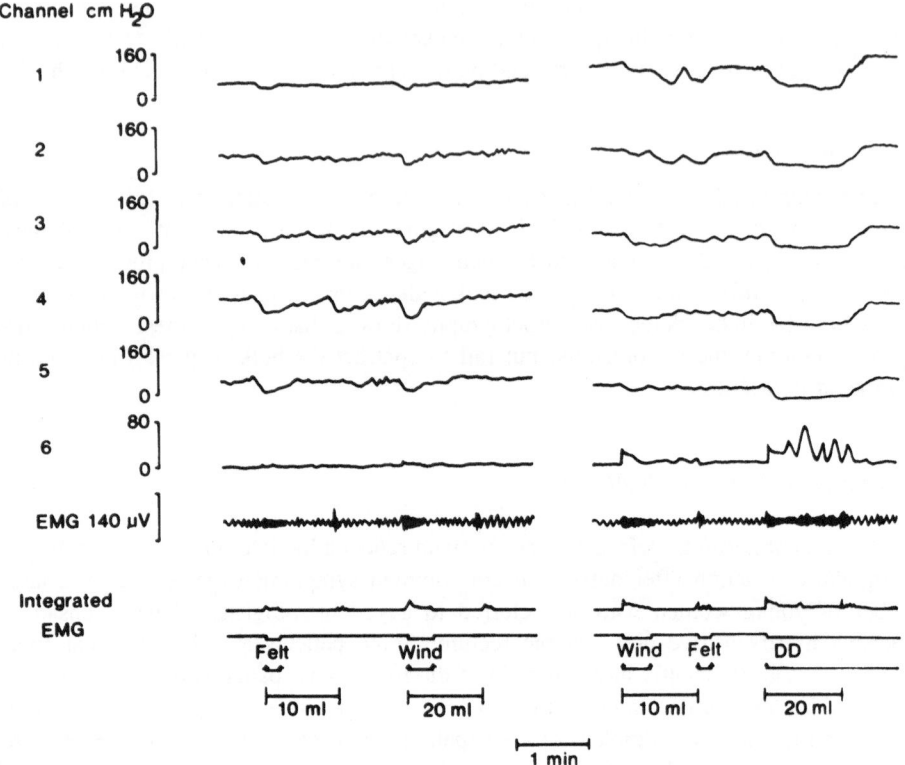

Figure 16. The anorectal pressure recorded during rectal distension in a normal subject (left) and a typical IBS patient (right). Channels 1–6 represent ports situated 0.5, 1.0, 1.5, 2.0, 2.5, and 4.5 cm from the anal verge. Note that rectal distension induces repetitive rectal contractions, sustained IAS relaxations, and a desire to defecate at lower volumes in the IBS patients.

that an enema containing as little as 1 m deoxycholic acid in 500 ml of saline could sensitize the rectum, producing all the manometeric features of IBS (Edwards and Read, unpublished observations), whereas increasing the concentration of deoxycholic acid to 3 mM generated large rectal contractions associated with severe urgency and at times incontinence.

About 25% of patients with IBS complain of episodes of incontinence.[82] These patients usually have the additional feature of EAS weakness, due often to obstetric trauma or pudendal neuropathy.[82,83] The association of large rectal contractions, rectal mucus, precipitous IAS relaxations, and a weak EAS is particularly difficult to treat.

REFERENCES

1. Bouvier M, Gonnella J: Nervous control of the internal anal sphincter of the cat. J Physiol (London) 310:457–469, 1981

2. Rayner V: Characteristic of the internal anal sphincter and the rectum of the vervet monkey. J Physiol (London) 286:383–399, 1979

3. Burleigh DE, D'Mello A: Physiology and pharmacology of the internal anal sphincter, in Henry MM, Swash M (eds): Coloproctology and the Pelvic Floor: Pathophysiology and Management. London, Butterworths, 1985, pp 22–41

4. Gonella J, Bouvier M, Blanquet F: The external innervation of motility of the small and large intestines and related sphincters. Physiol Rev 67:902–961, 1987

5. Shepherd JJ, Wright PG: The response of the internal anal sphincter in man to stimulation of the presacral nerve. Am J Dig Dis 13:421–427, 1968

6. Gibbons CP, Bannister JJ, Trowbridge EA, et al: An analysis of anal sphincter pressure and anal compliance in normal subjects. Int J Colorect Dis 1:231–237, 1986

7. Gibbons CP, Trowbridge EA, Bannister JJ, et al: The mechanics of the anal sphincter complex. J Biomech 21:601–604, 1988

8. Read MG, Read NW, Haynes WG, et al: A prospective study of the effect of haemorrhoids on sphincter function and faecal continence. Br J Surg 69:396–398, 1982

9. Whitehead WE, Orr WC, Engel BT, et al: External anal sphincter response to rectal distension: Learned response or reflex? Psychophysiology 19:57–72, 1982

10. Duthie HL, Bennett RC: The relation of sensation in the anal canal to the functional anal sphincter; a possible factor in anal continence. Gut 4:179–182, 1963

11. Swash M: Histopathology of the pelvic floor muscles, in Henry MM, Swash M (eds): Coloproctology and the Pelvic Floor. London Butterworths, 1985, pp 138–143

12. Salducci J, Planche D, Naudy B: Physiological role of the internal anal sphincter and the external anal sphincter during micturition, in Weinbeck M (ed): Motility of the Digestive Tract. New York, Raven Press, 1982, pp 513–520

13. Sun WM, Donnelly TC, Read NW: Anorectal function in normal subjects: Effect of gender. Gastroenterology 94:A449, 1988

14. Monges HO, Salducci J, Naudy B, et al: The electrical activity of the internal anal sphincter: A comparative study in man and in cats, in Christensen L (ed): Gastrointestinal Motility. New York, Raven Press, 1980, pp 495–501

15. Henry MM, Parks AG, Swash M: The pelvic floor musculature in the descending perineum syndrome. Br J Surg 69:470–472, 1982

16. Read NW, Bannister JJ: Anorectal manometry: Techniques in health and anorectal disease, in Henry MM, Swash M (eds): Coloproctology and the Pelvic Floor. London, Butterworths, 1985, pp 65–87

17. Bartolo DCC, Jarratt JA, Read NW: The use of conventional EMG to assess external sphincter neuropathy in man. J Neurol Neurosurg Psychiatry 46:1115–1118, 1983

18. Kiff ES, Swash M: Slowed conduction in the pudendal nerves in idiopathic (neurogenic) faecal incontinence. Br J Surg 71:614–616, 1984

19. Snooks SJ, Swash M, Setchell M, et al: Injury to innervation of pelvic floor sphincter musculature in childbirth. Lancet 2:546–550, 1984

20. Bartolo DCC, Read NW, Jarratt JA, et al: The role of partial denervation of the puborectalis in idiopathic faecal incontinence. Br J Surg 70:664–667, 1983

21. Read NW, Bartolo DCC, Read MG: Differences in anal function in patients with incontinence to solids and in patients with incontinence to liquids. Br J Surg 71:39–42, 1984

22. Schuster MM: The riddle of the sphincters. Gastroenterology 69:249–262, 1979

23. Parks AG: Anorectal incontinence. Proc R Soc Med 68:681–690, 1975

24. Schiller LRA, Santa Ana CA, Schmulen AC, et al: Pathogenesis of faecal incontinence in diabetes mellitus. N Engl J Med 207:1666–1671, 1982

25. Sun WM, Donnelly TC, Read NW: Impaired internal sphincter function in patients with idiopathic faecal incontinence. Gastroenterology 94:A449, 1988

26. Aaronson I, Nixon HH: A clinical evaluation of anorectal pressure studies in the diagnosis of Hirschsprung's disease. Gut 13:138–146, 1972

27. Faverdom C, Dornic C, Ahran P: Quantitative analysis of anorectal pressures in Hirschsprung's disease. Dis Colon Rectum 24:422–427, 1981

28. Meunier P, Marechal JM, Jaubert de Beaujeu M: Recto-anal pressures and rectal sensitivity in childhood constipation. Gastroenterology 77:330–336, 1979

29. Lennard-Jones JE: Constipation: Pathophysiology, clinical features and treatment, in Henry MM, Swash M (eds): Coloproctology and the Pelvic Floor: Pathophysiology and Management. London, Butterworths, 1985, pp 350–375

30. Baldi F, Ferrarini F, Corinadesi R, et al: Function of the internal anal sphincter and rectal sensitivity in idiopathic constipation. Digestion 24:14–22, 1982

31. Frenckner B, Ihre T: Influence of autonomic nerves on the internal anal sphincter in man. Gut 17:306–312, 1976

32. Dent J, Dodds WJ, Friedman RH, et al: Mechanism of gastroesophageal reflux in recumbent asymptomatic human subjects. J Clin Invest 65:256–267, 1980

33. Dodds WJ, Dent J, Hogan JF, et al: Mechanism of gastroesophageal reflux in patients with reflux esophagitis. N Engl J Med 307:1547–1552, 1982

34 Sun WM, Donnelly TC, Read, NW: Inappropriate transient anal relaxations: A cause of faecal incontinence? Gastroenterology 94:A449, 1988

35. Callaghan RP, Dixon HH: Megarectum: Physiological observation. Arch Dis Child 39:153–157, 1984

36. Denny-Brown D, Robertson EG: An investigation of the nervous control of defaecation. Brain 58:256–310, 1935

37. Meunier P, Mollard P: Control of the internal anal sphincter (manometric study with human subjects). Pflügers Arch 370:233–239, 1977

38. Naudy B, Planche D, Monges B, et al: Relaxations of the internal anal sphincter elicited by rectal distension and extrarectal distension in man, in Roman C (ed): Gastrointestinal Motility. Lancaster, MTP Press, 1983, pp 451–458

39. Sun WM, Read NW: Anorectal manometry and rectal sensation in patients with the irritable bowel syndrome. Gastroenterology 94:A450, 1988

40. Rao SSC, Holdsworth CD, Read NW: Anorectal sensitivity and reactivity in patients with ulcerative colitis. Gastroenterology 93:1270–1275, 1987

41. Whitehead WE, Engel BT, Schuster MM: Irritable bowel syndrome. Dig Dis Sci 25:404–413, 1980

42. Gonella J, Bouvier M, Blanquet F: Extrinsic nervous control of motility of small and large intestine and related sphincters. Physiol Rev 67:903–961, 1987

43. Schiller LR, Santa Ana CA, Schmulen AC, et al: Pathogenesis of faecal incontinence in diabetes mellitus. N Engl J Med 307:1666–1671, 1982

44. Sasaki H, Yoshida T, Noda K, et al: Urethral pressure profiles following radical hysterectomy. Obstet Gynecol 59:101–104, 1982

45. Wald A, Tunuguntla AK: Anorectal sensation dysfunction in faecal incontinence and diabetes mellitus. N Engl J Med 310:1282–1287, 1984

46. Buser WD, Miner PB Jr: Delayed rectal sensation with faecal incontinence; successful treatment using anorectal manometry. Gastroenterology 91:1186–1191, 1986

47. Guttmann L: Spinal Cord Injuries. London, Blackwell, 1976

48. Melzak J, Porter NH: Studies of the reflex activity of the external sphincter ani in spinal man. Paraplegia 1:277–296, 1964

49. Frenckner B: Function of the anal sphincters in spinal man. Gut 16:638–644, 1975

50. Wheatley IC, Hardy KJ, Dent J: Anal pressure studies in spinal patients. Gut 18:488–490, 1977

51. White JC, Verlot MG, Ehrentheil O: Neurogenic disturbances of the colon and their investigation by the colonmetrogram. Ann Surg 112:1042–1056, 1940

52. Phillips SF, Edwards DAW: Some aspects of anal continence and defaecation. Gut 6:396–405, 1965

53. Parks AG, Porter NH, Melzack J: Experimental study of the reflex mechanism controlling the muscles of the pelvic floor. Dis Colon Rectum 5:507–414, 1962

54. Finlay IG, Brown D: Posterior pelvic floor repair—A new surgical approach for outlet obstruction constipation (obstructed defaecation). Gut 29: A1546, 1988

55. Brown DC, Lauder JC, Poon FW, et al: Outlet obstruction constipation (obstructed defaecation)—a failure of the posterior pelvic floor? Gut 29:A734, 1988

56. Preston DM, Lennard-Jones JE: Severe chronic constipation of young women: Idiopathic slow transit constipation. Gut 27:41–48, 1986

57. Read NW, Timms JM, Barfield LJ, et al: Impairment of defaecation in young women with severe constipation. Gastroenterology 90:53–60, 1986

58. Barnes PRH, Lennard-Jones JE: Balloon expulsion from the rectum in constipation of different types. Gut 25:1049–1052, 1985

59. Barnes PRH, Hawley PR, Preston DM, et al: Experience of posterior division of the puborectalis muscle in the management of chronic constipation. Br J Surg 72:475–477, 1985

60. Smith B: Effect of irritant purgatives on the myenteric plexus in man and the mouse. Gut 9:139–143, 1968

61. Kamm MA, Hawley PR, Lennard-Jones JE: Outcome of colectomy for severe idiopathic constipation. Gut 29:969–973, 1988

62. Preston DM, Lennard-Jones JE: Pelvic colon motility and response to intraluminal bisacodyl in slow transit constipation. Dig Dis Sci 30:289–294, 1985

63. Wood JD: Physiology of the enteric nervous system, in Johnson LR (ed): Physiology of the Gastrointestinal Tract, ed 2. New York, Raven Press, 1987, pp 67–109

64. Brocklehurst JC, Khan MY: A study of fecal stasis in old age and the use of Dorbanex in its prevention. Gerontol Clin 11:293–300, 1969

65. Banks S, Marks, IN: The aetiology, diagnosis and treatment of constipation and diarrhoea in geriatric patients. S Afr Med J 51:509–414, 1977

66. Read NW, Abouzekry L, Read MG, et al: Anorectal function in elderly patients with faecal impaction. Gastroenterology 89:959–966, 1985

67. Read NW, Abouzekry L: Why do patients with faecal impaction have faecal incontinence? Gut 27:283–287, 1986

68. Gibbons CP, Bannister JJ, Read NW: Role of constipation and anal hypertonia in the pathogenesis of haemorrhoids. Br J Surg 75:656–660, 1988

69. Sun WM, Donnelly TC, Read NW, et al: Is the high anal pressure in patients with haemorrhoids of vascular origin? Gastroenterology 94:A449, 1988

70. Thompson WHF: The nature of haemorrhoids. Br J Surg 62:542–555, 1975

71. Hancock BD: Internal sphincter and the nature of haemorrhoids. Gut 18:651–6756, 1976

72. Womack NR, Williams NS, Holmfield JHM, et al: Pressure and prolapse—the cause of solitary rectal ulceration. Gut 28:1228–1233, 1987

73. Bartolo DCC, Read NW, Jarratt JA, et al: Differences in anal sphincter function and clinical presentation in patients with pelvic floor descent. Gastroenterology 85:68–75, 1983

74. Sun WM, Read NW: Rectal prolapse, anterior mucosal prolapse, solitary rectal ulcer: Are they caused by rectal herniation through a weak sphincter? Gut 28:A1363, 1987

75. Mahieu P, Pringot J, Bodart P: Defaecography II. Contribution to the diagnosis of defaecation disorders. Gastrointest Radiol 9:253–261, 1984

76. Manning AP, Thompson WG, Heaton KW, et al: Towards positive diagnosis of irritable bowel. Br Med J 2:653–654, 1978

77. Bannister JJ, Davison P, Timms JM, et al: Effect of the stool size and consistency of defaecation. Gut 28:1246–1250, 1987

78. Sullivan MA, Cohen S, Snape WJ: Colonic myoelectrical activity in the irritable bowel syndrome; effect of eating and anticholinergics. N Engl J Med 298:878–883, 1978

79. Harvey RF, Read AE: Effect of cholecystokinin on colonic motility and symptoms in patients with irritable bowel syndrome. Lancet 1:1–3, 1973

80. Taylor I, Basu P, Hammond P, et al: Effect of bile acid perfusion on colonic motor function in patients with irritable bowel syndrome. Gut 21:843–847, 1980

81. Merrick MV, Eastwood MA, Ford MJ: Is bile and malabsorption under diagnosed? An evaluation of accuracy of diagnosis by measurement of SeHCAT retention. Br Med J 290:665–668, 1985

82. Cann A, Read NW, Brown C, et al: The irritable bowel syndrome (IBS) relationship of disorders in the transit of a single solid meal to symptom patterns. Gut 24:405–411, 1983

83. Cann PA, Read NW, Holdsworth CD, et al: The role of loperamide and placebo in the management of the irritable bowel syndrome (IBS). Dig Dis Sci 29:239–247, 1984

15

Functional Bowel Disturbances in Childhood

Paul E. Hyman

Children or their advocates may seek medical attention for a number of functional gastrointestinal disorders. Most functional disorders of childhood are relatively transient, and specific for a particular stage of development. Several are common conditions, frequently managed successfully by practicing pediatricians and only occasionally requiring more extensive evaluations and interventions by the pediatric gastroenterologist. These conditions include infantile colic, chronic nonspecific diarrhea of infancy, and recurrent abdominal pain of childhood. Two other conditions—constipation and gastroesophageal reflux—are found in adults, but require a different diagnostic approach and treatment for children. One functional disorder is serious but rare: chronic intestinal pseudoobstruction. In common, all of the conditions to be discussed (with the possible exception of infantile colic) are considered to be related to disturbances in gastrointestinal motility.

The emphasis of this chapter is on the physiology of these disorders. Such an emphasis is consistent with the intent of this volume, but may not reflect the weight of investigation into the psychological aspects of several functional gastrointestinal disorders of childhood. Indeed, authorities have suggested that psychological factors trigger infantile colic, recurrent abdominal pain of childhood, and encopresis in susceptible individuals. The major morbidity from those three physically benign conditions is psychological, with the potential for disturbing both the affected child and the family. For a more extensive discussion of the psychological aspects of functional bowel disorders in childhood, the reader is referred elsewhere.[1,2]

1. INFANTILE COLIC

Colic is characterized by intractable fussing without failure to thrive in an otherwise healthy infant. Typical paroxysms are apparently unprovoked, unexplained periods of

Paul E. Hyman • Division of Pediatric Gastroenterology, Harbor–UCLA Medical Center, Torrance, California 90502.

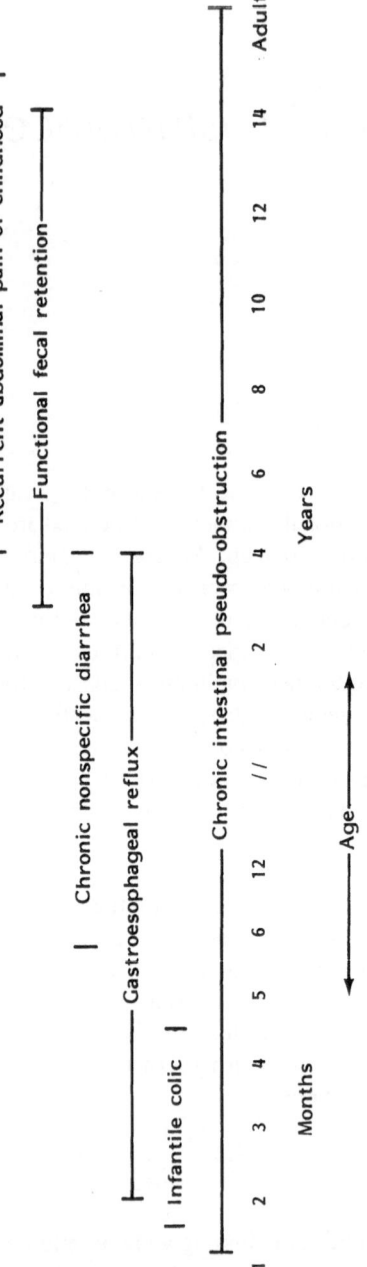

Figure 1. Age of vulnerability to functional bowel disorders in childhood.

inconsolable crying, frequently occurring at the same time of day, most often during the late afternoon or evening. The onset of infantile colic occurs after the first weeks of life, and is limited in duration to the first 3–4 months of life (see Fig. 1). Variable features include high-pitched screaming, a tense abdomen, flatulence, borborygmi, and facial flushing. Although it is assumed that the symptoms are a response to abdominal pain, there is little objective evidence that affected infants actually have physical discomfort. Infantile colic is common, with an incidence of about 10% of all infants, but as high as 23% in one study.[3] Sex and birth order do not appear to influence the occurrence of colic.

1.1. Pathophysiology

Over the years a heterogeneous group of physiological and psychological disturbances have been suggested as causes for colic. "Intestinal hyperperistalsis" and "colonic spasms" were postulated to be responsible for colic by pediatricians making behavioral observations, but gastrointestinal motor function was not evaluated objectively. Central nervous system,[4] endocrine,[5,6] and immune[7,8] functions have been indicted as responsible for intestinal symptoms, but arguments for each of these have been unconvincing. For example, several investigators provided data supporting a role for cow milk allergy in the pathogenesis of colic.[7–9] However, Thomas et al., in a study of a large population of infants, found no greater prevalence of colic in infants fed commercial formula than in those fed human milk.[10] Further, stool concentrations of α_1-antitrypsin and hemoglobin were not increased in infants with colic. These data suggest that in colic there is no mucosal injury. It seems likely that milk allergy may cause abdominal pain during infancy, but milk allergy is responsible for only a minority of infants diagnosed as having "infantile colic." Colic the symptom must be differentiated from infantile colic the diagnosis. A number of organic conditions of infancy may cause the symptom, but the diagnosis is dependent upon finding the symptom without evidence of organic disease and in the absence of "failure-to-thrive."

1.2. Treatment

Remedies suggested for the treatment of colic lack satisfactory documentation of efficacy. In recent studies, sedatives and antispasmodics,[11,12] and simethicone[13] failed to change the symptoms of infantile colic. Because colic is a physically benign and relatively brief affliction, the best treatment appears to be providing emotional support and effective reassurance to the parents of the affected infant. Taking the time for a detailed history and scrupulously complete physical examination, preferably with the anxious parent in attendance, is a necessity. When the physician is confident of the diagnosis and prognosis, that confidence must be communicated to the parent. Communication is best achieved by an unhurried explanation in a relaxed setting.

2. GASTROESOPHAGEAL REFLUX

Gastroesophageal reflux is defined as gastric contents moving into the esophagus. All infants "spit up" or "wet burp," so, by definition, all infants have gastroesophageal reflux. In a few infants, gastroesophageal reflux has consequences that result in clinical symptoms. Morbidity from gastroesophageal reflux occurs in six areas: (1) recurrent vomiting and failure to thrive, (2) aspiration pneumonia, (3) apnea, (4) asthma, (5) esophagitis, (6) psychosocial adaptation.

2.1. Pathophysiology

Lower esophageal sphincter (LES) pressures gradually increase over the first weeks of life to reach adult values within a month or two.[14,15] In one carefully designed study of infants, reflux episodes were associated most often (54% of episodes) with increased intraabdominal pressure, compared to 34% associated with inappropriate LES relaxation, and only 12% associated with prolonged decreases in sphincter pressure.[16] During infancy, normal crying increases intraabdominal pressure, and predisposes to reflux. Children with moderate to severe symptoms related to reflux frequently have delayed gastric emptying,[17,18] as well as decreased amplitude of peristaltic contractions of the esophagus, and an increased number of nonperistaltic contractions.[18]

Infants with bronchopulmonary dysplasia, a chronic lung disease associated with prematurity and treatment with mechanical ventilation and high concentrations of oxygen, seem at especially high risk for developing clinically important gastroesophageal reflux (Fig. 2). Reflux episodes may be increased because of the inspiratory effort of these infants, which results in intraabdominal pressure that is often higher than that of the LES. Infants with recurrent pneumonia and reflux often had increased sphincter pressure.[19] There is speculation that refluxed material may be aspirated in small quantities, contributing to the lung disease. Repeated regurgitation may result in loss of calories sufficient to cause retarded growth. Finally, larger amounts of refluxed material may occlude the airway, and cause apnea.[20]

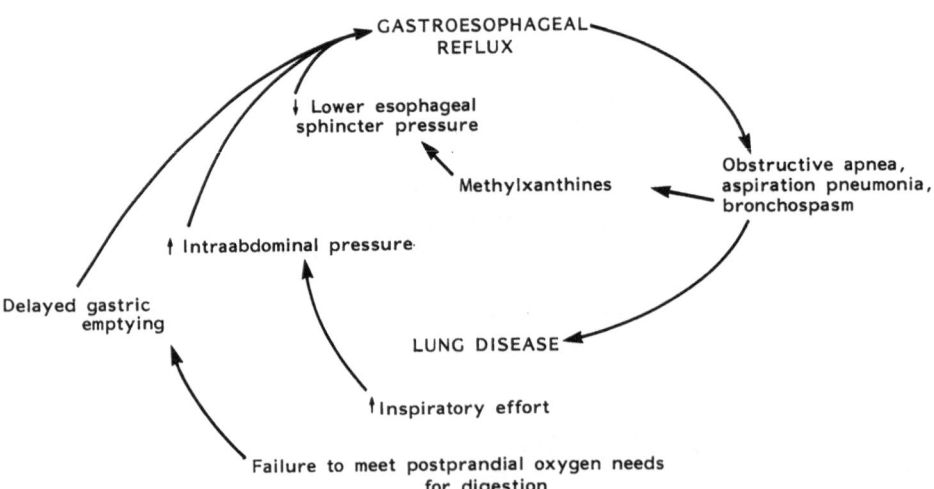

Figure 2. Possible interrelationships between gastroesophageal reflux and chronic lung disease in infants with bronchopulmonary dysplasia.

Gastroesophageal reflux may contribute to the pathogenesis of asthma in some affected children.[21] As in bronchopulmonary dysplasia, a predisposition to increased episodes of reflux may exist because of an increased intraabdominal pressure with inspiration. Hypotheses to explain the mechanism for reflux-induced asthma in children include: (1) bronchospasm due to acid reflux stimulation of receptors located in the esophagus, hypopharynx, or trachea, (2) protein sensitivity to minute quantities of aspirated material, and (3) aspiration of large amounts of refluxed material.

Gastroesophageal reflux and apnea are seldom associated.[22] However, in unusual but well-documented instances, apnea occurred in direct temporal relationship with prolonged reflux episodes, and disappeared following an effective fundoplication.[23] Intraesophageal perfusion of acid induced apnea in a group of preterm infants.[24] The possibility that gastroesophageal reflux may induce apnea has stimulated discussion that reflux may be one of the causes of the sudden infant death syndrome.[25]

Children with severe psychomotor retardation have a high incidence of complications related to gastroesophageal reflux, including esophagitis, recurrent regurgitation, and repeated aspiration pneumonia.[26,27]

2.2. Diagnosis

A history suggesting the possibility of reflux-related complications should stimulate investigations to confirm or refute the clinical impression.

Barium studies of the esophagus, stomach, and small bowel are useful in assessing the possibility of anatomic abnormalities.

Esophageal manometry does not assess reflux, but may prove useful when there is clinical evidence of reflux. Only a few infants will have LES pressures less than 10 mm Hg, but these infants are less likely to improve with time, have a higher incidence of reflux-related complications, and are more likely than those with normal sphincter pressures to require fundoplication.[28,29] Abnormalities in the contraction of the esophageal body are common when esophagitis is present.[30]

The best test for esophagitis is endoscopy and biopsies.[31] Children may develop Barrett's esophagus.[32,33]

Intraesophageal pH monitoring is helpful in defining the temporal relationships between reflux events and symptoms such as wheezing or cough in patients with asthma, and apnea in patients with a history of "missed" sudden infant death syndrome. Studies repeated before and after drug treatment or fundoplication provide an objective evaluation of the efficacy of the intervention.

Isotope scintiscanning of ^{99m}Tc sulfur colloid added to a meal may be most useful for evaluating two different reflux-related issues: assessment of the rate of gastric emptying and the documentation of pulmonary aspiration of refluxed material.

2.3. Treatment

Regurgitation in the first months of life can usually be reduced by a combination of careful feeding technique and appropriate postprandial positioning. Excessive air swallowing and overfeeding may predispose to regurgitation. Recent studies have shown that reflux is minimized in infants placed prone with the head elevated 30°.[34] Postprandial reflux was reduced by decreasing the volume of the feeding.[35]

Thickening the feedings by adding dry cereal did not alter the episodes of reflux monitored by intraesophageal pH electrode in infants with failure-to-thrive.[36] However, in another study the total volume of emesis decreased with thickened feedings, due to a decrease in vomiting episodes, suggesting that thickened feedings may be an effective treatment for replacing the calories lost in regurgitated gastric contents.[37] Feedings were thickened by the addition of 15 ml dry rice cereal to each 30 ml of infant formula. This addition did not affect the volume of the feeding, but increased the caloric density from 0.67 to 1.0 kcal/ml.

Esophagitis associated with reflux in infants requires a more aggressive management which usually includes drug therapy. Bethanechol, which in infants increased LES pressure[38] without altering gastric emptying,[39] was the first drug used commonly for treatment of reflux in children.[40,41] Metoclopramide, which increased LES pressure [42] and improved gastric emptying,[39] is used frequently. Disadvantages to metoclopramide include a low therapeutic index, with frequent central nervous system side effects, and the development of tolerance within several months of initiation. Cisapride appears to be an effective drug for treating esophagitis in infants,[43] and has had a more acceptable safety profile than metoclopramide. Elimination of acid would seem to be another means of treating esophagitis. Antacids have been advocated,[44] but the amount and frequency of administration necessary for efficacy are not well studied in children. Similarly, the use of histamine H_2 receptor antagonists seems reasonable for treating peptic esophagitis, but there is little experience to document drug efficacy in children.[45]

Fundoplication is an effective means of treating the complications of gastroesophageal reflux which do not respond to medical management.[46] When reflux and apnea are temporally associated, fundoplication to prevent all reflux episodes may be lifesaving. In severely retarded children, fundoplication with feeding gastrostomy improves the supportive care by decreasing aspiration pneumonias and providing a simple means for nutritional support. Fundoplication has been advocated for the treatment of intractable asthma associated with reflux,[47] and for bronchopulmonary dysplasia.[48] Prior to surgical intervention, it is prudent to assess esophageal motility and gastric emptying, since severe motility disorders presenting as gastroesophageal reflux may cause even more troublesome symptoms after fundoplication.[49]

3. CHRONIC NONSPECIFIC DIARRHEA (TODDLER'S DIARRHEA)

Between the ages of 6 months and 3 years some children develop a pattern of defecation that is different from their earlier pattern, and distinctly bothersome to the child's caregivers. Watery stools, often containing identifiable bits of undigested matter from the preceding meal, run over the diaper material three to six times daily. There are no associated signs or symptoms; the affected children do not complain, and if left alone will grow and develop normally. Chronic nonspecific diarrhea (CNSD) ends with toilet training. No one knows if the stool pattern changes.

Although there is often a history of acute gastroenteritis immediately preceding the onset of chronic diarrhea, there is no evidence to support an infectious cause for CNSD. Stools are watery, but the strict definition for diarrhea in childhood—20 g/kg per day—is not achieved. Blood, leukocytes, and reducing substances (reflecting carbohydrate malabsorption) are not found in the stool.

3.1. Pathophysiology

CNSD has been attributed to abnormally fast gastrointestinal transit, and to an exaggerated gastrocolonic reflex.[50,51] The migrating motor complex (MMC) persisted in affected infants, but was replaced by a fed pattern in control infants when both groups were given an intraduodenal glucose meal.[52] These results were interpreted to suggest that feeding did not inhibit the MMC in affected infants, and that persistent cycling moved food along rapidly, resulting in the clinical condition. In another study, a high-fat diet decreased the number of stools in affected children.[53] It was suggested that increases in dietary fat delayed gastric emptying and thus slowed overall transit. It also seems possible that dietary fat may be an effective inducer of a fed motility pattern.

3.2. Diagnosis

The diagnosis is strongly sugggested by the history. Confirmation of the diagnosis may require a number of negative laboratory studies, including stool examinations for ova and parasites, blood, white cells, reducing substances, and fecal fat. A normal erythrocyte sedimentation rate indicates the absence of serious inflammatory disease.

Occasionally confounding the diagnosis, a reduced rate of growth, termed "failure-to-thrive," is due to the misuse of elimination diets.[54] In many cases, the level of parental anxiety is directly proportional to the number of dietary manipulations and medical interventions.

3.3. Treatment

CNSD is a benign condition. Parents must be provided with effective reassurance that their child is in no danger, and that no specific treatment is necessary. In fact, a high-fat diet, high-fiber diet, aspirin, and loperamide[55] have all been effective in some patients. However, symptomatic improvement is variable, and it seems most prudent to avoid prescribing medication which may reinforce sick-role behavior, and instead to educate the family about the natural history of the disorder.

4. CONSTIPATION AND FUNCTIONAL FECAL RETENTION

Constipation occurs when the stool is hard. Passage of stool may be a cause of pain or blood-streaked bowel movements. Constipation may be best defined by the character of the stool and by associated symptoms, and not necessarily by the length of time between bowel movements.

Constipation is a common complaint, found in 3% of all pediatric outpatient visits.[56] Ten to twenty percent of children referred to pediatric gastroenterologists have a disorder of defecation. Infants have little difficulty with chronic constipation because they make no attempt to exercise control over the act of defecation. With time, a child begins to perceive the urge to defecate, and to develop skill to temporarily withhold the passage of stool. Toilet training reinforces this retentive function as part of socially acceptable behavior.

Children with constipation may develop an exaggerated retentive response to the urge to defecate. If defecation is painful, a child may consciously or unconsciously decide to postpone defecation. When such decisions are consistent and chronic, the result is functional fecal retention, one of the most common conditions seen by the pediatric gastroenterologist.[57] The clinical features of functional fecal retention include: (1) passage of enormous stools at intervals of 1 week or more, (2) retentive posturing, (3) overflow fecal soiling, (4) irritability, (5) abdominal pain, (6) anorexia. A dramatic disappearance of symptoms 2–6 follows immediately the passage of the big, hard stool.

Encopresis or fecal soiling, the deposition of stool in places that are socially inappropriate, may be a consequence of functional fecal retention, neural and muscular disorders causing incontinence, or psychiatric disorders.

The physician must differentiate the unusual causes of chronic constipation from functional fecal retention, and then provide an effective means of treatment.

Up to 10% of children at some time require medical attention because of constipation that is most often due to diet and a constitutional tendency to make hard stools. Hirschsprung's disease occurs in 1 in 5000 births, but the majority of those affected present in infancy with diarrheal disease or bowel obstruction. Only a few patients with Hirschsprung's disease present with chronic constipation. The chances that a constipated child has short segment Hirschsprung's disease are small.

The many unusual causes of chronic constipation and fecal soiling in childhood are listed in Ref. 58.

4.1. Physiology of Childhood Constipation and Functional Fecal Retention

Evidence for a genetic influence on the incidence of childhood constipation was found in twin studies.[59] Monozygotic twins were concordant for constipation four times more often than dizygotic twins. In monozygotic twins the coincidence of constipation was 70%. Further support for hereditary tendency to constipation came from the discovery that specific dermatoglyphic (fingerprint) patterns correlate with the childhood onset of constipation and abdominal pain.[60]

Largely because of ethical problems in studying healthy infants and children, there is limited knowledge of normal colonic motility and absorption during childhood. Therefore, a number of studies investigating children with chronic constipation are of interest but remain inconclusive with respect to elucidating the underlying physiological basis for constipation. It seems likely that a number of different abnormal motility patterns are associated with the clinical condition. A clear classification system is not yet developed.

Sigmoid and rectal motility indices were decreased in children with constipation and encopresis compared to healthy control children.[61] This finding might be explained by the reversible dilation of the lumen that occurs in children with chronic fecal retention, since the motility indices reverted to normal in posttreatment testing.

There are alterations in anorectal sensation and motor function in children with functional fecal retention, but the findings are inconsistent, with different children having different abnormalities. In one study, 97% of constipated children had at least one abnormal test of defecation dynamics.[62] However, results have been contradictory. One group found decreased resting anal sphincter pressure in encopretic children.[63,64] Another described failure of the anus to relax, termed *anal achalasia*.[65] Other investigators studying children without encopresis found no difference between control and constipated subjects in resting anal sphincter pressure.[66] Others suggested that encopretic children frequently had hypertensive anal sphincter pressures.[67,68] Thresholds of internal sphincter relaxation have been higher than[67,68] or similar to[61,69] control children. Conscious rectal sensitivity threshold, the perception of distension, decreased in some studies[58,67] but not in others.[69,70] These variable results suggest that many of the differences in anorectal function are a response to rather than cause of encopresis, or a result of rather than cause of rectal dilation.

Another possible mechanism, for functional fecal retention is an inability to properly relax the involved musculature. In one study, 43% of encopretic boys had external sphincter contractions during attempted defecation.[69] Electromyography showed that 42% of encopretic children did not relax the pelvic floor muscles during defecation.[71]

The persistence of decreased rectal conscious sensitivity threshold following clinical improvement and return of the rectum to normal size in some patients,[70] and the inability to defecate water-filled balloons following treatment in others,[72] suggest that in some patients organic abnormalities of anorectal function may be a predisposing factor for constipation and encopresis.

4.2. Diagnosis

A history including the criteria for the functional fecal retention syndrome is usually sufficient to make invasive diagnostic tests unnecessary. In school-age boys with encopresis of short duration, it is often possible to obtain a history of a specific incident prompting the retentive behavior. Hirschsprung's disease is not associated with encopresis or retentive posturing. During the physical examination of a patient with functional fecal retention, it is common to palpate a midline fecal mass, sometimes extending superior to the umbilicus.

Rectal suction biopsies are the most effective means of establishing the absence of ganglion cells, and so the diagnosis of Hirschsprung's disease in infants and toddlers.[73] Biopsies are often unnecessary when the history and physical examination are characteristic for functional fecal retention. In "short segment" Hirschsprung's disease, the barium enema may not show an unrelaxed segment and transition zone distal to dilated bowel. Anal manometry may be useful in problem cases, since the rectoanal inhibitory reflex is present in functional fecal retention, but absent in Hirschsprung's disease.

4.3. Treatment

There are effective treatments for functional fecal retention emphasizing the physical aspects,[58] psychological aspects,[74] or biofeedback.[75] One attractive plan emphasizes patient and parent education, and allows the affected child to assume responsibility for relearning good bowel habits. Education consists of explanations of normal defecation and of fecal accumulation and the mechanism for encopresis in the patient. These explanations are accomplished with the aid of simple, sequential diagrams (Fig. 3) using words that the child understands. These patients often believe that they alone suffer from encopresis, and are greatly relieved to learn how common, how well understood, and how benign their condition is. Next, they are ready to relearn normal bowel habits. In the agreement or contract, each participant has specific duties and responsibilities. The physi-

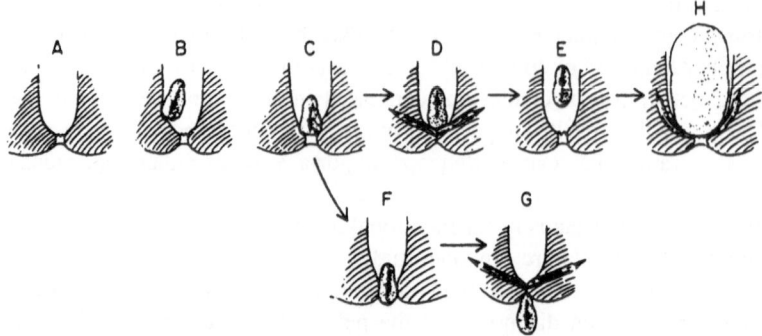

Figure 3. Events during defecation, fecal continence, and chronic fecal retention. (A) The rectum is empty. The levator ani holds the sides of the anal canal in apposition. (B) Stool enters the rectum. (C) Distension of the rectal wall causes transient reflex relaxation of the internal sphincter, allowing stool to contact the anoderm. There is a conscious awareness of the stool. (D) In order to preserve continence, the levator ani contracts, shifting the stool cephalad. (E) Stool is no longer in contact with the rectoanal junction. The defecatory urge decreases. (F) Relaxation of the levators opens the anal canal. The accompanying Valsalva maneuver increases intrarectal pressure, propelling stool down the anal canal. (G) Contraction of the pelvic floor follows the passage of stool through the canal. (H) If a patient responds to the defecatory urge by repeatedly withholding ("C" to "D"), a fecal mass accumulates in the rectum. As the puborectalis muscles fatigue, the anal sphincter becomes incompetent, resulting in leakage of liquid stool. The patient resorts to retentive posturing, attempting to preserve continence by contracting the gluteal and pelvic floor muscles. From Fleisher.[57]

cian provides continuing guidance and prescribes mineral oil (1 to 4 ounces daily, depending initially on the size of the child and modified as indicated by the clinical response) to keep the stool soft. The parent agrees to provide the child with encouragement and private time in the family lavatory, usually for 15 min after breakfast and dinner, and to make sure mineral oil is available. The patient agrees to take the mineral oil as prescribed and to respond appropriately to the urge to defecate and not to hold back. Close follow-up is essential to provide reinforcement, because compliance is critical for early success.

It appears that in the majority of cases, chronic childhood constipation tends to resolve with age.[76]

5. FUNCTIONAL RECURRENT ABDOMINAL PAIN

Functional recurrent abdominal pain of childhood is defined by a history of at least three paroxysmal episodes of abdominal pain severe enough to limit activity, occurring over a period longer than 3 months.[77] Recurrent abdominal pain is common, affecting 10 to 15% of 5- to 13-year-old children.[77,78]

5.1. Pathophysiology

A major question is whether functional recurrent abdominal pain of childhood is the latency age equivalent of the irritable bowel syndrome of adulthood. In a preliminary report, eight children with functional recurrent abdominal pain underwent antroduodenal manometry while not acutely ill.[79] When compared to healthy adolescent controls, the patients had higher mean amplitude of contractions, and more frequent episodes of shorter duration of phase III of the MMC. These results might be expected to cause a decrease in transit time in affected children, but in a different study, the transit of carmine red was delayed in children with recurrent abdominal pain compared to controls.[80] A study evaluating colonic motility described increases in the amplitude and duration of contractions in the sigmoid and rectum following prostigmine in 78% of children with recurrent abdominal pain, but in only 33% of control patients.[81]

In contrast to those who suspect a motility disorder as the cause of functional recurrent abdominal pain, others believe that malabsorption of lactose is the cause,[82,83] with subsequent distension of the bowel producing pain. Other investigators were unable to confirm lactose intolerance as a cause of pain,[84–86] but the possibility exists that lactose or some other undigested carbohydrate such as sorbitol[87] may be resposible for abdominal pain in some patients. In only one study did increases in breath hydrogen coincide with episodes of abdominal pain.[88]

5.2. Diagnosis

A diagnosis of functional recurrent abdominal pain is based on careful history, physical examination, and prudent laboratory testing. Because there is no specific clinical marker for the condition, a program of routine follow-up is a necessity. Rarely there may be an evolution of signs and symptoms after the initial diagnosis.

Patients present between 5 and 13 years of age, with a peak at 9–10 years. The pain is most often crampy (50%) or dull and aching (30%), and is periumbilical (61%) or epigastric (16%).[89] In general, the farther from the umbilicus, the more likely the pain is not functional. The duration of pain is variable: less than 30 min in 22%, 30–60 min in 20%, 1–3 hr in 43%, and over 3 hr or "continuous" in 15%. The pain occurs daily in 51%, more than once weekly in 24%, and less than once weekly in 25%. The pain is not related to meals, bowel movements, position, activity, and does not awaken the patient from sleep. Headaches (25–50%), pallor (40%), nausea (40%), anorexia (35%), constipation (34%), fatigue (26%), dizziness (25%), and vomiting (22%) frequently accompany the pain.[89] Nearly half of the patients have immediate family members who complain of abdominal pain. Medical illness was present in 56% of mothers and 44% of fathers of children with recurrent abdominal pain. In two-thirds of the patients, the onset of pain was associated with an important psychosocial event such as a death in the family, divorce, or starting a new school.

The physical examination is normal. There may be some tenderness to deep palpation of the abdomen, especially in the lower quadrants. There is no blood in the stool.

Provided that the history and physical examination are consistent with functional rather than organic causes of the pain, the initial laboratory tests include a complete blood count and erythrocyte sedimentation rate, urinalysis and culture, and stool examinations for blood, leukocytes, and ova and parasites. In pubescent females a pregnancy test should be included.

About 1 in 20 patients presenting with recurrent abdominal pain has an organic cause for the pain. Half of the organic causes are due to disorders of the genitourinary system such as ovarian cysts, pelvic inflammatory disease, nephrolithiasis, hydronephrosis, and pyelonephritis. Some of the gastrointestinal conditions which may cause recurrent abdominal pain include peptic ulcer disease, inflammatory bowel disease, lactose intolerance, functional fecal retention, and parasites (for a complete differential diagnosis see Refs. 89–91).

5.3. Treatment

When the physician is confident of the diagnosis of functional recurrent abdominal pain, that confidence must be communicated to the patient and the parents. The most important aspect of treatment involves returning the affected child to "normal" functioning for age. To accomplish this task it is necessary to provide an explanation for and a plan to cope with the pain. Parents are asked to accept the pain as real, just like a headache or leg cramp: each of these is painful, but not a disease. Disease has been excluded by the history, physical examination, and laboratory tests. The child must return to regular daily activity, including school. Often the most effective way of dealing with pain is to allow the child to lie down in a quiet, dimly lit room until the pain is gone. The school authorities are asked to stop sending the child home, but instead to allow respite in "the nurse's office" until the episode passes.

If a specific triggering psychosocial stress was identified, its relationship to the pain should be explained. Stresses such as school problems or changing peer relationships may be reversible. The physician must be ready to provide continuing support, and reassurance that he or she will be available if the symptoms change.

Dietary changes are controversial. One study concluded that a high-fiber diet resulted in symptomatic improvement in children with recurrent abdominal pain.[92] Several investigators demonstrated lactose intolerance in a higher percentage of affected patients than in control children,[82,83] and a trial of lactose elimination has been advocated for patients failing a lactose breath test with 1 g/kg lactose.[91]

There are no data on treatment of functional recurrent abdominal pain with drugs.

The outcome of children with functional recurrent abdominal pain has been observed longitudinally in several studies.[93–96] In 30 to 50% of patients, symptoms resolve 2 to 6 weeks after diagnosis. However, it appears that Apley's warning[90] that "little bellyachers become big bellyachers" may be accurate. Half of those followed had functional complaints as adults, and half of these complaints were of abdominal pain. Patients who were male, who had a father or mother with functional abdominal pain, who had onset of symptoms before 6 years of age, or duration of symptoms longer than 6 months prior to evaluation were more likely than others to have symptoms persist into adult life.[96]

6. CHRONIC INTESTINAL PSEUDOOBSTRUCTION

Chronic intestinal pseudoobstruction occurs when a child has signs or symptoms of bowel obstruction without evidence of an obstructing lesion. Such a broad definition reflects an evolving understanding of the diverse group of disorders comprising pseudoobstruction. Diagnoses such as Hirschsprung's disease, prolonged postoperative ileus, and gastroparesis of prematurity are distinguished from primary pseudoobstruction by specific clinical or pathological features, but may be thought of as secondary intestinal pseudoobstruction or pseudoobstruction associated with another disorder.

Intestinal pseudoobstruction is the clinical expression of a wide spectrum of disturbances in gut motility which differ in pathophysiology, genetics, natural history, and response to treatment. Pseudoobstruction occurs as a primary disease, or as a secondary manifestation of other diseases which may transiently (e.g., hypothyroidism) or permanently (e.g., scleroderma or amyloid) alter bowel motility. Primary pseudoobstruction may be congenital, or present at any time during life. The onset may be precipitous or slowly progressive. Symptoms may progress, persist, or remit spontaneously. The disease may affect small or large areas of the gastrointestinal tract, from esophagus to rectum. Assorted patterns of Mendelian inheritance occur, with variable expressivity within families. The histopathology of the affected bowel may reveal immaturity, inflammation, or noninflammatory degeneration of either nerve or muscle.[97]

Because of this heterogeneity, many similar patients have been described under different terms, such as "functional intestinal obstruction,"[98] "chronic idiopathic intestinal pseudoobstruction,"[99] "hereditary hollow visceral myopathy,"[100] "familial visceral myopathy,"[101] "familial megaduodenum,"[102] or "megacystis intestinal hypoperistalsis syndrome."[103]

6.1. Clinical Disease in Childhood

Eighty-seven children were reported in a survey study of patients with intestinal pseudoobstruction.[104] The onset of symptoms occurred at birth in 22%, within the first month in 43%, and by the end of the first year in 65%. The most common symptoms were abdominal distension (85%), constipation (60%), vomiting (59%), failure to gain weight (27%), and diarrhea (25%). Urological abnormalities, most often a dilated, atonic bladder, were found in 33%.

Two-thirds of the children were diagnosed at the time of exploratory laparotomy. Full thickness biopsies and histological techniques including silver stains[105] were helpful in differentiating abnormalities of nerve from smooth muscle. Radiological studies were frequently abnormal but nonspecific. Gastroesophageal reflux (52%), generalized dilation of the small bowel (36%), delayed gastric emptying of barium (26%), and megaduodenum (24%) were the most common abnormalities.

Esophageal manometry performed in only 16% of patients was abnormal in all. Anal manometry was normal in those tested. No other motility tests of the small bowel or colon were done in this series of patients.

Dietary management with total parenteral nutrition (15%), a combination of enteral and parenteral support (31%), or dietary restrictions only (44%) was effective in 90%. Ten percent of the children required surgery to reverse intractable pain or massive secretory diarrhea. Metoclopramide and bethanechol had no effects on symptoms in 57 patients tested. Antibiotics were useful for treating diarrhea due to bacterial overgrowth. However, after treatment of bacterial overgrowth with antibiotics, many patients developed constipation and abdominal distension that were more uncomfortable and incapacitating than the diarrhea had been.

In several small series,[106,107] and numerous case reports[103,108-113] there are detailed descriptions of individual infants and kindreds with pseudoobstruction.

6.2. Pathophysiology

Patterns of fasting and postprandial antroduodenal motility have been established for normal infants.[114,115] In normal subjects the fasting record consists of the MMC, which cycles in four "phases" about ever 2 hr. During phase III of the MMC, repetitive, high-amplitude contractions move slowly from proximal to distal, sweeping undigestible luminal contents and bacteria out of the small bowel. In the absence of an effective phase III, bacterial overgrowth is common.[116] The MMC is interrupted by meals. The fed pattern consists of variable-amplitude intermittent contractions, some of which are propagated. In the absence of contractions following meals, the luminal contents do not move, and fluid pools in the lumen. Patients develop distension, nausea, and vomiting. In the largest series to date, 13 children with chronic intestinal pseudoobstruction had qualitative abnormalities in either fasting or fed antroduodenal contractions or both.[117] The abnormalities in antroduodenal motility were found when the patients were not acutely ill, and, in several instances, when colonic (not small bowel) motility was the main clinicial concern. Antroduodenal motility was studied in several smaller series of children.[113,118] In three case reports, serosal electromyography revealed arrhythmias in gastric and/or small bowel electrical activity in children with pseudoobstruction.[119,120]

Previous studies have shown an assortment of distinctive abnormalities of the myenteric plexus and smooth muscle in many but not all children with chronic intestinal pseudoobstruction.[97] It is apparent that studies such as antroduodenal manometry and electromyography complement pathological studies, and provide another means of differentiating many of the conditions which present with the clinical signs and symptoms of pseudoobstruction.

6.3. Treatment

The medical management of pseudoobstruction consists of optimizing nutritional support, minimizing the risks of infectious complications, and treating any underlying or complicating illness. Drug therapy, except in rare cases, has not restored function. Cisapride, which improved the symptoms of pseudoobstruction in a group of adults,[121] increased the postcibal motility index of children with pseudoobstruction.[117] Further studies are required to determine if clinical improvement will attend the objective manometric improvement changes in children treated with cisapride.

Surgery has been useful not only in the diagnosis of pseudoobstruction, but also in the elective, palliative treatment of some children and adults with disabling and medically unresponsive symptoms.[122–124] Pitt et al.[123] advocated elective gastrostomy as a means of decompressing a distended bowel whenever symptoms of pain or vomiting occurred. This group found that hospitalizations were decreased in number following venting enterostomies. Restrictions or bypass of the affected bowel are frequently unsuccessful. With time, disease may recur in portions of the bowel thought to be unaffected at the time of surgery.

Surgery should be reserved for those patients incapacitated by symptoms that are unmangeable by medical means. Infants may require emergency surgery not only for diagnosis but for decompression of a dilated bowel which impairs diaphragmatic movement and compromises respiration.

In the near future looms the possibility of bowel transplantation. Well-nourished patients with primary pseudoobstruction may be superior candidates for transplantation, when compared to adults with a short bowel from atherosclerotic vascular or inflammatory bowel diseases. Bowel transplantation will provide the possibility for total correction of pseudoobstruction.

REFERENCES

1. Apley J, MacKeith R, Meadow R: The Child and His Symptoms. Oxford, Blackwell, 1978
2. Schaefer CE, Millman HL, Levine GF (eds): Therapies for Psychosomatic Disorders in Children. San Francisco, Jossey–Bass, 1979, pp 41–112
3. Paradise JL: Maternal and other factors in the etiology of infantile colic. J Am Med Assoc 197:123–131, 1966
4. Brazelton TB: Crying in infancy. Pediatrics 29:579–588, 1962
5. Clark RL, Ganis FM, Bradford WL: A study of the possible relationship of progesterone to colic. Pediatrics 31:65–71, 1963
6. Lothe L, Ivarsson SA, Lindberg T: Motilin, vasoactive intestinal polypeptide and gastrin in infantile colic. Acta Paediatr Scand 76:316–320, 1987
7. Lothe L, Lindberg T, Jakobsson I: Cow's milk formula as a cause of infantile colic: A double-blind study. Pediatrics 70:7–10, 1982
8. Jakobsson I, Lindberg T: Cow's milk proteins cause infantile colic in breast-fed infants: A double-blind crossover study. Pediatrics 71:268–271, 1983
9. Harris MJ, Petts V, Penny R: Cow's milk allergy as a cause of infantile colic: Immunofluorescent studies of jejunal mucosa. Aust Paediatr J 13:276–280, 1977
10. Thomas DW, McGilligan K, Eisenberg LD, et al: Infantile colic and type of milk feeding. Am J Dis Child 141:451–453, 1987
11. Hwang CP, Danielsson B: Dicyclomine hydrochloride in infantile colic. Br Med J 291:1014, 1985
12. O'Donovan JC, Bradstock AS: The failure of conventional drug therapy in the management of infantile colic. Am J Dis Child 133:999–1001, 1979
13. Danielsson B, Hwang CP: Treatment of infantile colic with surface active substance (simethicone). Acta Paediatr Scand 74:446–450, 1985
14. Gryboski JD, Thayer WR, Spiro HM: Esophageal motility in infants and children. Pediatrics 31:382–388, 1963
15. Boix-Ochoa J, Canals J: Maturation of the lower esophagus. J Pediatr Surg 11:749–752, 1979
16. Werlin S, Dodds W, Hogan W, et al: Mechanisms of gastroesophageal reflux in children. J Pediatr 97:244–249, 1980
17. Hillimeier AC, Lange R, Seashore J, et al: Delayed gastric emptying in infants with gastroesophageal reflux. J Pediatr 98:190–194, 1981
18. Hillimeier AC, Grill RB, McCallum R, et al: Esophageal and gastric motor abnormalities in gastroesophageal reflux during infancy. Gastroenterology 84:741–746, 1983
19. Herbst J, Book LS, Johnson P, et al: The lower esophageal sphincter in gastroesophageal reflux. J Clin Gastroenterol 1:119–123, 1979
20. Menon AP, Schefft GL, Thach BT: Apnea associated with regurgitation in infants. J Pediatr 106:625–629, 1985
21. Berquist W, Rachelefsky G, Kadden M, et al: Gastroesophageal reflux, associated recurrent pneumonia, and chronic asthma in children. Pediatrics 68:29–34, 1981
22. Walsh JK, Farrell MK, Keenan WJ: Gastroesophageal reflux in infants: Relation to apnea. J Pediatr 99:197–199, 1981
23. Berquist WE, Ament ME: Upper GI function in sleeping infants. Am Rev Respir Dis 131 (suppl.):S26–S29, 1985
24. Herbst JJ, Book LS, Minton SD: Gastroesophageal reflux causing respiratory distress and apnea in newborn infants. J Pediatr 95:763–769, 1979

25. Herbst J, Book LS, Bray P: Gastroesophageal reflux in the "near miss" sudden infant death syndrome. J Pediatr 92:73–75, 1978
26. Cadman D, Richards J, Feldman W: Gastroesophageal reflux in severely retarded children. Dev Med Child Neurol 20:95–97, 1978
27. Sondheimer JM, Morris BA: Gastroesophageal reflux among severely retarded children. J Pediatr 94:710–714, 1979
28. Euler AR, Ament ME: Value of esophageal manometric studies in the gastroesophageal reflux of infancy. Pediatrics 59:58–60, 1977
29. Hyams JS, Ricci A, Litchner AM: Clinical and laboratory correlates of esophagitis in young children. J Pediatr Gastroenterol Nutr 7:52–56, 1988
30. Cucchiara S, Staiano A, DiLorenzo C, et al: Esophageal motor abnormalities in children with gastroesophageal reflux and peptic esophagitis. J Pediatr 108:907–910, 1986
31. Biller JA, Winter HS, Grand RJ, et al: Are endoscopic changes predictive of histologic esophagitis in children? J Pediatr 103:215–218, 1985
32. Dahms BB, Rothstein FC: Barrett's esophagus in children: A consequence of chronic gastroesophageal reflux. Gastroenterology 86:318–323, 1984
33. Hassall E, Weinstein WM, Ament ME: Barrett's esophagus in childhood. Gastroenterology 89:1331–1337, 1984
34. Orenstein SR, Whittington PF: Positioning for prevention of infant gastroesophageal reflux. J Pediatr 103:534–537, 1983
35. Sutphen JL, Dillard VL: Effect of feeding volume on early postcibal gastroesophageal reflux in infants. J Pediatr Gastroenterol Nutr 7:185–188, 1988
36. Bailey DJ, Andres JM, Danek GD, et al: Lack of efficacy of thickened feeding as a treatment for gastroesophageal reflux. J Pediatr 110:187–189, 1987
37. Orenstein SR, Magill HL, Brooks P: Thickening of infant feedings for therapy of gastroesophageal reflux. J Pediatr 110:181–186, 1987
38. Sondheimer JM, Arnold GL: Early effect of bethanechol on the esophageal motor function of infants with gastroesophageal reflux. J Pediatr Gastroenterol Nutr 5:47–51, 1986
39. Hyman P, Abrams C, Dubois A: Effect of metoclopramide and bethanechol on gastric emptying in infants. Pediatr Res 19:1029–1032, 1985
40. Euler AR: Use of bethanechol for the treatment of gastroesophageal reflux. J Pediatr 96:321–324, 1980
41. Strickland AD, Chang JHT: Results of treatment of gastroesophageal reflux with bethanechol. J Pediatr 103:311–313, 1983
42. Machida HM, Forbes DA, Gall DG, et al: Metoclopramide in gastroesophageal reflux of infancy. J Pediatr 112:483–487, 1988
43. Cucchiara S, Staiano A, Capozzi C, et al: Cisapride for gastroesophageal reflux and peptic oesophagitis. Arch Dis Child 62:454–457, 1987
44. Sutphen JL, Dillard VL, Pipan ME: Antacid and formula effects on gastric acidity in infants with gastro esophageal reflux. Pediatrics 78:55–57, 1986
45. Cucchiara S, Staiano A, Romaniello G, et al: Antacids and cimetidine treatment for gastroesophageal reflux and peptic esophagitis. Arch Dis Child 59:842–847, 1984
46. Fonkalsrud EW, Berquist W, Vargas J, et al: Surgical treatment of the gastroesophageal reflux syndrome in infants and children. Am J Surg 154:11–18, 1987
47. Berquist WE, Rachelefsky GS, Kadden M, et al: Gastroesophageal reflux-associated recurrent pneumonia and chronic asthma in children. Pediatrics 68:29–35, 1981
48. Giuffre RM, Rubin S, Mitchell I: Antireflux surgery in infants with bronchopulmonary dysplasia. Am J Dis Child 141:648–651, 1987
49. Hyman PE: Absent postprandial duodenal motility in a child with cystic fibrosis: Correction of the symptoms and manometric abnormality with cisapride. Gastroenterology 90:1274–1279, 1986
50. Davidson M, Wasserman R: The irritable colon of childhood (chronic nonspecific diarrhea syndrome). J Pediatr 69:1027–1038, 1966
51. Davidson M, Sleisinger MH, Almy TP, et al: Studies of distal colonic motility in children. II. Propulsive activity in diarrheal states. Pediatrics 17:820–830, 1956
52. Fenton TR, Harries JT, Milla PJ: Disordered intestinal motility: A rational basis for toddler diarrhea. Gut 24:897–903, 1983

53. Cohen SA, Hendricks KM, Mathis RK, et al: Chronic nonspecific diarrhea: Dietary relationships. Pediatrics 64:402–407, 1979
54. Lloyd-Still JD: Chronic diarrhea of childhood and the misuse of elimination diets. J Pediatr 95:10–14, 1979
55. Hamdi I, Dodge JA: Toddler diarrhea: Observations on the effects of aspirin and loperamide. J Pediatr Gastroenterol Nutr 4:362–365, 1985
56. Levine MD: Children with encopresis: A descriptive analysis. Pediatrics 56:412–416, 1975
57. Fleisher DR: Diagnosis and treatment of disorders of defecation in children. Pediatr Ann, November 1976
58. Silverman A, Roy CC: Pediatric Clinical Gastroenterology. St. Louis, Mosby, 1983, pp 398–399
59. Bakwin H, Davidson M: Constipation in twins. Am J Dis Child 121:179–181, 1971
60. Gottlieb SH, Schuster MM: Dermatoglyphic (fingerprint) evidence for a congenital syndrome of early onset constipation and abdominal pain. Gastroenterology 91:428–432, 1986
61. Loening-Baucke VA, Younoszai MK: Effect of treatment on rectal and sigmoid motility in chronically constipated children. Pediatrics 73:199–205, 1984
62. Meunier P, Louis D, deBeaujeu MJ: Physiologic investigation of primary chronic constipation in children: Comparison with barium enema study. Gstroenterology 87:1351–1357, 1984
63. Loening-Baucke VA, Younoszai MK: Abnormal anal sphincter response in chronically constipated children. J Pediatr 100:213–218, 1982
64. Loening-Baucke VA: Abnormal rectoanal function in children recovered from chronic constipation and encopresis. Gastroenterology 87:1299–1304, 1984
65. Davidson M, Bauer CH: Studies of distal colonic motility in children. iv. Achalasia of the distal rectal segment despite presence of ganglia in the myenteric plexuses of this area. Pediatrics 21:746–761, 1958
66. Corazziari E, Cucchiara S, Staiano A, et al: Gastrointestinal transit time, frequency of defecation, and anorectal manometry in healthy and constipated children. J Pediatr 106:379–382, 1985
67. Meunier P, Marechal JM, deBeaujeu MJ: Rectoanal pressures and rectal sensitivity in chronic childhood constipation. Gastroenterology 77:330–336, 1979
68. Arhan P, Devroede G, Jehannin B, et al: Idiopathic disorders of fecal continence in children. Pediatrics 71:774–779, 1983
69. Wald A, Chandra R, Gabel S, et al: Anorectal manometric and continence studies in childhood encopresis. Dig Dis Sci 29:554–559, 1984
70. Loening-Baucke VA: Sensitivity of the sigmoid colon and rectum in children treated for chronic constipation. J Pediatric Gastroenterol Nutr 3:454–459, 1984
71. Loening-Baucke VA: Pelvic floor dysfunction in encopresis. Gastroenterology 88:1479–1483, 1985
72. Loening-Baucke VA: Factors responsible for persistence of childhood constipation. J Pediatr Gastroenterol Nutr 6:915–922, 1987
73. Venugopal S, Mancer K, Shandling B: The validity of rectal biopsy in relation to morphology and distribution of ganglion cells. J Pediatr Surg 16:433–437, 1981
74. Taitz LS, Wales JKH, Urwin OM, et al: Factors associated with outcome in management of defecation disorders. Arch Dis Child 61:472–477, 1986
75. Wald A, Chondra R, Gabel S, et al: Evaluation of biofeedback in childhood encopresis. J Pediatr Gastroenterol Nutr 6:554–558, 1987
76. Abrahamian FP, Lloyd-Still JD: Chronic constipation in childhood: A longitudinal study of 186 patients. J Pediatr Gastroenterol Nutr 3:460–467, 1984
77. Apley J, Naish N: Recurrent abdominal pains: A field survey of 1,000 school children. Arch Dis Child 33:165–170, 1958
78. Oster J: Recurrent abdominal pain, headache, and limb pains in children and adolescents. Pediatrics 50:429–436, 1972
79. Pineiro-Carrero VM, Andres JM, Davis RH, et al: Altered gastroduodenal motility in children with recurrent abdominal pain. Gastroenterology 90:1586, 1986 abstr
80. Dinson SB: Transit time related to clinical findings in children with recurrent abdominal pain. Pediatrics 47:666–668, 1972
81. Kopel FB, Kim IC, Barbero G: Comparison of rectosigmoid motility in normal children, children with RAP, and children with ulcerative colitis. Pediatrics 39:539–545, 1967
82. Barr RG, Levine MD, Watkins JB: Recurrent abdominal pain of childhood due to lactose intolerance. A prospective study. N Engl J Med 300:1449–1452, 1979

83. Liebman WM: Recurrent abdominal pain in children: Lactose and sucrose intolerance, a prospective study. Pediatrics 64:43–45, 1979
84. Lebenthal E, Rossi TM, Nord KS, et al: Recurrent abdominal pain and lactose absorption in children. Pediatrics 67:828–832, 1981
85. Blumenthal I, Kelleher J, Littlewood JM: Recurrent abdominal pain and lactose intolerance in childhood. Br Med J 282:2013–2014, 1981
86. Wald A, Chandra R, Fisher SE, et al: Lactose malabsorption in recurrent abdominal pain of childhood. J Pediatr 100:65–68, 1982
87. Hyams JS: Sorbitol intolerance: An unappreciated cause of functional gastrointestinal complaints. Gastroenterology 84:30–33, 1983
88. Kneepkens CMF, Bijleveld CMA, Vonk RJ, et al: The daytime breath hydrogen profile in children with abdominal symptoms and diarrhoea. Acta Paediatr Scand 75:632–638, 1986
89. Silverman A, Roy CC: Pediatric Clinical Gastroenterology. St. Louis, Mosby, 1983, pp 418–430
90. Apley J: The Child with Abdominal Pain. Oxford, Blackwell, 1964
91. Boyle JT: Functional abdominal pain in childhood, in Cohen S, Soloway RD (eds): Functional Disorders of the Gastrointestinal Tract. Edinburgh, Churchill Livingstone, 1987, pp 189–209
92. Feldman W, McGrath P, Hodgson C, et al: The use of dietary fiber in the management of simple, childhood, idiopathic, recurrent abdominal pain. Am J Dis Child 139:1216–1218, 1985
93. Magni G, Pierri M, Donzelli F: Recurrent abdominal pain in children: A long term follow-up. Eur J Pediatr 146:72–74, 1987
94. Christensen MF, Mortensen O: Long-term prognosis in children with recurrent abdominal pain. Arch Dis Child 50:110–114, 1975
95. Stickler GB, Murphy DB: Recurrent abdominal pain. Am J Dis Child 133:486–490, 1979
96. Apley J, Hale B: Children with recurrent abdominal pain: How do they grow up? Br Med J 3:7–8, 1973
97. Krishnamurthy S, Schuffler MD: Pathology of neuromusclar disorders of the small intestine and colon. Gastroenterology 93:610–639, 1987
98. Rack FJ, Crouch WL: Functional intestinal obstruction in the premature newborn infant. J Pediatr 40:579–583, 1982
99. Maldonado JE, Gregg JA, Green PA, et al: Chronic idiopathic intestinal pseudoobstruction. Am J Med 49:203–213, 1970
100. Faulk DL, Anuras S, Gardner D: A familial visceral myopathy. Ann Intern Med 89:600–606, 1987
101. Schuffler MD, Lowe MC, Bill AH: Studies of idiopathic intestinal pseudoobstruction: I. Heredity hollow visceral myopathy: Clinical and pathological studies. Gastroenterology 73:327–338, 1977
102. Law DH, Eyck EAT: Familial megaduodenum and megacystis. Am J Med 33:911–921, 1962
103. Berdon WE, Baker DH, Blanc WA, et al: Megacystis-microcolon intestinal hypoperistalsis syndrome: A new cause of intestinal obstruction in the newborn—report of radiologic findings in five newborn girls. Am J Roentgenol 126:957–964, 1976
104. Vargas JH, Ament ME: Chronic intestinal pseudo-obstruction syndrome (CIPS) in pediatrics—Results of a North American survey. Clin Res 35:210A, 1987
105. Smith B: The Neuropathology of the Alimentary Tract. London, Edward Arnold, 1972
106. Anuras S, Mitros FA, Soper RT, et al: Chronic intestinal pseudo-obstruction in young children. Gastroenterology 91:62–70, 1986
107. Byrne W, Cipel L, Euler A, et al: Chronic idiopathic intestinal pseudoobstruction syndrome in children: Clinical characteristics and prognosis. J Pediatr 90:585–589, 1977
108. Tanner MS, Smith B, Lloyd J: Functional intestinal obstruction due to deficiency of argyrophil neurons in the myenteric plexus. Arch Dis Child 51:837–841, 1976
109. Wiswell T, Rawlings J, Wilson J, et al: Megacystis-microcolon-intestinal hypoperistalsis syndrome. Pediatrics 63:805–808, 1979
110. Waterfall WE, Cameron OG, Sarna SH, et al: Disorganized electrical activity in a child with idiopathic intestinal pseudo-obstruction. Gut 22:77–83, 1981
111. Puri P, Lake BD, Gorman F, et al: Megacystis-microcolon-intestinal hypoperistalsis syndrome: A visceral myopathy. J Pediatr Surg 18:64–69, 1983
112. Anuras S, Mitros FA, Milano A, et al: A familial visceral myopathy with dilatation of the entire gastrointestinal tract. Gastroenterology 90:385–390, 1986
113. Tomomasa T, Itoh Z, Koizumi T, et al: Manometric study on the intestinal motility in a case of megacystis-microcolon-intestinal hypoperistalsis syndrome. J Pediatr Gastroenterol Nutr 4:307–310, 1985

114. Tomomasa T, Itoh Z, Koizumi T, et al: Non-migrating rhythmic activity in the stomach and duodenum of neonates. Biol Neonate 48:1–9, 1985

115. Tomomasa T, Hyman PE, Itoh K, et al: Gastroduodenal motility in neonates: Response to human milk compared to cow milk formula. Pediatrics 80:434–438, 1987.

116. VanTrappen G, Janssens J, Hellemans J: The interdigestive motor complex of normal subjects and patients with bacterial overgrowth of the small intestine. J Clin Invest 59:1158–1166, 1977

117. Hyman PE, McDiarmid SV, Napolitano JA, et al: Antroduodenal motility in children with chronic intestinal pseudo-obstruction. J Pediatr 112:899–905, 1988

118. Boige N, Cargill G, Mashako L, et al: Trimebutine induced phase III-like activity in infants with intestinal motility disorders. J Pediatr Gastroenterol Nutr 6:548–553, 1987

119. Telander RL, Morgan KG, Kreolen DL, et al: Human gastric atony with tachygastria and gastric retention. Gastroenterology 75:497–501, 1978

120. Cucchiara S, Janssens J, VanTrappen G, et al: Gastric electrical dysrhythmias (tachygastria and tachyarrhythmia) in a girl with chronic intractable vomiting. J. Pediatr. 108:264–267, 1986

121. Camilleri M, Brown ML, Malagelada JR: Impaired transit of chyme in chronic intestinal pseudo-obstruction connection by cisapride. Gastroenterology 91:619–626, 1986

122. Schuffler MD, Deitch EA: Chronic idiopathic intestinal pseudo-obstruction: A surgical approach. Ann Surg 192:752–761, 1980

123. Pitt HA, Mann LL, Berquist WE, et al: Chronic intestinal pseudo-obstruction: Management with total parenteral nutrition and a venting enterostomy. Arch Surg 120:614–618, 1985

124. Shaw A, Shaffer HA, Anuras S: Familial visceral myopathy: The role of surgery. Am J Surg 150:102–108, 1985

16

Surgical Approach to Functional Bowel Disease

Sean J. Mulvihill and Haile T. Debas

1. INTRODUCTION

Nowhere in surgery must greater caution be exercised nor a more deliberate course of action taken than in the management of motility disorders of the gastrointestinal tract. The main reason for this is that their pathophysiology is poorly understood and appropriate corrective surgical procedures are, therefore, difficult to design. Indeed, poorly conceived surgical decisions can result in sequelae that are worse than the original disease. The success of surgical treatment varies with different disorders of motility. Best results are obtained when a defined, well-understood problem, such as Zenker's diverticulum or achalasia, is treated. The worst results can be expected in such poorly understood conditions as biliary dyskinesia, chronic idiopathic intestinal obstruction, or postgastrectomy syndromes. The indication for surgery in such disorders must be either extreme functional impairment or the development of complications that must be corrected. Surgery is usually considered only after all conservative measures fail.

In the discussion below, we shall identify what is known of the pathophysiology and outline the indications and the principles of surgical treatment. The following conditions will be discussed: (1) motility disorders of the esophagus, including achalasia, diffuse spasm, and diverticula; (2) motility disorders of the stomach, including tachygastria and postgastrectomy syndromes; (3) biliary dyskinesia; (4) chronic and acute forms of intestinal pseudoobstruction; and (5) colon dysmotility syndromes, including diverticular disease, chronic constipation, and Hirschsprung's disease.

Sean J. Mulvihill and Haile T. Debas • Department of Surgery, University of California–San Francisco, San Francisco, California 94143.

2. MOTILITY DISORDERS OF THE ESOPHAGUS

Esophageal motor disorders are rare but can be debilitating. Their pathophysiology is poorly understood but is thought to be due to disruption of the neurohumoral muscular control of peristalsis and the functions of the upper and lower esophageal sphincters. Detailed discussion of pathophysiology is given in Chapter 7 by Richter. In this section, we will focus on three conditions: diffuse esophageal spasm, achalasia, and esophageal diverticula.

2.1. Diffuse Esophageal Spasm

2.1.1. Pathophysiology and Clinical Presentation

Diffuse esophageal spasm is a condition in which normal peristalsis in the body of the esophagus is absent. Instead, there is simultaneous contraction of high amplitude over a variable length of the esophagus, usually the distal third. The resting pressure of the esophageal sphincter may be normal or elevated, but its pattern of relaxation is usually normal.[1,2] Variants of diffuse esophageal spasm that have been described include the nutcracker esophagus and isolated elevation of the lower esophageal sphincter pressure.[3] Diffuse esophageal spasm may evolve into achalasia in 3–5% of patients.[4] An intermediate form may be the so-called vigorous achalasia. Most patients with diffuse esophageal spasm are middle-aged or elderly. The dominant symptoms are chest pain and dysphagia in nearly all patients. The pain is substernal and may be severe and colicky. Aspiration is uncommon.

2.1.2. Surgical Management

Although medical management, including nitrites and calcium channel blockers, may temporarily improve symptoms, there is no effective long-term treatment. Since surgery is not uniformly successful either, it is indicated only in severely disabled patients and after all conservative measures have been exhausted. Surgical management most commonly entails long myotomy of the esophagus. Controversies exist as to the length of myotomy and whether the lower esophageal sphincter should be included. Manometric assessment is critical to the choice and extent of surgical intervention. Manometry should determine: (1) the length of esophagus involved in diffuse spasm and (2) whether a hypertensive lower esophageal sphincter is present, or whether abnormalities of relaxation are present. The length of involved esophagus in diffuse spasm determines the length of myotomy. The presence or absence of lower esophageal sphincter dysfunction dictates the inclusion of the sphincter in the myotomy. Barium swallow and endoscopy are required to exclude associated lesions.

A second controversy in surgical management is whether or not an antireflux procedure should be preformed concurrent with the myotomy. Our choice is to avoid the addition of an antireflux procedure except in the setting where reflux is a prominent presenting symptom. When an antireflux procedure is indicated, the classic Nissen fundoplication should be avoided, as disabling dysphagia may result. Instead, the Belsey procedure, using a 270° wrap of the gastric fundus around the lower esophagus, is preferable. Although a modified short Nissen fundoplication has been advocated by

Table I. Results of Extended Myotomy
in Diffuse Esophageal Spasm

Study	No. of patients	% Success
Ellis, 1964[5]	40	78
Ferguson, 1969[6]	13	92
Flye, 1975[7]	11	100
Leonardi, 1977[8]	11	91
Henderson, 1987[2]	34	88

some,[2] long-term results are not available. The operation is best approached through the left chest.

Results of surgery have been variable, probably explained by differences in patient selection. In more recent reports, the outcome has been satisfactory (Table I). Good to excellent results can be expected in 90% of patients treated as outlined above.

2.2. Achalasia

2.2.1. Pathophysiology and Clinical Presentation

Achalasia is a disease of unknown etiology characterized by abnormal or absent peristalsis in the body of the esophagus, and failure of normal lower esophageal sphincter relaxation. This functional obstruction of the lower esophagus results in progressive dilation of the body, culminating in megaesophagus. The incidence is estimated to be 0.6 per 100,000 patients.[9] Progressive, painless dysphagia is the primary symptom. Few patients experience pain and, as mentioned above, the presence of pain may indicate an intermediate form of diffuse spasm. Retention of food and regurgitation of sweet-tasting material are characteristic of advanced achalasia. Weight loss becomes prominent in the advanced stages of the disease. Nocturnal aspiration may occur in up to 30% of patients.[2] Eight to ten percent of patients develop esophageal carcinoma.[10,11]

2.2.2. Surgical Management

Barium swallow and upper gastrointestinal endoscopy are required for the investigation of dysphagia. The characteristic radiologic features include absence of organized peristalsis, failure of lower esophageal sphincter relaxation, esophageal dilatation, and a distal bird's beak deformity. Endoscopy is particularly important to exclude an associated carcinoma. Additionally, it may show a dilated esophagus, tapering down distally. When gentle pressure is applied to the lower esophageal sphincter region, a characteristic "give" is experienced. In advanced cases, it may be difficult to pass the endoscope into the stomach. Although achalasia is readily diagnosed by these studies, manometry is useful in defining the motility abnormality. The findings include an aperistaltic esophagus with feeble or absent contractions, and incomplete sphincter relaxation on deglutition, often with premature contraction. Elevated resting lower esophageal sphincter pressure may be present.

Most patients will be successfully treated with drug therapy and bougienage. More

Table II. Results of Distal Esophageal Myotomy in Achalasia

Study	No. of patients	Mortality rate	Satisfactory outcome	Follow-up (years)
Ellis and Olsen, 1969[20]	336	0.3%	94%	5
Okike et al., 1979[13]	200	0	94%	6.5
Jara et al., 1979[19]	145	0	81%	10
Ellis et al., 1984[16]	113	0	91%	6.7
Henderson, 1987[2]	50	0	98%	Unstated

advanced cases require forceful balloon dilatation.[12–14] The results in 879 patients so treated at the Mayo Clinic have been summarized by Okike et al.[13] Excellent results were achieved in 65% of patients, and fair results in an additional 16%. Nearly 20% of patients required repeated dilatations. Serious complications occurred in 5% of patients. Surgical intervention was required in 10 patients for major distal esophageal rupture during the dilation.

Surgical treatment is indicated in patients who fail forceful balloon dilatation. However, some believe that surgery should be the primary form of therapy in severe cases, as it provides a higher success rate and longer-lasting relief from dysphagia.[15–17] The operation of choice is a short lower esophageal myotomy, usually performed through a left thoracotomy. In elderly patients, and in those with respiratory compromise, the myotomy can be performed through the abdomen. The myotomy is performed in the contracted esophageal segment, extending for a short distance proximally and for a few millimeters onto the stomach distally. A useful landmark for terminating the distal myotomy is the appearance of the highest submucosal vein plexus in the cardia as the last circular muscle fibers are divided. Extension of the myotomy more distally results in postoperative gastroesophageal reflux. The muscle layer is dissected off the submucosa for at least 50% of the esophageal circumference. We agree with Ellis et al.[16] that routine performance of an antireflux procedure is unnecessary, as the incidence of postoperative reflux when myotomy is performed as described is only 3%.[18] Results of surgery are largely good. The outcome in the largest recent series reported is given in Table II. We recommend repeat myotomy in patients with first-recurrent dysphagia who are found manometrically to have had an incomplete initial myotomy. Resection is indicated in the presence of carcinoma, and if the patient has recurrent symptoms following two adequate myotomies.

2.3. Zenker's Diverticulum

2.3.1. Pathophysiology and Clinical Presentation

The most prominent presenting symptom of Zenker's diverticulum is dysphagia. Regurgitation of undigested food, halitosis, and, on occasion, a swelling in the left neck may be present. The pathogenesis of this disorder is dysfunction of the upper esophageal sphincter mechanism, leading to a pulsion diverticulum between the inferior constrictor muscle of the pharynx and the cricopharyngeus muscle. Esophageal manometric studies demonstrate normal to increased upper esophageal sphincter pressure and, more importantly, dyscoordinated or incomplete relaxation upon deglutition. This is often associated with some degree of diffuse esophageal dysmotility. The high pharyngeal pressure generated on swallowing causes gradual herniation of mucosa and submucosa, usually into the left paravertebral space. A few patients, with neurologic dysfunction following stroke or head injury, will have the typical symptoms and clinical presentation of Zenker's diverticulum, although no diverticulum is present. Manometric study in these patients reveals decreased pharyngeal peak pressure (pharyngeal pump failure), with normal upper esophageal sphincter pressure. Sphincter relaxation with deglutition is usually normal.[21]

2.3.2. Surgical Treatment

The diagnosis of pharyngoesophageal diverticulum is usually suspected from the typical symptoms, and the only confirmatory test necessary is a barium swallow. Esophagoscopy poses the risk of inadvertent perforation of the thin-walled diverticulum. It is unnecessary unless the presence of malignancy is suspected. In patients with symptoms of upper esophageal dysphagia without evidence of diverticulum on barium swallow, manometry is essential to define the nature of the abnormality. In the presence of a diverticulum, manometry does not add useful information.

All patients with Zenker's diverticulum should be considered for surgical treatment, irrespective of the size of the diverticulum or the duration of symptoms. In the presence of recurrent aspiration or cachexia, surgery should not be postponed, as no other treatment is likely to be successful. The options in surgical management include diverticulectomy alone, cricopharyngeal myotomy alone, or diverticulectomy and myotomy. In the Mayo Clinic experience with 164 patients undergoing diverticulectomy alone and followed from 5 to 14 years after operation, only 4% of patients developed recurrent diverticulae, and another 3% had continued symptoms.[22] Since that time, however, esophageal motility studies have established the etiologic role of sphincter dysmotility, and the trend has been toward cricopharyngeal myotomy. Although this operation has greater physiologic rationale, the long-term results have generally not been better that with diverticulectomy alone. In patients with small diverticulae, diverticulectomy is technically difficult, and myotomy alone is the preferred treatment. Patients with recurrent diverticulae appear to have excellent results from myotomy and diverticulectomy, although the operation is technically more difficult.[23,24]

In patients with pharyngoesophageal dysmotility without diverticulum, the outcome of surgical treatment has been mixed. In one review, only 64% of patients had a successful outcome.[25] The best results are achieved in patients with documented incomplete or discoordinated relaxation of the upper esophageal sphincter upon deglutition.[21] Cricopharyngeal myotomy has a role in those patients with pharyngeal pump failure, such as following neurologic injury, as it is the best treatment available, but the outcome does not appear as good.[21]

2.4. Lower Esophageal (Epiphrenic) Diverticulum

2.4.1. Pathophysiology and Clinical Presentation

Lower esophageal diverticula are often called pulsion diverticula implying that increased intraesophageal pressure may be etiologic. Indeed, in 65 patients with lower esophageal diverticula reported by Debas et al., investigated by manometry, 50 had evidence of abnormal motility, most often diffuse spasm or achalasia.[26] Even in those 15 patients considered to have no dysmotility, 13 had hiatal hernia and 5 high-grade distal esophageal stricture. The symptoms in patients with lower esophageal diverticula are most often those of the underlying motility disorder. In the above-mentioned study of 65 cases from the Mayo Clinic, the most common presenting symptoms were dysphagia, chest pain, and regurgitation. Of 46 patients with dysphagia, 36 were due to the motility disorder and only 10 due to mechanical obstruction. Similarly, of 32 patients with chest pain, 30 were due to the motility abnormality and only 2 due to ulceration in the diverticulum. When symptoms are due to the diverticulum itself, the causes are either diverticulitis, often with ulceration, or obstruction of the distal esophagus due to displacement by a filled diverticulum.

2.4.2. Surgical Management

An esophagogram, especially with cinefluoroscopy, may show not only the diverticulum but also the underlying motility disturbance. All patients require upper gastrointestinal endoscopy in order to (1) exclude more common diseases such as carcinoma or reflux esophagitis, (2) visualize the diverticulum to determine if inflammation, ulceration, or esophageal displacement and obstruction are present, and (3) to exclude the presence of an associated hiatal hernia. Rarely, a carcinoma has been discovered in lower esophageal diverticula with or without coexistent esophagitis. The best way to assess the underlying motility disorder is by esophageal manometry. Careful attention should be paid to the amplitude and propagation of the constriction waves in the body of the esophagus, and the resting pressure, pattern, and completeness of relaxation of the distal esophageal sphincter.

The indication for surgery is clear when the diverticulum has caused a mechanical obstruction of the esophagus or when severe inflammation and ulceration are present within the diverticulum. In the absence of these, the treatment of lower esophageal diverticulum is the treatment of the underlying disease. The indications for surgery are then those described for diffuse esophageal spasm and achalasia. On occasion, a distal esophageal stricture due to reflux esophagitis is present and surgical treatment is indicated when esophageal dilatation and medical therapy fail. When surgical treatment is indicated, the diverticulum should be excised and the underlying motor disturbance or mechanical obstruction corrected.

3. MOTILITY DISORDERS OF THE STOMACH

3.1. Gastric Dysrhythmias

3.1.1. Pathophysiology and Clinical Presentation

A variety of gastric dysrhythmias, including tachygastria, bradygastria, and gastric arrhythmia, have been described in association with disorders of gastric emptying in human patients. Although unproven, there is good reason to suspect that these identified abnormalities of gastric electrical activity are the cause of the disordered motility patterns and symptoms of nausea, bloating, and vomiting.

The electrical patterns of the normal stomach are characterized by sustained, non-phasic activity in the fundus and proximal corpus, and well-defined, phasic activity in the distal fundus and antrum. This distal phasic activity appears to arise from a pacemaker area on the mid-greater curvature of the stomach, and has been termed the "basic electrical rhythm," "slow-wave activity," or "pacemaker potential." These slow waves propagate at a rate of 3 cycles/sec in humans[27] and 5 cycles/sec in dogs[28] circumferentially and longitudinally from the pacemaker to the pylorus. Gastric smooth muscle contraction does not appear to occur in response to slow waves, but is more closely correlated with increases in plateau potentials, which can be induced by stimulants such as acetylcholine and pentagastrin, and inhibited by norepinephrine and prostaglandin E_2.[29]

Code and Marlett[30] and Telander et al.[31] were the first to describe disturbances in normal gastric electrical activity in dogs and humans, respectively. They observed absence of the plateau potential, decreased responsiveness of smooth muscle to stimulation, and the presence of an ectopic pacemaker which generated electrical cycles at an increased rate. This has been referred to as tachygastria. This electrical pattern is observed transiently in normal patients, in those in the postoperative period, and in motion sickness.[32–34] There is accumulating evidence that this, and other gastric dysrhythmias, are associated with abnormalities of gastric emptying in patients with diabetic gastroparesis, anorexia nervosa, unexplained vomiting, and others.[35–38] The underlying mechanism is unclear, but there is evidence in dogs that it may be prostaglandin-mediated.[39]

3.1.2. Surgical Management

Treatment options for gastric dysrhythmias are limited. Most patients are unresponsive to pharmacologic treatment, although newer and more potent agents such as cisapride have shown promise. A few have benefited from subtotal gastrectomy.[31,40] Gastric drainage procedures have been largely unsuccessful, except in children.[41] Before undertaking such procedures, it is crucial to have as complete an understanding of the pathology as possible. Ill-conceived operations have the risk of making matters worse. Self-limiting causes of dysmotility, such as electrolyte imbalance, pancreatitis, and narcotic abuse, can easily be excluded. A quantitative radionuclide-labeled gastric emptying study of both a solid and liquid meal is helpful in defining the degree of impairment and assessing the response to various therapeutic maneuvers. It is of interest that only about 50% of those patients thought to have delayed gastric emptying on clinical grounds will actually have objective abnormalities upon testing.[42] When segmental gastric dysmotility is identified, our initial approach is to attempt to increase gastric emptying with a trial of metoclopramide or cisapride. If the patient remains symptomatic, and repeated quantitative gastric emptying studies show persistent delayed emptying, pyloroplasty is indicated. For those patients who remain symptomatic following pyloroplasty, subtotal gastrectomy with Billroth II reconstruction may be warranted. In rare instances, total gastrectomy may be required.

3.2. Postgastrectomy Syndromes

3.2.1. Dumping

3.2.1a. Pathophysiology and Clinical Presentation. Dumping syndrome refers to the presence of troublesome gastrointestinal and cardiovascular symptoms following gastric surgery. The most common gastrointestinal symptoms include epigastric pain, abdominal bloating, nausea, and vomiting. These may be associated with cardiovascular manifestations, including dizziness, weakness, sweating, and palpitations. Typically, these symptoms begin a few minutes following ingestion of a meal and subside within an hour. Because of the early temporal relationship with eating, this has been known as early dumping. Late dumping refers to symptoms of hypoglycemia occurring an hour or more following a meal. The incidence of dumping depends on the type of gastric procedure which has been performed. Following truncal vagotomy with either antrectomy, pyloroplasty, or gastroenterostomy, the incidence is about 15%. Following highly selective vagotomy, however, the incidence is 1%. About two thirds of patients who initially suffer from dumping eventually become symptom-free without any specific treatment.[43]

Rapid gastric emptying seems to be an important factor in the pathogenesis of dumping. In the normal stomach, emptying of a mixed meal occurs slowly over 3–4 hr. Following partial gastrectomy, the rate increases to 10–30 min, and within 3–5 min in some patients.[44] The severity of symptoms, however, does not appear to directly correlate with the rate of gastric emptying.[45] Total gut transit time is unaltered by gastrectomy.[46] In the absence of a normally functioning pylorus, rapid gastric emptying delivers a large volume of hypertonic fluid into the proximal jejunum. This luminal hyperosmolality is diluted by an outpouring of fluid, which distends the jejunum.[47] There is a corresponding decrease in circulating plasma volume and a paradoxical increase in peripheral vascular resistance.[48] Jejunal motor activity is increased[49] and there is elevation in the serum concentrations of a number of gut hormones, including serotonin, kinins, substance P, neurotensin and enteroglucagon.[50–52]

3.2.1b. Surgical Management. Most patients with dumping improve with dietary management alone. The major modifications include avoidance of simple sugars, ingestion of liquids 30–45 min following the solid portions of the meal, and utilizing six small feedings per day. In patients in whom these maneuvers fail, drug therapy may be tried. There are three classes of drugs available at present: anticholinergics, such as atropine, which delay gastric emptying; hypoglycemic agents, such as tolbutamide, to prevent postprandial hyperglycemia; and serotonin antagonist, such as methysergide, to block the effects of endogenous postprandial serotonin release. None of these drugs has had striking success, although they have been valuable in some cases. Recently, there have been reports of amelioration of symptoms by the long-acting somatostatin analogue, octreotide.[53]

Only about 1% of all patients with dumping require operation. There are three major options in the management, depending mainly on what the previous procedure has been. If a resection and Billroth II reconstruction have been performed, this can be converted to a Billroth I anastomosis. In some series, this has resulted in success in 80–90% of patients.[54] The theoretic advantage is restoration of flow of gastric contents through the duodenum, which may result in improved osmotic regulation. The second major approach to operative therapy is the placement of an antiperistaltic jejunal segment between the gastric remnant and the duodenum. This has the rationale of decreasing the rate of gastric emptying. Its success appears critically dependent on the length of the antiperistaltic segment. A segment too short fails to relieve symptoms, whereas a longer segment can result in gastric stasis and ulceration. Sawyers and Herrington report that improvement in symptoms occurs in about 75% of patients treated with short reversed jejunal segments, but that 25% of patients have late complications such as stasis or ulceration, which sometimes requires remedial surgery.[55] In patients who have previously undergone pyloroplasty, there is evidence that reversal of the pyloroplasty may ameliorate symptoms of dumping. A variety of reports indicate that success can be expected in 75–80% of patients with this approach.[56–58] Given its simplicity, it is probably the best initial form of surgical treatment in patients who have previously undergone pyloroplasty.

3.2.2. Diarrhea

3.2.2a. Pathophysiology and Clinical Presentation. Diarrhea can be a troublesome symptom following gastric surgery. It appears to be more closely related to the performance of a vagotomy rather than to a gastric resection or drainage procedure. The incidence is greatest following truncal vagotomy (25–35%), and less following selective (8%) and highly selective (1–2%) vagotomy.[59] Fortunately, less than 1% of patients are disabled by their symptoms. The cause of diarrhea following operations upon the stomach is not understood. There is some evidence that it results from a disturbance of small bowel motility, the nature of which is controversial.[60] Other abnormalities identified in patients with postvagotomy diarrhea include increased excretion of chenodeoxycholic acid in the stool.[61] Stool electrolyte, water, and sugar absorption are unaltered by vagotomy, and jejunal biopsies are usually unrevealing, with normal disaccharidase and lactase activity.

3.2.2b. Surgical Management. The great majority of patients with diarrhea following vagotomy improve spontaneously, or with dietary and medical management. A variety of surgical procedures have been devised to correct the diarrhea, and none are completely satisfactory. The most popular operation has been insertion of a reversed 10-cm jejunal segment 50–100 cm distal to the ligament of Treitz. Herrington reported that 13 of 19 patients in whom he performed this operation have had excellent results, 4 have been improved, and 2 are considered failures.[62] If the patient has had a pyloroplasty, there is some evidence that the diarrhea can be ameliorated by pyloric reconstruction.[58] Inasmuch as the pathophysiology of postvagotomy diarrhea is poorly understood, the most logical corrective procedure is not clear.

4. BILIARY DYSKINESIA

4.1. Pathophysiology and Clinical Presentation

Biliary dyskinesia represents an ill-defined group of disorders characterized manometrically by either (1) elevated sphincter of Oddi pressure (spasm), (2) abnormally rapid phasic contractions of the sphincter (tachyoddia), or (3) dyscoordinate bile duct motility. The very existence of these disorders historically has been met with skepticism, which has lessened with the advent of endoscopic techniques that have enabled direct measurement of sphincter and bile duct pressures. Even so, the categorization of these disorders and the understanding of their relationship to clinical symptoms remain incomplete. The term *postcholecystectomy syndrome* has unfortunately been used to group all patients with persistent or recurrent symptoms following cholecystectomy. For many of these patients, a defined cause of their symptoms is known, such as gastroesophageal reflux, peptic ulcer disease, or residual common bile duct stone. Others may have fibrotic stenosis of the sphincter (papillary stenosis) amenable to sphincteroplasty.[63,64] A small number of patients probably have residual symptoms due to a dyskinesia of the biliary tract. Indeed, it has been suggested that one cause of common bile duct stones may be failure of antegrade bile duct contractions.[65]

The single most useful diagnostic test is upper gastrointestinal endoscopy with cannulation of the ampulla of Vater and retrograde cholangiopancreatography. At that time, esophagitis, peptic ulcer disease, papillary stenosis, and retained common bile duct stone can all be excluded with reasonable certainty. If these conditions are not present, biliary manometric studies are indicated. Several studies have documented a high incidence of abnormal biliary manometrics in this group of patients.[66,67] The common abnormalities are elevated resting sphincter pressures and increased frequency of retrograde propagation of phasic contractions. These patients also appear to have a paradoxical response to stimulation with cholecystokinin and cerulein.[68]

4.2. Surgical Management

If biliary dyskinesia is identified in the setting of recurrent abdominal pain, endoscopic sphincterotomy is the procedure of choice. Excellent short-term results have been reported by several groups.[67,69,70] With longer-term follow-up, however, up to 50% of patients may have recurrent symptoms.[71] It appears, however, that the physiologic consequences of endoscopic papillotomy on sphincter function are retained for at least 2 years,[72] so the cause of the late failure is unclear. An alternative procedure is transduodenal sphincteroplasty, which is thought to have more permanent effect on sphincter function. Little data are available, however, and there have been no controlled trials comparing endoscopic sphincterotomy with operative sphincteroplasty.

5. INTESTINAL PSEUDOOBSTRUCTION

5.1. Chronic Idiopathic Intestinal Pseudoobstruction

5.1.1. Pathophysiology and Clinical Management

Chronic idiopathic intestinal pseudoobstruction is a puzzling syndrome mimicking mechanical intestinal obstruction without the presence of a physical, obstructing, lesion. It occurs in patients of all ages and of both sexes. The usual presentation includes multiple attacks of nausea, vomiting, abdominal distension, and pain. Both constipation and diarrhea are common. Intestinal bacterial overgrowth due to stasis leads to malabsorption and steatorrhea, worsening the chronic malnutrition. The extent of involvement in the gut is variable, ranging from isolated segments to the entire gastrointestinal tract. Abnormalities in esophageal motility are commonly present, although dysphagia is only rarely a complaint. The pathophysiology is poorly understood, but is accepted to be a disorder of intestinal motility resulting in ineffective propulsion. A variety of abnormalities of visceral neurons have been identified and implicated in the pathogenesis of the disorder.[73] At least one form appears to be familial, with probable autosomal dominant transmission.[74]

5.1.2. Surgical Management

Differentiation of mechanical intestinal obstruction, which is relatively frequent in surgical practice, from the rare instance of the patient presenting with pseudoobstruction can be exceedingly difficult. Some radiologic features, such as dilatation of the duodenum, colonic redundancy, and absent haustral markings, may aid in the diagnosis of pseudoobstruction,[75] but these are not always present. Indeed, most patients with pseudoobstruction have previously undergone multiple prior laparotomies in an unsuccessful search for a mechanical cause of obstruction.

Operation is only rarely indicated in patients known to have chronic idiopathic intestinal pseudoobstruction. A number of procedures, including lysis of adhesions, intestinal plication, and gastrojejunostomy, have been shown to be ineffective. A select number of patients, however, may benefit from operations designed to address specific, segmental motility defects. Rarely, patients will have megaduodenum, with normal gastric and small intestinal motility, and in these cases, duodenojejunostomy has been beneficial.[76] Similarly, patients with isolated colonic symptoms have benefited from subtotal colectomy, although it has been noted that some of these patients later develop symptoms related to small bowel involvement.[76,77] Radical small bowel resection has been reported to benefit the rare patient debilitated by small bowel involvement.[78,79] The decision to pursue this course must be carefully balanced against the risk of creating a short bowel syndrome with attendant problems of malnutrition and diarrhea. Pitt et al.[80] described a series of 20 patients managed with long-term total parenteral nutrition and "venting" enterostomy. In these patients, the presence of a gastrostomy, jejunostomy, or cecostomy tube allowed relief of intermittent episodes of distension at home, reducing the periods of hospitalization. In their patients, total parenteral nutrition was required to maintain adequate caloric intake.

5.2. Acute Colonic Pseudoobstruction

5.2.1. Pathophysiology and Clinical Presentation

In 1948, Sir Heneage Ogilvie first described a syndrome strongly suggestive of mechanical colonic obstruction with normal barium enema examination.[81] In both of his cases, no obstructing lesions were found at laparotomy; however, in each patient, extensive malignant processes were present in the celiac ganglia and diaphragmatic crural regions. Ogilvie hypothesized that the symptoms of obstruction in these patients were due to malignant inhibition of colonic sympathetic innervation with unopposed sacral parasympathetic innervation.

Since that time, numerous other reports have confirmed the existence of the syndrome as a distinct clinical entity. A variety of names, including idiopathic colonic obstruction, acute colonic pseudo-obstruction, colonic ileus, and others, have been applied, but the disease is more commonly referred to as Ogilvie's syndrome. Characteristically, patients are elderly, and present with several days of progressive abdominal distension and obstipation. Shortness of breath due to limited diaphragmatic excursion is common. Nausea and vomiting are usually present, but may not be prominent symptoms. Mild, diffuse abdominal tenderness is present, but peritonitis is absent, unless perforation has occurred. Bowel sounds are characteristically absent, which may help distinguish the process from mechanical obstruction, such as volvulus or neoplasm. Abdominal radi-

Table III. Associated Conditions
in Ogilvie's Syndrome
(Collected Series)

Condition	% of patients
Sepsis or inflammation	15%
Abdominal surgery	12%
Idiopathic	12%
Trauma	10%
Cardiac disease	10%
Pregnancy	10%
Retroperitoneal disease	7%
Neurologic disorders	6%
Orthopedic surgery	5%
Alcoholism	5%
Burns	2%
Other	6%

ographs demonstrate massive distension which, in the presence of a competent ileocecal valve, may be limited to the colon. In many cases, the colonic distension appears segmental, with a cutoff sign at the splenic or hepatic flexure, which may suggest mechanical obstruction.

The syndrome has been associated with a variety of underlying disorders, including abdominal malignancy, orthopedic injury or operation, narcotic use, kidney transplantation or dialysis, massive blunt trauma, myocardial infarction, neurologic impairment, and pregnancy (Table III). In a few cases, no underlying disorder has been identified. The pathophysiology has not been studied in detail, but is generally accepted to be an adynamic ileus of the colon, predominantly on the right side. This may be due to inhibition of parasympathetic innervation or stimulation of sympathetic inhibitory fibers. In at least two case reports, elevated prostaglandin E levels have been associated with acute colonic pseudoobstruction, with levels returning to normal with resolution of the ileus.[82,83] Given the variety of associated abnormalities, it is likely that the underlying pathophysiology is complex. As the colon distends, the risk of perforation increases. It is generally accepted that the risk of perforation is highest in those patients in whom the cecal diameter is increasing at a rapid rate, and in those in whom the absolute diameter is greater than 12 cm. The perforation generally occurs on the anterior, antimesenteric wall of the cecum, and initiates diffuse peritoneal inflammation and infection.

5.2.2. Surgical Management

Initial management of uncomplicated Ogilvie's syndrome includes correction of fluid and electrolyte abnormalities, nasogastric suction, avoidance of narcotics, and treatment of any underlying disorder. Although the use of rectal tubes has been advocated, they usually are not therapeutic. A variety of pharmacologic maneuvers, including cholinergic agents and metoclopramide, have been tried without success. Serial abdominal radiographs should be obtained to ascertain the rate of increase in distension, and the response to treatment. If no improvement is observed, colonoscopic decompression should be performed. Since the first report by Kukora and Dent,[84] it has become clear that, in many patients, even severe distension can be treated colonoscopically. In a further report in 1983, Strodel et al. reported results of such treatment in 44 patients.[85] In their patients, the mean cecal diameter was reduced from 12.8 to 8.7 cm with a 73% initial success rate. Eight patients required repeated procedures. Perforation occurred during colonoscopy in 1 patient (2%). Operation was required in 9 patients (20%) for continued or recurrent colonic dilation. The overall mortality in their series was 32%.

Operation is indicated in patients in whom colonoscopic decompression is unsuccessful, for those with recurrent dilation, and in the presence of perforation. Several surgical options are available, including cecostomy, transverse loop colostomy, and resection. The decision as to which of these options to pursue is individualized, depending on the general condition of the patient, the extent of involved colon, the presence of peritoneal contamination, and the presence of cecal necrosis. Cecostomy has generally been the most commonly used operation. It has the advantage of being a minimally invasive procedure, which, if necessary, can be performed through a limited right lower quadrant incision under local anesthesia. In the presence of a pinpoint perforation, the tube can be placed through the cecal defect. The decompression afforded by cecostomy is usually adequate, but meticulous care is required to ensure continued patency of the tube. No large series of patients are available for critical analysis of results. Adams reported one of the larger series of 20 patients, 14 of whom required operation.[86] A cecostomy was performed in each, under local anesthesia in 9, general anesthesia in 4, and epidural anesthesia in 1. Of the operatively treated patients, 3 died, for a mortality rate of 21%. No operatively treated patients had recurrent dilation. Resection is indicated when intestinal ischemia is present, or when an extensive perforation has occurred. The mortality rate in the presence of perforation rises to approximately 45%.[87]

The outcome in patients with Ogilvie's syndrome is critically dependent on their underlying disorder. Of patients with severe distension, colonoscopy is successful in decompression in about 80%. As shown in Table IV, the overall mortality rate from selected publications since 1971 is 18%. Although colonoscopic decompression has not significantly reduced the mortality rate for this condition, fewer patients are requiring operative intervention.

Table IV. Treatment and Outcome of Patients with Ogilvie's Syndrome

| First author | Year | N | Final treatment | | | Mortality |
			Medical	Colonoscopic	Operation	
Wanebo	1971	23	14	0	9	26%
Adams	1974	20	6	0	14	30%
Bachulis	1978	35	24	2	9	6%
Baker	1979	11	11	0	0	9%
Nivatvongs	1982	22	—	19	3	0%
Strodel	1983	44	—	31	13	32%
Nakhgevany	1984	10	—	9	1	10%
Geelhoed	1985	12	3	3	6	17%
Total		177	58	64	55	18%

6. COLONIC DYSMOTILITY SYNDROMES

6.1. Colonic Diverticular Disease

6.1.1. Pathophysiology and Clinical Presentation

Diverticular disease of the colon is quite prevalent in Western countries, with a lifetime risk of nearly 50%.[88] This has been generally attributed to a decline in daily crude fiber intake in these countries.[89] Diverticulosis represents the formation of pulsion-type outpouchings of mucosae and muscularis mucosae through weak areas of the colon at sites of perforation of intramural blood vessels. In order for these diverticula to develop, a pressure gradient must exist across the bowel wall. There is evidence that this pressure gradient arises as a result of disordered colonic motility.[90] In 1964, Painter found elevated intraluminal colonic pressure in patients with diverticular disease, especially upon stimulation with morphine or prostigmine.[91] There is also evidence that segmentation is increased in the sigmoid colon, and that pressures as high as 90 mm Hg can be achieved within these cells.[92,93] An increase in the colonic myoelectric pattern from the normal of 3 cycles/min to 12–18 cycles/min has been identified in patients with symptomatic diverticular disease. This pattern returns toward normal with the ingestion of bran.[94] These and a number of other lines of evidence have suggested that colonic dysmotility is an important basis for the development of colonic diverticular disease.[95]

6.1.2. Surgical Management

In 1964, Reilly was the first to advocate longitudinal colonic myotomy as a treatment for uncomplicated diverticular disease, with the rationale that myotomy would reduce the increased intraluminal pressure.[96] The short-term results with this operation appeared promising, with symptomatic improvement and decreased intraluminal pressures and motility indices.[97,98] Unfortunately, the long-term results have been less satisfactory, with recurrence rates of approximately 40%.[99,100] Other forms of myotomy[101–103] have not been greeted enthusiastically. This has been due, in large part, because myotomy is technically difficult, poses a significant risk of postoperative fistulas, and achieves long-term results which do not appear superior to resection.[104] Inasmuch as 75% of patients with acute diverticulitis treated medically recover without recurrent symptoms or attacks[105] and that this percentage is not increased by early operation, surgery is now reserved for patients with recurrent bouts of acute diverticulitis or complications such as perforation, obstruction, or bleeding.[106,107] The number of potential candidates for myotomy is thus small, and it is unlikely that myotomy will supplant resection as the standard surgical treatment for complicated diverticular disease.

6.2. Chronic Constipation

6.2.1. Pathophysiology and Clinical Presentation

Sir W. Arbuthnot Lane is generally credited as being the first to advocate operation for certain severe cases of ''chronic intestinal stasis,'' and reported on 39 cases. Excellent results were achieved following colectomy in 29. Since that time, the syndrome of chronic slow-transit constipation in young women has been known by the eponym, Arbuthnot Lane's disease. It has been only recently, however, that constipation has been adequately defined and measured. Generally, spontaneous defecation less than once every 3 days may be taken as abnormal.[108] A more reliable measure is the rate of passage of radio-paque markers through the gut, with normal limits being clearance of 80% of markers by 5 days and 100% by 7 days.[109]

At least three different patterns of constipation have been identified.[110] Recognition of the various types of possible abnormalities is particularly important when considering an operative strategy. Approximately one third of patients have what is termed "colonic inertia," which appears to be a generalized atonicity of the colonic musculature. Another one third of patients have a motility disorder limited to the hindgut, particularly the rectosigmoid junction. The final one third have isolated anal sphincter dysfunction. The pathophysiology of these disorders is poorly understood. In some patients with idiopathic constipation, decreased colonic concentrations of vasoactive intestinal polypeptide, an important nonadrenergic, noncholinergic inhibitory neurotransmitter, has been found.[111] It is unknown whether this is secondary to the long-standing constipation, or an etiologic factor. Other studies have demonstrated decreased numbers of ganglion cells and axons in the colonic myenteric plexus from patients with idiopathic constipation, but the etiologic significance is unknown.[112]

6.2.2. Surgical Management

Surgical management is considered only after all conservative measures have failed and after careful review of the medical history to exclude the presence of systemic disorders or the use of drugs implicated in constipation. Although operations for constipation have been looked upon with disfavor, there are clearly patients with marked disability who have dramatic relief following surgery. Any operation for constipation must fulfill three criteria: (1) there must be a physiologic rationale for the procedure, (2) it must be effective, and (3) it must be free of significant morbidity.

For patients with colonic inertia, total abdominal colectomy with ileorectal anastomosis has had favorable results (Table V). Although the number of patients in each reported series is small, overall about 90% of appropriately selected patients can be expected to achieve normal evacuation without morbidity. Although others have advocated sparing of the cecum with cecorectal anastomosis, this appears to result in a high rate of recurrent symptoms.[115] In a few patients with segmental hypomotility, segmental colectomy has been successful.[119] In that it can be difficult to assess normal from abnormal colon, the desire to prevent recurrent symptoms, and the lack of increased morbidity, total abdominal colectomy is probably the better operation for most patients.

When anal sphincter dysfunction is present, colectomy is inappropriate, as it does not address the physiologic abnormality. Instead, the best option in surgical management appears to be rectal myectomy. Other options, such as anal dilatation and posterior division of the puborectalis muscle, are less effective. In rectal myectomy, a narrow, submucosal resection of rectal muscle is performed in the posterior midline. The resection is begun in the intersphincteric groove, including the internal sphincter, and extends proximally up to 10 cm. In a small, randomized trial, Yoshioka and Keighley found rectal myectomy to be superior to anal dilatation.[120] In this study, rectal pressures were signifi-

Table V. Results of Total Abdominal Colectomy and Ileorectal Anastomosis for Colonic Inertia

Study	No. of patients	Mean follow-up (years)	Operative mortality (%)	Successful outcome (%)
McCready and Beart, 1979[113]	6	2.4	0	100
Klatt, 1983[114]	9	2.1	0	100
Preston et al., 1984[115]	8	5.7	0	88
Beck et al., 1987[116]	14	1.2	0	100
Walsh et al., 1987[117]	19	3.3	0	63
Gasslander et al., 1987[118]	6	—	0	100

cantly reduced and rectal emptying was significantly increased following myectomy. Only 54% of their patients were considered successfully palliated, however. Similar findings have been reported by others.[121] Factors that appear to predict good results following rectal myectomy include higher preoperative resting rectal pressures, normal colonic transit time, and shorter history of constipation.[120]

6.3. Hirschsprung's Disease

6.3.1. Pathophysiology and Clinical Presentation

Although Hirschsprung's disease is the most common cause of colonic obstruction in the neonate, it is a rare cause of chronic constipation in the adult patient. The disorder is characterized by absence of intramural ganglion cells in the most distal intestine. The proximal extent of involvement is variable. It is thought that the etiology is failure of distal migration of intestinal neuroblasts, a process which is normally complete by the 12th week of gestation.[122] Adult patients with the disease usually have involvement limited to the rectum, with occasional involvement of the distal sigmoid. The colon proximal to the aganglionic segment becomes dilated, sometimes to gigantic proportions. The typical adult patient presents with a history of intermittent constipation since birth, but without the malnutrition and vomiting seen in the infant. In most, the diagnosis of Hirschsprung's disease will not have been suspected during childhood and adolescence because of the mild degree of symptoms.

6.3.2. Surgical Management

The diagnosis of Hirschsprung's disease can be confirmed with full-thickness or suction biopsy of the posterior rectal wall, which demonstrates the absence of ganglion cells. Anorectal manometry and barium enema are useful in defining the extent of dysmotility. The usual surgical approach consists of two stages. In the first operation, the extent of proximal colonic involvement is assessed with multiple biopsies. Decompression of the distended colon is accomplished by end colostomy in the most distal colon containing ganglion cells. Over the next 2 to 6 months, the dilated proximal bowel returns to normal caliber, and any impaction in the distal bowel is evacuated. Reconstruction is achieved by one of three operations: the Swenson procedure, the Duhamel procedure, or the Soave procedure. All have satisfactory results in children. The Swenson procedure has the disadvantage of the greatest amount of pelvic dissection, which increases the risk of impotence. The Soave procedure, in which the proximal colon is pulled through a muscular sleeve of the distal rectum, minimizes the pelvic dissection, but can be difficult to perform if the diameter of the limbs of colon are discrepant. The Duhamel procedure is preferable in this situation. Other operations, such as posterior sphincterotomy and rectal myomectomy, have limited usefulness, except in the rare case of short-segment Hirschsprung's disease.

There are few published reports of outcome of treatment of adult Hirschsprung's disease.[123–125] Starling et al.[123] obtained excellent results in seven of eight patients and good results in one patient with a mean follow-up of 6.1 years. Most of their patients were treated with the Soave procedure. As in children, relief from constipation can be expected, and the operative risks are low.

7. SUMMARY

The role of surgery in the management of motility disorders of the gastrointestinal tract remains poorly defined. For certain disorders, such as Zenker's diverticulum and Hirschsprung's disease, well-understood abnormalities can be addressed with specific operations with a high degree of success. In settings where the underlying pathophysiology is poorly understood, the clinician should recommend operation with caution, and generally only after all other measures have failed to provide relief. When applied to such carefully selected patients, surgery has the greatest chance of relieving what might otherwise be disabling symptoms.

REFERENCES

1. Cohen S: Motor disorders of the esophagus. N Engl J Med 301:184–192, 1979
2. Henderson RD: Esophageal motor disorders. Surg Clin North Am 67:455–474, 1987
3. Benjamin SB, Richter JE, Cordova CM, et al: Prospective manometric evaluation with pharmacologic provocation of patients with suspected esophageal motility disorders. Gastroenterology 84:893–899, 1983
4. Vantrappen G, Janssens H, Hellmans J, et al: Achalasia, diffuse esophageal spasm, and related motility disorders. Gastroenterology 76:450–457, 1979
5. Ellis FH Jr, Schlegel JF, Code CF, et al: Surgical treatment of esophageal hypermotility disturbances. JAMA 188:862–865, 1964
6. Ferguson TB, Woodbury JD, Roper CL, et al: Giant muscular hypertrophy of the esophagus. Ann Thorac Surg 8:209, 1969
7. Flye ME, Sealy WC: Diffuse spasm of the esophagus. Ann Thorac Surg 19:677, 1975
8. Leonardi HK, Shea JA, Crozier RE, Ellis FH Jr: Diffuse spasm of the esophagus. Clinical, manometric and surgical considerations. J Thorac Cardiovasc Surg 74:736–743, 1977
9. Earlam RJ, Ellis FH Jr: Achalasia of the esophagus in a small urban community. Mayo Clin Proc 44:478–482, 1969
10. Just-Viera JO, Morris JD, Haight C: Achalasia and esophageal carcinoma. Ann Thorac Surg 3:526, 1967
11. Hankins JR, McLaughlin JS: The association of carcinoma of the esophagus with achalasia. J Thorac Cardiovasc Surg 69:355–360, 1975
12. Sanderson DR, Ellis FH Jr, Olsen AM: Achalasia of the esophagus: Results of therapy by dilation, 1950–1967. Chest 58:116, 1970

13. Okike N, Payne WS, Neufeld DM, et al: Esophagomyotomy versus forceful dilation for achalasia of the esophagus: Results in 899 patients. Ann Thorac Surg 28:119–125, 1979
14. Dellipiani AW, Hewetson KA: Pneumatic dilatation in the management of achalasia: Experience of 45 cases. Q J Med 58:253–258, 1986
15. Ellis FH Jr: Surgical management of esophageal motility disturbances. Am J Surg 139:752–759, 1980
16. Ellis FH Jr, Crozier RE, Watkins E Jr: Operation for esophageal achalasia. Results of esophagomyotomy without an antireflux operation. J Thorac Cardiovasc Surg 88:344–351, 1984
17. Donahue PE, Schlesinger PK, Bombeck CT, et al: Achalasia of the esophagus. Treatment controversies and the method of choice. Ann Surg 203:505–511, 1986
18. Ellis FH Jr, Kiser JC, Schlegel JF, et al: Esophagomyotomy for esophageal achalasia. Experimental, clinical, and manometric aspects. Ann Surg 166:640–656, 1967
19. Jara FM, Toledo-Pereyra LH, Lewis JW, et al: Long-term results of esophagomyotomy for achalasia of esophagus. Arch Surg 114:935–936, 1979
20. Ellis FH Jr, Olsen AM: Achalasia of the Esophagus. Philadelphia, Saunders, 1969, p 196
21. Bonavina L, Khan NA, DeMeester TR: Pharyngoesophageal dysfunctions. The role of cricopharyngeal myotomy. Arch Surg 120: 541–549, 1985
22. Welsh GF, Payne WS: The present status of one-stage pharyngo-esophageal diverticulectomy. Surg Clin North Am 53:953–958, 1973
23. Huang B, Payne WS, Cameron AJ: Surgical management for recurrent pharyngoesophageal (Zenker's) diverticulum. Ann Thorac Surg 37:189–191, 1984
24. Payne WS, King RM: Pharyngoesophageal (Zenker's) diverticulum. Surg Clin North Am 63:815–824, 1983
25. Hurwitz AL, Duranceau A: Upper esophageal sphincter dysfunction: Pathogenesis and treatment. Dig Dis Sci 23:275–281, 1978
26. Debas HT, Payne WS, Cameron AJ, et al: Physiopathology of lower esophageal diverticulum and its implications for treatment. Surg Gynecol Obstet 151:593–600, 1980
27. Hinder RA, Kelly KA: Human gastric pacesetter potential: Site of origin, spread, and response to gastric transection and proximal gastric vagotomy. Am J Surg 133:29–33, 1977
28. Kelly KA, Code CF, Elveback LR: Patterns of canine gastric electrical activity. Am J Physiol 217:461–470, 1969
29. Szurszewski JH: Electrical basis for gastrointestinal motility, in Johnson LR (ed): Physiology of the Gastrointestinal Tract. New York, Raven Press, 1981, Vol 2, pp 1435–1466
30. Code CF, Marlett JA: Canine tachygastria. Mayo Clin Proc 49:325–332, 1974
31. Telander RL, Morgan KG, Kreulen DL, et al: Human gastric atony with tachygastria and gastric retention. Gastroenterology 75:497–501, 1978.
32. Stoddard CJ, Smallwood RH, Duthie HL: Electrical arrhythmias in the human stomach. Gut 22:705–712, 1981
33. Bertrand J, Dorval ED, Metman EH, et al: Electrogastrography and serosal electrical recording of the antrum after proximal vagotomy in man. Gastroenterology 86:1026, 1984 (abstr)
34. Stern RM, Koch KL, Stewart WR, et al: Spectral analysis of tachygastria recorded during motion sickness. Gastroenterology 92:92–97, 1987
35. Abell TL, Malagelada JR, Lucas AR, et al: Gastric electromechanical and neurohormonal function in anorexia nervosa. Gastroenterology 93:958–965, 1987
36. Abell TL, Camilleri M, Malagelada JR: High prevalence of gastric electrical dysrhythmias in diabetic gastroparesis. Gastroenterology 86:1299, 1984 (abstr)
37. You CH, Lee KY, Chey WY, et al: Electrogastrographic study of patients with unexplained nausea, bloating, and vomiting. Gastroenterology 79:311–314, 1980
38. Kim CH, Malagelada JR: Electrical activity of the stomach: Clinical implications. Mayo Clin Proc 61:205–210, 1986
39. Kim CH, Zinmeister AR, Malagelada JR: Mechanisms of canine gastric dysrhythmia. Gastroenterology 92:993–999, 1987
40. You CH, Chey WY, Lee KY, et al: Gastric and small intestinal myoelectric dysrhythmia associated with chronic intractable nausea and vomiting. Ann Intern Med 95:449–451, 1981
41. Mulvihill SJ, Fonkalsrud EW: Pyloroplasty in infancy and childhood. J Pediatr Surg 18:930–936, 1983
42. Pellegrini CA, Broderick WC, Van Dyke D, et al: Diagnosis and treatment of gastric emptying disorders: Clinical usefulness of radionuclide measurements of gastric emptying. Am J Surg 145:143–151, 1983

43. Chaimoff C, Dintsman M, Tigva P: The long-term fate of patients with dumping syndrome. Arch Surg 105:554–556, 1972
44. Owren PA: The pathogenesis and treatment of iron deficiency anemia after partial gastrectomy. Acta Chir Scand 104:206, 1952
45. Silver D, Anlyan WG, Postlethwait RW, et al: Serotonin metabolism and the dumping syndrome. Ann Surg 161:995, 1965
46. Welbourn RB, Hallenback GA, Bollman JL: Effect of gastric operations on loss of fecal fat in the dog. Gastroenterology 23:441, 1953
47. Machella TE: Mechanism of post-gastrectomy dumping syndrome. Gastroenterology 14:237, 1950
48. Hinshaw DB, Joergenson EJ, Davis HA, et al: Peripheral blood flow and blood volume studies in the dumping syndrome. AMA Arch Surg 74:686, 1957
49. Glazebrook AJ, Welbourn RB: Some observations on the function of the small intestine after gastrectomy. Br J Surg 40:111, 1952
50. Reichle FA, Brigham MP, Riechle RM, et al: The effects of gastrectomy on serotonin metabolism in the human portal vein. Ann Surg 172:585, 1970
51. Zeitlin IJ, Smith AN: 5-Hydroxyindoles and kinins in the carcinoid and dumping syndromes. Lancet 2:986, 1966
52. Bloom SR, Roystan CMS, Thomson JPS: Gastric operations and glucose homeostasis. Gastroenterology 62:1109, 1972
53. Hopman WP, Wolberink RG, Lamers CB, et al: Treatment of the dumping syndrome with the somatostat-in analogue SMS 201-995. Ann Surg 207:155–159, 1988
54. Reber HA, Way LW: Surgical treatment of late postgastrectomy syndromes. Am J Surg 129:71–77, 1975
55. Sawyers JL, Herrington JL Jr: Superiority of antiperistaltic jejunal segments in management of severe dumping syndrome. Ann Surg 178:311–321, 1973
56. Cheadle WG, Baker PR, Cuschieri A: Pyloric reconstruction for severe vasomotor dumping after vagotomy and pyloroplasty. Ann Surg 202:568–572, 1985
57. Ebeid FH, Ralphs DNL, Hobsley M, et al: Dumping symptoms after vagotomy treated by reversal of pyloroplasty. Br J Surg 69:527–528, 1982
58. Christiansen PM, Hansen OH, Pedersen T: Reconstruction of the pylorus for postvagotomy diarrhoea and dumping. Br J Surg 61:519–520, 1974
59. Johnston D, Humphrey CS, Walker BE, et al: Vagotomy without diarrhea. Br Med J 3:788–790, 1972
60. Strauss R, Wise L: New concepts in the prevention, causes, and treatment of postgastrectomy diarrhea. Curr Surg 35:77–84, 1978
61. Allen JG, Gerskowitch VP, Russell R: The role of bile salts in the pathogenesis of postvagotomy diarrhea. Br J Surg 61:516, 1974
62. Herrington JL: The postgastrectomy syndrome. Contemp Surg 29:13–22, 1986
63. Warshaw AL, Simeone J, Schapiro RH, et al: Objective evaluation of ampullary stenosis with ultra-sonography and pancreatic stimulation. Am J Surg 149:67–72, 1985
64. Nardi GL, Michelassi F, Zannini P: Transduodenal sphincteroplasty. 5–25 year follow-up of 89 patients. Ann Surg 198:453–461, 1983
65. Toouli, J, Geenen JE, Hogan WG, et al: Sphincter of Oddi motor activity: A comparison between patients with common bile duct stones and controls. Gastroenterology 82:111–117, 1982
66. Meshkinporir H, Mollot M, Eckerling GB, et al: Bile duct dyskinesia. Clinical and manometric study. Gastroenterology 87:759–762, 1984
67. Hogan WG, Geenen JE, Dodds WJ: Dysmotility disturbances of the biliary tract: Classification, diagnosis, and treatment. Semin Liver Dis 7:302–310, 1987
68. Rolny P, Arleback A, Funch-Jensen P, et al: Paradoxical response of sphincter of Oddi to intravenous injection of cholecystokinin or ceruletide. Manometric findings and results of treatment in biliary dyskinesia. Gut 27:1507–1511, 1986
69. Rolny P, Arleback A, Jarnerot G, et al: Endoscopic manometry of the sphincter of Oddi and pancreatic duct in chronic pancreatitis. Scand J Gastroenterol 21:415–421, 1986
70. Lempinen M: Biliary dyskinesia. Scand J Gastroenterol 20(suppl 109):103–106, 1985
71. Roberts-Thomson IC: Endoscopic sphincterotomy of the papilla of Vater: An analysis of 300 cases. Aust NZ J Med 14:611–617, 1984
72. Geenen JE, Toouli J, Hogan WJ, et al: Endoscopic sphincterotomy: Follow-up evaluation of effects on the sphincter of Oddi. Gastroenterology 87:754–758, 1984

73. Schuffler MD, Lowe MC, Bill AH: Studies of idiopathic intestinal pseudoobstruction. I. Hereditary hollow visceral myopathy. Clinical and pathologic studies. Gastroenterology 73:327–338, 1977

74. Schuffler MD, Bird TD, Sumi SM, et al: A familial neuronal disease presenting as intestinal pseudoobstruction. Gastroenterology 75:889–898, 1978

75. Byrne WJ, Cipel L, Ament ME, et al: Chronic idiopathic intestinal pseudo-obstruction syndrome. Radiologic signs in children with emphasis on differentiation from mechanical obstruction. Diagn Imag 50:294–304, 1981

76. Schuffler MD, Deitch EA: Chronic idiopathic intestinal pseudo-obstruction. A surgical approach. Ann Surg 192:752–761, 1980

77. McCready RA, Beart RW: The surgical treatment of incapacitating constipation associated with idiopathic megacolon. Mayo Clin Proc 54:779–783, 1979

78. Schuffler MD, Leon SH, Krishnamurthy S: Intestinal pseudoobstruction caused by a new form of visceral neuropathy: Palliation by radical small bowel resection. Gastroenterology 89:1152–1156, 1985

79. Paul CA, Tomiyasu U, Mellinkoff SM: Nearly fatal pseudo-obstruction of the small intestine. A case report of its relief by subtotal resection of the small bowel. Gastroenterology 40:698–704, 1961

80. Pitt HA, Mann LL, Berquist WE, et al: Chronic intestinal pseudo-obstruction. Management with total parenteral nutrition and a venting enterostomy. Arch Surg 120:614–618, 1985

81. Ogilvie H: Large-intestine colic due to sympathetic deprivation: A new clinical syndrome. Br Med J 2:671–673, 1948

82. Luderer JR, Demers LM, Bonnem EM, et al: Elevated prostaglandin E in idiopathic intestinal pseudo-obstruction. N Engl J Med 295:179, 1976

83. Chousterman M, Petite JP, Housset E, et al: Prostaglandins and intestinal pseudo-obstruction (letter). Lancet 2:138–139, 1977

84. Kukora JS, Dent TL: Colonoscopic decompression of massive nonobstructive cecal dilation. Arch Surg 112:512–517, 1977

85. Strodel WE, Nostrant TT, Eckhauser FE, et al: Therapeutic and diagnostic colonoscopy in nonobstructive colonic dilation. Ann Surg 197:416–421, 1983

86. Adams JT: Adynamic ileus of the colon. An indication for cecostomy. Arch Surg 109:503–507, 1974

87. Nanni G, Garbini A, Luchetti P, et al: Ogilvie's syndrome (acute colonic pseudo-obstruction): Review of the literature (October 1948 to March 1980) and report of four additional cases. Dis Colon Rectum 25:157–166, 1982

88. Parks TG: Post-mortem studies on the colon with special reference to diverticular disease. Proc R Soc Med 61:30–32, 1968

89. Almy TP, Howell DA: Diverticular disease of the colon. N Engl J Med 302:324–331, 1980

90. Hackford AW, Veidenheimer MC: Diverticular disease of the colon. Current concepts and management. Surg Clin North Am 65:347–363, 1985

91. Painter NS: The aetiology of diverticulosis of the colon with special reference to the action of certain drugs on the behaviour of the colon. Ann R Coll Surg Engl 34:98–119, 1964

92. Arfwidsson S, Dock NG: Pathogenesis of multiple diverticula of the sigmoid colon in diverticular disease. Acta Chir Scand 342 (suppl):5–68, 1964

93. Painter, NS: Diverticular disease of the colon. Br Med J 3:475–479, 1968

94. Taylor I, Duthie HL: Bran tablets and diverticular disease. Br Med J 1:988–990, 1976

95. Smith AN: Colonic muscle in diverticular disease. Clin Gastroenterol 15:917–935, 1986

96. Reilly M: Sigmoid myotomy. Proc R Soc Med 57:556–559, 1964

97. Janson JHG, Lawrence LR, Localio SA: Colomyotomy; a new approach to surgery for colonic diverticular disease. Am J Surg 123:185, 1972

98. Attisha RP, Smith AN: Pressure activity of the colon and rectum in diverticular disease before and after sigmoid myotomy. Br J Surg 56:891–894, 1969

99. McGinn, FP: Distal colomyotomy; follow-up of 37 cases. Br J Surg 63:309–312, 1976

100. Smith, AN, Wistar RP, Clarke S: Motility after colomyotomy and resection of the colon for diverticular disease. Am J Dig Dis 16:72–76, 1971

101. Hodgson J: Colonic diverticular disease: Transverse taeniamyotomy. Dis Colon Rectum 18:555–559, 1975

102. Landi E, Fianchini A, Landa L, et al: Multiple transverse taeniamyotomy for diverticular disease. Surg Gynecol Obstet 148:221–226, 1979

103. Correnti FS, Pappalardo G, Mobarhan S, et al: Follow-up results of a new colomyotomy in the treatment of diverticulosis. Surg Gynecol Obstet 156:181–186, 1983
104. Almy TP, Howell DA: Medical progress. Diverticular disease of the colon. N Engl J Med 302:324–331, 1980.
105. Larson DM, Masters SS, Spiro HM: Medical and surgical therapy in diverticular disease. A comparative study. Gastroenterology 71:734–737, 1976
106. Hackford AW, Veidenheimer MC: Diverticular disease of the colon. Current concepts and management. Surg Clin North Am 65:347–363, 1985
107. Rodkey GV, Welch CE: Changing patterns in the surgical treatment of diverticular disease. Ann Surg 200:466–478, 1984
108. Poisson J, Devroede G: Severe chronic constipation as a surgical problem. Surg Clin North Am 63:193–217, 1983
109. Martelli H, Devroede G, Arhan P, et al: Some parameters of large bowel motility in normal man. Gastroenterology 75:612–618, 1978
110. Reynolds JC, Ouyang A, Lee PA, et al: Chronic severe constipation. Prospective motility studies in 25 consecutive patients. Gastroenterology 92:414–420, 1987
111. Koch TR, Carney JA, Go L, et al: Idiopathic chronic constipation is associated with decreased colonic vasoactive intestinal peptide. Gastroenterology 94:300–310, 1988
112. Ariel I, Hershlag A, Lernan OZ: Hypoganglionosis of the myenteric plexus with normal Meissner's plexus. A new variant of colonic ganglion cell disorders. J Pediatr Surg 20:90–92, 1985
113. McCready RA, Beart RW: The surgical management of incapacitating constipation associated with idiopathic megacolon. Mayo Clin Proc 54:779–783, 1979
114. Klatt GR: Role of subtotal colectomy in the treatment of incapacitating constipation. Am J Surg 145:623–625, 1983
115. Preston DM, Hawley PR, Lennard-Jones JE, et al: Results of colectomy for severe idiopathic constipation in women (Arbuthnot Lane's disease). Br J Surg 71:547–552, 1984
116. Beck, DE, Jagelman DG, Fazio VW: The surgery of idiopathic constipation. Gastro Clin North Am 16:143–156, 1987
117. Walsh PV, Peebles-Brown DA, Watkinson G: Colectomy for slow transit constipation. Ann R Coll Surg Engl 69:71–75, 1987
118. Gasslander T, Larsson J, Wetterfors J: Experience of surgical treatment for chronic constipation. Acta Chir Scand 153:553–555, 1987
119. DeLorimier AA, Benzian SR, Gooding CA: Segmental dilatation of the colon. Am J Radiol 112:100, 1971
120. Yoshioka K, Keighley MR: Randomized trial comparing anorectal myectomy and controlled anal dilatation for outlet obstruction. Br J Surg 74:1125–1129, 1987
121. Martelli H, Devroede G, Arhan P, et al: The mechanisms of idiopathic constipation: Outlet obstruction. Gastroenterology 75:623–631, 1978
122. Okamoto E, Ueda T: Embryogenesis of intramural ganglia of the gut and its relation to Hirschsprung's disease. J Pediatr Surg 2:437, 1967
123. Starling JR, Croom RD III, Thomas CG Jr: Hirschsprung's disease in young adults. Am J Surg 151:104–109, 1986
124. Fairgrieve J: Hirschsprung's disease in the adult. Br J Surg 223:506–514, 1963
125. Todd IP: Adult Hirschsprung's disease. Br J Surg 64:331–342, 1967

Index